D1023948

Stedman's

ALTERNATIVE
MEDICINE
WORDS

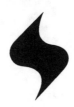

Stedman's
ALTERNATIVE
MEDICINE
WORDS

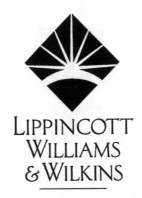

LIPPINCOTT
WILLIAMS
&WILKINS

Series Editor: Beverly Wolpert
Database Content Editor: Jennifer Schmidt
Art Direction: Jonathan Dimes
Art Coordinator: Jennifer Clements
Associate Marketing Manager: John Trader
Production Manager: Tricia Smith
Typesetter: Peirce Graphic Services, Inc.
Printer & Binder: Victor Graphics

Copyright © 2000 Lippincott Williams & Wilkins
530 Walnut Street
Philadelphia, Pennsylvania 19106-3620 USA

Printed in the United States of America

2000

Library of Congress Cataloging-in-Publication Data

Stedman's alternative medicine words.
    p. ; cm. -- (Stedman's word books)
    ISBN 0-7817-2161-X
    1. Alternative medicine-Terminology. I. Title: Alternative medicine words. II.
Stedman, Thomas Lathrop, 1853-1938. III. Series.
    [DNLM: 1. Alternative Medicine--Terminology--English. WB 15 S812 1999]
R733 .S835 1999
615.5'01'--dc21

                                                                99-057675

                                                                00
                                              2 3 4 5 6 7 8 9 10

Contents

Acknowledgments

An important part of our editorial process is the involvement of medical transcriptionists — as advisors, reviewers and/or editors.

We extend special thanks to Ellen Atwood; Jeanne Bock, CSR, MT; and Nicole G. Peck for editing the manuscript, helping to resolve many difficult content questions, and contributing material for the appendix sections. We also extend special thanks to our Editorial Advisory Board members, including Lee Bean, NCTMBW, Baltimore Holistic Health Center Clinic Director; Janie Gilbert, CMT; Kathryn Mason, CMT; Mary Jo Molloy, Raincross Medical Group Supervisor/Trainer; Wendy Ryan, ART; Karen L. Thomas-Bates, CMT; and Tina Whitecotton, CMT, who were instrumental to the development of this reference. They recommended sources, gathered new content, and offered the many benefits of their experience, including their very valuable judgment, insight, and perspective.

Other important contributors to this edition include Phyllis J. Campbell, CMT; Susan Couper, CMT; Charlotte Glenn; Robin Koza; Lee Ann O'Brien; Jenifer Walker, MA; Peg Nelson, CMT; and Velta Jo Reider.

Barb Ferretti played an integral role in the process by reviewing the content files for format, updating the database, and providing a final quality check. Also integral to the development of this reference were the advice and assistance of our Lippincott Williams & Wilkins colleagues, including Tim Hiscock, Joyce Murphy, Dana Jackson, and Susan Stern.

As with all our *Stedman's* word references, this resource incorporates the suggestions and expertise of our many contacts in the medical transcriptionist community. Thanks to all of our advisory board participants, reviewers, and editors; AAMT meeting attendees; and others who have written us with requests and comments — keep talking, and we'll keep listening.

Editor's Preface

In many cultures, traditional remedies and therapies have been studied and implemented for centuries. To this day, members of these cultures believe in and treat ailments, both physical and mental, with acupressure, acupuncture, reflexology, massage, and meditation, as well as herbal therapies. In the 1800s, the practice of homeopathy was utilized in Europe and in the United States but was, however, considered an alternative form of therapy.

In this century, scientists researched and managed to prove the connection between our minds and bodies. A large part of the medical community has come to acknowledge, and even endorse, the value of many treatments once considered alternative or, even worse, quackery. But now, homeopathy and other traditional remedies and therapies, previously segregated and even dismissed as a group under the dubious "alternative medicine" heading, are gaining increasing acceptance and integration with the standard allopathic approaches to healing. Every day, more patients turn again toward holistic medicine and its various treatment options, either in place of, or in conjunction with, standard medical practices.

As allusions to alternative therapies occur more and more frequently in the language of the public, patient records, and healthcare professionals, a reference containing the terms from the various alternative treatment modalities has become a necessary tool. That need has sparked the development of this book.

When I was first asked to work on this project initially as a researcher and eventually as an editor, I readily accepted out of curiosity. I had experienced some of these treatments from the patient's perspective and was hungry to learn more. Our work on this book has fed that curious hunger.

In the beginning stages, I had no idea how many nuances there might be in the terminology related to the Chinese practices of acupuncture and acupressure or how many variant spellings we might encounter for many of these terms. Likewise, I was amazed to discover the variations in the spellings of scientific and common herb names, thereby prompting the need to choose the "most common" spelling for inclusion in this first edition of *Stedman's Alternative Medicine Words*. Additionally, I was surprised to discover how critical and integral a role herbal therapy plays in all of the fields of alternative medicine included in this book; herbal therapy stands alone as a form of treatment, but also works very much in concert with the other modalities of what we, in the United States, call alternative medicine.

Terms for *Stedman's Alternative Medicine Word Book* were collected and organized only through the special talents of many individuals, two of whom, Ellen Atwood and Nicole G. Peck, provided invaluable assistance with the manuscript. Along with these gifted editors, countless other extraordinary individuals have contributed their talents to make this book what it is, and to them I express my sincere thanks.

Jeanne Bock, CSR, MT

Publisher's Preface

Stedman's Alternative Medicine Words offers an authoritative assurance of quality and exactness to the wordsmiths of the healthcare professions — medical transcriptionists (MTs), medical and copy editors, health information management personnel, court reporters, and the many other users and producers of medical documentation.

In the specialty of alternative medicine, authoritative references are difficult to identify. Time-consuming Internet searches may yield results, but "we can't be sure that what we find is correct," in the words of one of many of the MTs who requested that Stedman's develop an alternative medicine wordbook. Over the past few years, as requests for such a reference continued to accumulate, we realized that medical language professionals needed a comprehensive, current reference for alternative medicine.

Terminology for this reference comes from some of the most respected print and electronic sources available, including *Stedman's Medical Dictionary* (please see list of References on page xvii). When discrepancies occurred in spellings, the editors considered the quality of each source and the number of sources using each spelling to determine which to include in this reference. We resorted to further research in many cases to reflect accurate spellings in accordance with current usage.

As a result of these efforts, users will find thousands of words encompassing acupuncture, osteopathy, bodywork, and massage techniques, plus the common and scientific names of herbs, among other alternative medicine terminology. This compilation of more than 40,000 entries, fully cross-indexed for quick access, was built from a base vocabulary of more than 30,000 medical words, phrases, abbreviations, and acronyms.

We at Lippincott Williams & Wilkins strive to provide you with the most up-to-date and accurate word references available. Your use of this wordbook will prompt new editions, which we will publish as often as updates and revisions justify. We welcome your suggestions for improvements, changes, corrections, and additions—whatever will make this Stedman's product more useful to you. Please complete the postpaid card at the back of this book, and send your recommendations care of *"Stedman's"* at Lippincott Williams & Wilkins.

Explanatory Notes

Medical transcription is an art as well as a science. Both are needed to correctly interpret the dictation of a physician, whose language is a product of education, training, and experience. This variety in medical language means there are several acceptable ways to express certain or similar terms, including jargon. *Stedman's Alternative Medicine Words* provides variant spellings and phrasings for many terms. These elements, in addition to complete cross-indexing, make *Stedman's Alternative Medicine Words* a valuable resource for determining the validity of terms as they are encountered.

Common and Scientific Herb Names

Genus names of herbs appear with initial capitals and italic typeface. Species names appear in lowercase italics. The typeface for common names is lowercase roman. All main entries also appear in boldface, but subentries do not appear in boldface. For example:

armeniaca	**main entry species**
Prunus a.	**subentry genus**
Artemisia	**main entry genus**
A. absinthium	**subentry species**

Alphabetical Organization

Alphabetization of main entries is letter-by-letter as spelled, ignoring punctuation, spaces, prefixed numbers, or other characters. For example:

D3
da
dabao
d'accoucheur
dachangshu
effusion
EGB 761
EGb

In subentry alphabetization, the abbreviated singular form or the spelled-out plural form of the noun main entry word is ignored.

Subentry terms starting with Greek letters fall under the spelled-out version of the Greek letter, which appears as a main entry with the symbol as a variant. For example:

gamma, γ
  g. aminobutyric acid transaminase
  g. camera
  g. globulin

Format and Style
All main entries are in **boldface** to expedite locating a sought-after term, to enhance distinction between main entries and subentries, and to relieve the textual density of the pages.

Irregular plurals and variant spellings are shown on the same line as the singular or preferred form of the word. For example:

G6PD, G-6-PD
meninx, pl. **meninges**, gen. **meningis**

Hyphenation
As a rule of style, multiple eponyms (e.g., Mears-Rubash approach) are hyphenated. Also, hyphens have been added between a manufacturer and one or more eponyms (e.g., Vital-Metzenbaum dissecting scissors). Please note that hyphenation is a question of style, not of accuracy, and thus is a matter of choice (as is also the case with the use of apostrophes and the possessive "s" on eponyms, as explained below).

Possessives
Possessive forms with eponyms have been dropped in this reference for the sake of internal consistency, as well as conformance to written guidelines of the American Association for Medical Transcription (AAMT) and the American Medical Association (AMA). Please note, however, that retaining the possessive is a question of style, not of accuracy, and

thus is a matter of choice; to form the possessive of a word, simply add the apostrophe or apostrophe "s" to the end of the word.

For this book, we have chosen to retain the possessives with common or traditional herb names, religious or biblically based herb names, and occupational descriptors:

Aaron's rod
angel's trumpet
ass's foot
bachelor's button
bear's grape
bowman's reflex
brewer's yeast
carpenter's herb
St. Bartholomew's tea
St. Mary's thistle fruit
tanner's bark

We have also chosen to retain the possessives and capitals with brand name remedies and nostrums:

Atkinson & Barker's Gripe Mixture
Bartlean's Vita Flax

Cross-indexing

The word list is in an index-like main entry-subentry format that contains two combined alphabetical listings:

(1) A *noun* main entry-subentry organization is typical of the A-Z section of medical dictionaries like *Stedman's:*

orientation
    facet o.
    spine o.
    vertebral o.

spine
    occipitoatlantal cervical s.
    s. orientation
    posterior superior iliac s.

(2) An *adjective* main entry-subentry organization lists words and phrases as you hear them. The main entries are the adjectives or modifiers in a multiword term. The subentries are the nouns around which the terms are constructed and to which the adjectives or modifiers pertain:

arachnoid
    a. granulation
    a. layer of meninges

granulation
    arachnoid g.
    tissue g.

This format provides the user with more than one way to locate and identify a multiword term. For example:

antioxidant
    a. defense system

system
    antioxidant defense s.

palpation
    diagnostic p.

diagnostic
    d. palpation

It also allows the user to see together all terms that contain a particular descriptor, as well as all types, kinds, or variations of a noun entity. For example:

biofeedback
    electroacupuncture b.
    b. exercise
    b. instrumentation
    kinesthetic b.

field
    f. block anesthesia
    human energy f.
    interference f.
    f. mallow

Wherever possible, abbreviations are separately defined and cross-referenced. For example:

BZLZ
    bian zheng lun zhi
bian
    b. zheng lun zhi (BZLZ)
zhi
    bian zheng lun z. (BZLZ)

References

In addition to the manufacturers' literature we gather at various medical meetings, scientific reports from hospitals, and the lists of our MT Editorial Advisory Board members (from their daily transcription work), we used the following sources of new words for *Stedman's Alternative Medicine Words:*

Books

Alternative medicine: expanding medical horizons. A report to the National Institutes of Health on alternative medical systems and practices in the United States. Washington DC: U.S. Government Printing Office [prepared under the auspices of the Workshop on Alternative Medicine, Chantilly, Virginia, September 14–16, 1992].

American Osteopathic Association. Foundations of osteopathic medicine. Baltimore: Williams & Wilkins, 1997.

Balch JF, Balch PA. Prescription for nutritional healing, 2nd ed. New York: Avery Publishing Group, 1997.

Blumenthal M., editor. The complete German Commission E monographs: therapeutic guide to herbal medicines. Austin: American Botanical Council, 1998.

Burton Goldberg Group. Alternative medicine: the definitive guide. Fife, WA: Future Medicine Publishing, 1994.

Calkins CC, editor. Reader's Digest illustrated guide to gardening. Pleasantville, NY: Readers's Digest Association, 1978 (14th printing 1992).

Cassileth B. The alternative medicine handbook. New York: Norton, 1998.

DerMarderosian A, editor. The review of natural products. St. Louis: Facts and Comparisons, 1996–1998.

DiGiovanna EL, Schiowitz S. An osteopathic approach to diagnosis and treatment, 2nd ed. Philadelphia: Lippincott-Raven, 1997.

Dorland's illustrated medical dictionary, 28th ed. Philadelphia: Saunders, 1994.

Fetrow CW, Avila JR. Professional's handbook of complementary & alternative medicines. Springhouse, PA: Springhouse Corporation, 1999.

Forbis P, Bartolucci SL. Stedman's medical eponyms. Baltimore: Williams & Wilkins, 1998.

Fugh-Berman A. Alternative medicine: what works. Baltimore: Williams & Wilkins, 1997.

Gardner-Abbate S. Holding the tiger's tail: an acupuncture techniques manual in the treatment of disease. Santa Fe: Southwest Acupuncture College Press, 1996.

Gottlieb B. New choices in natural healing. New York: Bantam Books, 1997 [original copyright Emmaus, PA: Rodale Press, 1995.]

Greenman PE. Principles of manual medicine. 2nd ed. Baltimore: Williams & Wilkins, 1996.

Jonas W, Levin JS. Essentials of complementary and alternative medicine. Baltimore: Lippincott Williams & Wilkins, 1999.

Lance LL. Quick look drug book. Baltimore: Lippincott Williams & Wilkins, 1999.

The medical advisor: the complete guide to alternative & conventional treatments. Alexandria, VA: Time Life, 1996.

PDR for herbal medicines, 1st ed. Montvale, NJ: Medical Economics Co., 1998.

Pyle V. Current medical terminology, 5th ed. Modesto: Health Professions Institute, 1994.

Robbers JE, Tyler VE. Tyler's herbs of choice: the therapeutic use of phytomedicinals. New York: Haworth Herbal Press, 1999.

Salvo SG. Massage therapy: principles & practice. Philadelphia: Saunders, 1999.

Sloane SB. Medical abbreviations & eponyms, 2nd ed. Philadelphia: Saunders, 1997.

Sloane SB. The medical word book, 3rd ed. Philadelphia: WB Saunders Company, 1991.

Spencer JW, Jacobs JJ. Complementary/alternative medicine: an evidence-based approach. St. Louis: Mosby, 1999

Stedman's abbreviations, acronyms & symbols, 2nd ed. Baltimore: Lippincott Williams & Wilkins, 1999.

Stedman's medical dictionary, 26th ed. Baltimore: Williams & Wilkins, 1995.

Stedman's orthopaedic & rehab words, 3rd ed. Baltimore: Lippincott Williams & Wilkins, 1999.

Stedman's pathology & lab medicine words, 2nd ed. Baltimore: Lippincott Williams & Wilkins, 1998.

Stux G, Pomeranz B. Basics of acupuncture [4th revised ed.; trans. by Sahm KA]. New York: Springer-Verlag, 1997.

Taber's cyclopedic medical dictionary, 17th ed. Philadelphia: F. A. Davis, 1997.

Tierra M. The way of herbs. New York: Pocket Books/Simon & Schuster, 1990.

Tyler VE. Tyler's honest herbal, 4th ed. Binghamton, NY: Haworth Herbal Press, 1999.

Electronic media

Stedman's electronic medical dictionary, version 4.0. Baltimore: Williams & Wilkins, 1998.

Merriam-Webster's collegiate dictionary, 10th & deluxe electronic ed. Springfield, MA: Merriam-Webster, Incorporated, 1996.

The Merck manual illustrated, 17th ed., CD-ROM, Whitehouse Station, NJ: 1999.

American heritage talking dictionary. Cambridge, MA: The Learning Company, 1998.

Webster's international encyclopedia 1999, CD-ROM. Springfield, MA: Merriam-Webster, Incorporated, 1999.

A guide to alternative medicine CD-ROM for Windows. Cambridge, MA: The Learning Company, 1996.

Blake S. Alternative remedies CD-ROM. St. Louis: Mosby, 1999.

Journals

Alternative Therapies in Health and Medicine. Aliso Viejo, CA: Innovision Communications, 1998–1999.

HerbalGram. Austin: American Botanical Council, 1995–1999.

The Journal of Alternative and Complementary Medicine: Research on Paradigm, Practice, and Policy. Larchmont, NY: Mary Ann Liebert, Inc., 1998–1999.

The Integrative Medicine Consult: The Essential Guide to Integrating Conventional and Complementary Medicine. Newton, MA: 1998–1999.

Journal of the American Association for Medical Transcription. Modesto: American Association for Medical Transcription, 1998–1999.

MT monthly. Gladstone, MO: Computer Systems Management, 1998–1999.

Perspectives on the medical transcription profession. Modesto: Health Professions Institute, 1998–1999.

Stedman's WordWatcher. Baltimore: Williams & Wilkins, 1995–1999.

The Latest Word. Philadelphia: Saunders, 1998–1999.

Websites

http://207.48.132.28/tldp.htm

http://altmed.od.nih.gov/nccam/clearinghouse/

http://altmed.od.nih.gov/nccam/what-is-cam/classify.shtml

http://altmed.od.nih.gov/nccam/what-is-cam/fields/

http://cpmcnet.columbia.edu/dept/rosenthal/

http://dir.yahoo.com/Health/Alternative.Medicine/

http://infoseek.go.com/WebDir/Health/Alternative_medicine?Ik=noframs&svx=related

http://medicalacupuncture.org/helmsarticle.htm#hist

http://www.altmedicine.com [*Alternative Health News Online*/Frank Grazian]

http://www.acupuncture.com

http://www.americanwholehealth.com/library/acupuncture/acufaq.htm

http://www.americanwholehealth.com/library/acupuncture/earframe.htm

http://www.anmp.org [Association of Natural Medicine]

http://www.ars-grin.gov/cgi-bin/npgs/html/econ.pl [USDA, ARS, National Genetic Resources Program. Germplasm Resources Information Network—GRIN. (Online Database) National Germplasm Resources Laboratory, Beltsville, MD]

http://www.arxc.com

http://www.bgbm.fu-berlin.de [names in current use for extant plant genera, copyright 1997 International Association for Plant Taxonomy]

http://www.bioterrain.com/brochure/page1.html#features

http://www.mtdesk.com

http://www.healthlink.com. au/nat

http://www.healthonline.com

http://www.healthwwweb.com/

http://www.healthy.net/clinic/therapy/index.html

http://www.healthy.net/library/articles/ayurvedic/pancha.htm

http://www.healthy.net/library/columns/ChineseMedicine/archive/2qigong.htm

http://www.healthy.net/library/columns/galland/index.html

http://www.healthy.net/library/columns/mindbody/index.html

http://www.healthy.net/LIBRARY/columns/Sahelian/archives.htm

http://www.herbalgram.org [American Botanical Council]

http://www.leeds.ac.uk/ahi/ [South Bank and Leeds Universities, *Alternative Health International*]

http://www.Liebertpub.com/

http://www.nih.gov

http://www.noah.cuny.edu/alternative/alternative.html

http://www.ohsu.edu/ohmig/cam.html

http://www.omsmedical.com

http://www.onemedicine.com/

http://www.pitt.edu/~cbw/altm.html

http://www.swiha.org

http://www.sph.uth.tmc.edu/utcam

http://www.thorne.com/altmedrev/index.html [Thorne Research, *Alternative Medicine Review*]

http://www.touchamerica.com

http://www.webmedlit.com/cgi/AT-wml2search.cgi

α (*var. of* alpha)
A fiber
AA
 acupuncture analgesia
AACOM
 American Association of Colleges of
 Osteopathic Medicine
AAHP
 American Association of
 Homeopathic Pharmacists
AAMA
 American Academy of Medical
 Acupuncture
AAMI
 American Association for Medical
 Instrumentation
Aangamik DMG
AANP
 American Association of
 Naturopathic Physicians
AAPB
 Association for Applied
 Psychophysiology and Biofeedback
Aaron's rod
abalone shell
Abana
abapical
abasia
 atactic a.
abasic
abatic
abaxial
ABC
 Aerobic Bulk Cleanse
 American Botanical Council
abdomen
 extra point on the chest
  and a. (Ex-CA)
 muscles of a.
 transverse muscle of a.
abdominal
 a. aneurysm
 a. aorta
 a. auscultation
 a. breath
 a. distention
 a. external oblique muscle
 a. internal oblique muscle
 a. muscle
 a. part of thoracic duct

abdominis
 musculi a.
 musculus obliquus externus a.
 musculus obliquus internus a.
abdominopelvic plexus of nerve
abdominothoracic arch
abducens nerve
abducent
abduct
abduction
 hip joint a.
 passive hip a.
 restricted a.
abduction-adduction
abductor
 a. brevis muscle
 a. digiti minimi magnus
  musculus
 a. digiti minimi muscle
 a. digiti minimi muscle of
  foot
 a. digiti minimi muscle of
  hand
 a. digiti minimi pedis
  musculus
 a. digiti quinti muscle
 a. hallucis muscle
 a. longus muscle
 a. magnus muscle
 a. muscle of great toe
 a. muscle of little finger
 a. muscle of little toe
 a. pollicis brevis muscle
 a. pollicis longus muscle
abductus
 pes a.
aberrant
 a. afferent impulse
 a. afferent stimulation
 a. ganglion
 a. stimulation
abhyanga massage
abietis
 Viscum a.
ability
 baseline hypnotic a.
 fantasy a.
 high hypnotic a.
 hypnotic a.

ability *(continued)*
   low hypnotic a.
   moderate hypnotic a.
Abkit
abnormal
   a. barrier
   a. behavior
   a. chewing
   a. feel
   a. muscle firing pattern
abnormality
   asymmetry, range of motion
    abnormality, tissue texture a.
    (ART)
   boggy tissue texture a.
   congenital a.
   doughy tissue texture a.
   hot-cold tissue texture a.
   range of motion a.
   soft-hard tissue texture a.
   soft tissue texture a.
   tissue texture a. (TTA)
abortifacient
above-elbow amputation (AEA)
above-knee amputation (AKA)
ABPH
   American Board of Psychological
   Hypnosis
abreaction
abrin
abscess
   acute a.
   bacterial a.
   bone a.
   bursal a.
   collar-button a.
   gummatous a.
   hot a.
   hypostatic a.
   metastatic a.
   migrating a.
   perforating a.
   periarticular a.
   periodontal a.
   phlegmonous a.
   Pott a.
   psoas a.
   residual a.
   satellite a.
   sterile a.
   stitch a.
   thecal a.

   tuboovarian a.
   wandering a.
abscissa
absconsio
absent healing
absinthe
absinthin
absinthism
absinthium
   Artemisia a.
absinthol
absolute
   a. humidity
   a. yin
   a. yin channel axis
absorbent
absorption
   intestinal a.
   percutaneous a.
   a. test
abterminal
abuse
   polydrug a.
abyssinica
   Commiphora a.
   Hagenia a.
ACA
   American Chiropractic Association
Acacia
   A. catechu
   A. gum
   A. senegal
acacia
Academy of Traditional Chinese Medicine
acampsia
acantha
Acanthea virilis
acanthias
   Squalus a.
acanthion
acanthoid
Acanthopanax senticosus
acanthosis nigricans
acaricidal
acaricide
acausal relationship
accelerated hypertension
accelerator
   a. factor
   a. globulin

accessoria
    glandula thyroidea a.
    thyroidea a.
accessorii
    pars spinalis nervi a.
    pars vagalis nervi a.
accessorius
    musculus flexor a.
accessory
    a. cuneate nucleus
    a. flexor muscle of foot
    a. gland
    a. ligament
    a. movement
    a. nerve [CN XI]
    a. plantar ligament
    a. process of lumbar vertebra
    a. volar ligament
accident
    industrial a.
    motor vehicle a.
    vertebrobasilar a.
accidental hypothermia
accommodation
accompanying vein
accordion-type movement
accoucheur hand
Accu-Band
accumbens
    nucleus a.
accumulation
Accu-Patch
Accutane
ACE
    angiotensin-converting enzyme
acemannin
ACES + Zinc
acetabula (*pl. of* acetabulum)
acetabular
    a. branch
    a. fossa
    a. labrum
    a. labrum and posterior
      capsule stretch technique
    a. lip
    a. notch

acetabulare
    labrum a.
acetabularis
    margo a.
acetabuli
    fossa a.
    protrusio a.
acetabulum, pl. acetabula
    lunate surface of a.
    margin of a.
    transverse ligament of a.
acetaminophen
acetate
    oxyphenisatin a.
acetosella
    Rumex a.
acetylcholine secretion
acetyl-L-carnitine (ALC)
acetylsalicylate
    lysine a.
achalasia
Achillea
    A. collina
    A. lanulosa
    A. millefolium
Achilles
    A. bursa
    A. deep tendon reflex
    A. pain
    A. reflex
    A. tendon
    A. tendon bursitis
    A. tendon reflex
Achillis
    tendo A.
achillobursitis
achondroplasia
    homozygous a.
acicularis
    Rosa a.
acid
    alpha lipoic a.
    amino a.
    aristolochic a.
    ascorbic a.
    aspartic a.
    azelaic a.

NOTES

acid *(continued)*
  benzoic a.
  bile a.
  boswellic a.
  botulinic a.
  caffeic a.
  caprylic a.
  carnosic a.
  cellulosic a.
  chlorogenic a.
  cis-linoleic a.
  conjugated linoleic a.
  crocinic a.
  crystalline free-form amino a.
  deoxyribonucleic a. (DNA)
  dihomogammalinolenic a.
    (DGLA, DHGA)
  docosahexaenoic a. (DHA)
  docosenoic a.
  edetic a.
  eicosapentaenoic a. (EPA)
  erucic a.
  essential fatty a. (EFA)
  ethylenediaminetetraacetic a.
    (EDTA)
  fatty a.
  folic a.
  folinic a.
  free-form amino a.'s
  gamma aminobutyric a.
    (GABA)
  gamma linolenic a. (GLA)
  gastric a.
  glutamic a.
  glycyrrhizinic a.
  hyaluronic a.
  kojic a.
  labiatic a.
  lactic a.
  L-aspartic a.
  L-glutamic a.
  L-glutamine pantothenic a.
  linoleic a.
  linolenic a. (LNA)
  lipoic a.
  nicotinic a.
  a. odor
  oleic a.
  omega-3 essential fatty a.
  omega-3 polyunsaturated
    fatty a.
  oxalic a.
  pangamic a.

  pantothenic a.
  paraaminobenzoic a. (PABA)
  p-coumaric a.
  pectinic a.
  phosphoric a.
  polyglycolic a.
  retinoic a.
  ribonucleic a. (RNA)
  sinapic a.
  tannic a.
  thioctic a.
  ursodeoxycholic a. (UDCA)
Acid-Ease
acid-fast bacilli
acidic urine
acidification
  urinary a.
acidophilus
  a. douche
  Lactobacillus a.
  a. milk
acidosis
  metabolic a.
ackee fruit
acknemia
aclasis
  tarsoepiphyseal a.
acnemia
acnes
  Propionibacterium a.
acne vulgaris
aconite
Aconitum
  A. carmichaeli
  A. napellus
Acorus
  A. americanus
  A. calamus
**acquired immunodeficiency
  syndrome (AIDS)**
acral
acrid lettuce
acrinol
acroarthritis
acroataxia
acrocontracture
acromelia
acromial
  a. articular facies of clavicle
  a. articular surface of clavicle
  a. end of clavicle
  a. extremity of clavicle
  a. process

acromiale
  os a.
acromioclavicular
  a. articulation
  a. disk
  a. joint
  a. joint dysfunction
  a. joint functional technique
  a. joint separation
  a. ligament
acromioclavicularis
  articulatio a.
  discus articularis a.
acromiocoracoid
acromiohumeral
acromion
  articular surface of a.
  a. drop test
acromioscapular
acromiothoracic
acromyotonia
acromyotonus
acroteric
acrotism
act
  Controlled Substance A. (CSA)
  Federal Food, Drug, and
    Cosmetic A.
Actaea
  A. alba
  A. arguta
  A. pachypoda
  A. racemosa
  A. rubra
  A. spicata
ACTH
  adrenocorticotrophic hormone
  adrenocorticotropic hormone
actinidia
action
  cumulative a.
  initiate muscle a.
  modulate muscle a.
  a. potential
  specific a.
  A. Super Saw Palmetto Plus

activated
  a. B vitamin
  a. charcoal
  a. quercetin
activating force
activation
  cough a.
  a. force technique
  sympathetic a.
activator technique
active
  a. direct technique
  a. energy
  a. indirect technique
  a. length-tension curve
  a. motion
  a. movement
  a. muscle relaxation technique
  a. myofascial technique
  a. potential
  a. principle
  a. range of motion
  a. splint
  a. trunk rotation
Activex 40 Plus
activity, pl. activities
  alkylating a.
  altered neural a.
  antihelminthic a.
  antimicrobial a.
  brain wave a.
  craniosacral a.
  activities of daily living
    (ADL)
  electrodermal a. (EDA)
  mental a.
  neuroanatomical a.
  parasympathetic a.
  patient a.
  pilomotor a.
  reflex a.
  restore coordinated a.
  secretomotor a.
  sweat gland a.
  sympathetic a.
  vagal a.

NOTES

activity *(continued)*
  voluntary respiratory a.
  yang a.
Act-On Rub
Actualize oil
Acuball technique
aculeatus
  Ruscus a.
Acu-Magnet
acuminata
  Cola a.
acumoxatherapy
acupoint
  body a.
  a. map
  meridian a.
  a. stimulator
acupressure
  Jin Shin Do Bodymind A.
  process a.
  pronounced a.
acupuncture
  American Academy of
    Medical A. (AAMA)
  a. analgesia (AA)
  a. anesthesia
  auricular a.
  body a.
  chakra a.
  a. channel
  classic a.
  classical a.
  a. clinic
  conventional a.
  a. detoxification
  ear a.
  Eastern a.
  endonasal a.
  a. energetics
  Five Elements a.
  homuncular a.
  hybrid a.
  a. indication
  Japanese meridian a.
  Korean hand a.
  laser a.
  manual needle a.
  a. meridian
  a. needle
  oral a.
  P6 a.
  a. point

  a. point skin patch
  a. practice
  scalp a.
  a. session
  sham a.
  traditional Chinese a.
  a. treatment
  a. treatment session
  Western a.
acupuncture-like TENS
acupuncturist
Acu-Stop 2000
acute
  a. abscess
  a. angulation
  a. attack
  a. back pain
  a. brachial radiculitis
  a. bronchiolitis
  a. cauda equina syndrome
  a. cellular rejection
  a. disorder
  a. emergency
  a. hemolytic anemia
  a. lumbar sprain
  a. lymphoblastic leukemia
    (ALL)
  a. necrotizing myelitis
  a. pain
  a. promyelocytic leukemia
    (APL)
  a. reflex bone atrophy
  a. renal failure
  a. rickets
  a. somatic dysfunction
  a. spastic torticollis
  a. transverse myelitis
  a. type
  a. urticaria
  a. viral hepatitis
acutely painful condition
acutifolia
  Cassia a.
Acutouch
  Jin Shin A.
acutum
  Sinomenium a.
acu-yoga
ad
  a. lib
  a. sat
adamantinoma of long bones

Adam's
  A. apple
  A. needle
adaptation
  a. phenomenon
  regulatory a.
adaptive
  a. change
  a. response
  a. self-statement
adaptogen
adaptogenic
adaxial
ADD
  attention deficit disorder
adderwort
addiction
  alcohol a.
  cocaine a.
  nicotine a.
  opiate a.
addictive drug
Addison disease
additive
  a. effect
  food a.
adducent
adduct
adducta
  coxa a.
adduction
  hip joint a.
  restricted a.
  restricted abduction and a.
adductor
  a. brevis
  a. brevis muscle
  a. canal
  a. hallucis muscle
  a. hiatus
  a. longus muscle
  a. magnus muscle
  a. minimus muscle
  a. muscle
  a. muscle of great toe
  a. muscle of thumb
  a. pollicis longus muscle

  a. pollicis muscle
  a. reflex
  a. stretch
  a. tubercle of femur
adductorius
  canalis a.
  hiatus a.
adductovarus
  metatarsus a.
adductus
  metatarsus a.
  pes a.
adelfa
Adelir
adenohypophysis
adenoid
adenoma
  colonic a.
  colorectal a.
  prostatic a.
adenomyosis
adenosine triphosphate
Adenostyles alliariae
Aden senna
adenylate
adeps
Adhayatma yoga
ADHD
  attention deficit hyperactivity
  disorder
adhesion
  fibrinous a.
  fibrous a.
adhesive capsulitis
A'Di
  A'Ra'R A.
adipokinetic
adipose tissue
adiposum
  corpus a.
aditus pelvis
adjunct
adjunctive
  a. aid
  a. hypnotherapy
adjustive technique

NOTES

adjustment
> chiropractic a.
> a. phenomenon
> spinal a.

adjutant ingredient
adjuvant
ADL
> activities of daily living

admedial
adminiculum lineae albae
administration
> Food and Drug A. (FDA, USFDA)
> United States Food and Drug A. (USFDA)

adneural
adnexa
adolescence
adolescentium
adolescent round back
Adonis vernalis
Adrenaid
adrenal
> a. function
> a. gland
> a. hormone
> a. system

adrenergic blockade
adrenocorticotrophic hormone (ACTH)
adrenocorticotropic hormone (ACTH)
adrenoleukodystrophy
adrenomyeloneuropathy
Adson test
adsternal
adterminal
adult
> a. hypophosphatasia
> a. pseudohypertrophic muscular dystrophy
> a. rickets

adult-onset diabetes
aduncus
> unguis a.

advance
> A. Defense System Tablets

advanced
> A. Carotenoid Complex
> a. genetics
> a. glycosylation end-product (AGE)

advancement
> cumulative phase a. (CPA)

adventitia
adventitial
adventitious bursa
adverse reaction
advice
> dietary a.

adynamic ileus
AEA
> above-elbow amputation

AE Mulsion Forte
aerial part
aerobic
> A. 07
> A. Bulk Cleanse (ABC)
> a. conditioning
> a. exercise

aerodynamic size
Aeromonas hydrophilia
aerosol generator
aeruginosa
> *Pseudomonas a.*

aescin
Aesculus hippocastanum
aesthenic state
aestivum
> *Triticum a.*

Aethereum
> Extractum Filicis A.

Aetheroleum
affect
> iatrogenic a.

affected area
affectivity
> negative a.

afferent
> a. fibers of vagus nerve
> a. impulse
> a. information
> a. nerve
> a. reduction procedure
> a. stimulus
> a. vessel

affinity
> a. cluster
> color a.
> negative flavor a.
> positive flavor a.

afghanica
> *Cannabis a.*

A

afra
  Plantago a.
African
  A. coffee tree
  A. myrrh
  A. plum tree
africana
  Prunus a.
  Pygeum a.
africanum
  Pygeum a.
Afrodex
aftercontraction
agalactiae
  Streptococcus a.
agar, agar-agar
Agarbil
agaricus
  Bryonia a.
agastache
Agastache rugosa
agathosma
Agathosma betulina
AGE
  advanced glycosylation end-product
age
  bone a.
  a. regression
aged garlic extract
Ageless Beauty
agenesis of odontoid process
agent
  antiinflammatory a.
  antioxidizing a.
  cooling a.
  euphoric a.
  herbal a.
  host-defense a.
  lipid lowering a.
  neuroleptic a.
  neuromuscular blocking a.
  nonsteroidal antiinflammatory a.
  oxidizing a.
  pharmaceutical a.
  reducing a.
agglomeration
agglutinant

aggregation
  platelet a.
agitation
  internal a.
aglossia-adactylia syndrome
agmen
agneau chaste
agni
  dhatu a.
  jathar a.
agnus-castus
  Vitex a.-c.
agonist-antagonist
agonistic muscle
agonist muscle
Agrimonia eupatoria
agrimony
  water a.
Agua del Carmen
ague
  a. grass
  a. root
  a. tree
agueweed
aguru
ah
  a. shi point
  a. shi point stimulation
AHA
  American Heart Association
ahamkar
AHEC
  Area Health Education Center
AHHA
  American Holistic Health
    Association
aid
  adjunctive a.
  Calms Forte Sleep a.
  PMS A.
  Stress A.
AIDS
  acquired immunodeficiency
    syndrome
Aigin
aim
  primary a.

NOTES

9

air
    fresh a.
    a. splint
airplane splint
airway
    anatomic a.
ai ye
Ajaka
ajenjo
Ajna
AKA
    above-knee amputation
akazie
    katechu a.
Akebia quinata
akinesia amnestica
aknemia
akruti
ala, pl. **alae**
    a. major ossis sphenoidalis
    a. minor ossis sphenoidalis
    a. ossis ilii
    a. sacralis
    a. temporalis
Alacer
alanine aminotransferase (ALT)
alant
alar
    a. chest
    a. ligament
alarm point
alata
    scapula a.
alatira
    goma a.
alba
    Actaea a.
    Brassica a.
    Bryonia a.
    Morus a.
    Salix a.
albae
    adminiculum lineae a.
albicans
    Candida a.
albidum
    Sassafras a.
albocinereous
albuginea
albugineous
album
    Arsenicum a.
    Santalum a.

    Veratrum a.
    Viscum a.
albumin
albuminuria
    lordotic a.
albus
    Dictamnus a.
ALC
    acetyl-L-carnitine
alcaptonuria
Alchemilla
    A. vulgaris
    A. xanthochlora
alcohol
    a. addiction
    octacosyl a.
    perillyl a.
alcoholic recidivism
alder
    a. buckthorn
    spotted a.
alehoof
alertness
    restful a.
Aletris farinosa
Aletris-Heel
Aleurites
    A. cordata
    A. moluccana
Alexander technique
alfalfa tonic
alga, pl. **algae**
    blue-green a.
    brown a.
    super blue-green a.
alginate
    calcium a.
algiomotor
algiomuscular
algodystrophy
algology
algorithm
alignment
alimentary osteopathy
aliquot
    ozonating a.
alisma
Alisma plantago-aquatica
alkaline urine
alkaloid
    belladonna a.
    harmala a.
    pyrrolizidine a.

quinolizidine a.
tropane a.
alkalosis
metabolic a.
alkanet
Alkanna tinctoria
alkylate
alkylating activity
alkylglycerol
ALL
acute lymphoblastic leukemia
allantoin
Allen test
Aller Bee-Gone
allergen
contact a.
allergenicity
Aller G Formula 25
allergic
a. conjunctivitis
a. contact dermatitis
a. contact eczema
a. eczema
a. rhinitis
allergy
A. Care
a. desensitization
food a.
A. Liquescence
Allerid
Allermed
alliariae
Adenostyles a.
allicin
Allium
A. *ampeloprasum*
A. *ascalonicum*
A. *cepa*
A. *pustulosum*
A. *sativa*
A. *sativum*
allium
All Natural Aloe Vera Gel
allocation
allodynia
allopath
allopathic medicine

allopathy
allovedic remedy
allowance
recommended daily a. (RDA)
recommended dietary a. (RDA)
All-Purpose Bactericide Spray
allspice
almond
Alocasia macrorrhizos
aloe
A. *barbadensis*
Barbados a.
Cape a.
Curaco a.
Dermaide A.
A. Grande
A. Herbal Horse Spray
a. root
socotrine a.
Venezuela a.
a. vera
a. vera gel
a. vera inner leaf capsule
a. vera jelly
a. vera juice
a. vera liquid
a. vera ointment
a. vera pulp
a. vesta perineal benzoin
compound tincture
A. *vulgaris*
Zanzibar a.
aloifolia
Yucca a.
alopecia
reversible a.
Aloysia triphylla
alpha, α
a. lipoic acid
a. motor neuron
a. tocopherol
a. wave
Alpha-Max
Alphamul
alpha-theta brainwave training
Alpinia officinarum

NOTES

ALS
  amyotrophic lateral sclerosis
ALT
  alanine aminotransferase
  anterolateral tract
  ALT cell
alta
  patella a.
alteration
  congenital a.
  inflammatory a.
  a. of motion
  traumatic a.
altered
  a. muscle balance
  a. muscle firing pattern
    sequence
  a. neural activity
alternating fashion
alternative
  a. medicine (AM)
  A. Medicine Program Advisory
    Council (AMPAC)
  natural a.
  a. practitioner
  a. therapy
alternifolia
  Melaleuca a.
Althaea
  A. officinalis
  A. rosea
althaea, althea
  a. root
Altoids
  Wintergreen A.
alum
  a. bloom
  a. root
aluminum
  a. free indigestion
  a. toxicity
alvei (*pl. of* alveus)
alveolar
  a. macrophage
  a. ventilation
alveolaria
  juga a.
alveolitis
  postextraction a.
alveolus, gen. and pl. **alveoli**
alveus, pl. **alvei**

Alzheimer
  A. dementia
  A. disease
Alzoon
AM
  alternative medicine
ama
Amanita
  A. muscaria
  A. phalloides
  A. poisoning
amantilla
amara
  Ignatia a.
Amara Formula
amaraja
amaranth
Amaranthus hybridus var.
  erythrostachys
Amaro Maffioli
amarus
  Phyllanthus a.
amber touch-and-heal
ambiguous
ambilateral
amblyopia
ambrosoides
  Chenopodium a.
Ambu bag
ambulation
ambulatory anesthesia
amebic dysentery
amebicidal
ameliorate
amelioration
amenorrhea
America
  Biofeedback Certification
    Institute of A. (BCIA)
  Bioforce of A.
  Wakunaga of A.
American
  A. Academy of Medical
    Acupuncture (AAMA)
  A. Academy of Osteopathy
  A. aspen
  A. Association of Colleges of
    Osteopathic Medicine
    (AACOM)
  A. Association of Homeopathic
    Pharmacists (AAHP)
  A. Association for Medical
    Instrumentation (AAMI)

A. Association of Naturopathic
Physicians (AANP)
A. Board of Dental Hypnosis
A. Board of Medical Hypnosis
A. Board of Psychological
Hypnosis (ABPH)
A. Boards of Hypnosis
A. Botanical Council (ABC)
A. Chiropractic Association
(ACA)
A. cone flower
A. cowslip
A. cranesbill
A. dwarf palm tree
A. elm
A. ginseng
A. Heart Association (AHA)
A. Herbalists Guild
A. Holistic Health Association
(AHHA)
A. kino
A. mandrake
A. Massage Therapy
Association (AMTA)
A. mistletoe
A. mullein
A. Osteopathic Association
(AOA)
A. pennyroyal
A. saffron
A. Society of Clinical
Hypnosis
A. Society of Clinical
Hypnosis
A. upland cotton
A. valerian
A. vervain
A. yew
americana .
Phytolacca a.
americanum
Zanthoxylum a.
americanus
Acorus a.
amine

amino
a. acid
a. acid analysis
aminoglycoside antibiotic
Amino-LIV
aminotransferase
alanine a. (ALT)
aspartate a. (AST)
amitriptyline
amla
AmlaPlex
Amma therapy
Ammi
A. majus
A. visagna
ammi
a. fruit
greater a.
toothpick a.
ammonium ion
Ammonium muriaticum
amnesia
posthypnotic a.
selective a.
amnestica
akinesia a.
Amomum
A. repens
A. sublatum
A. villosum
amorphous ground substance
AMPAC
Alternative Medicine Program
Advisory Council
ampeloprasum
Allium a.
amphiarthrodial
amphiarthrosis
ampicillin
amplitude
cranial rhythmic impulse a.
CRI a.
low a.
pulse a.
pulse recording of a.
A.M./P.M. Ultimate Cleanse

NOTES

ampoule, ampule
ampulla, gen. and pl. ampullae
ampullar
ampullary aneurysm
ampullula
amputation
    above-elbow a. (AEA)
    above-knee a. (AKA)
    aperiosteal a.
    below-elbow a. (BEA)
    below-knee a. (BKA)
    bloodless a.
    central a.
    cinematic a.
    cineplastic a.
    circular a.
    consecutive a.
    a. in continuity
    double flap a.
    dry a.
    eccentric a.
    elliptical a.
    excentric a.
    flap a.
    flapless a.
    forequarter a.
    guillotine a.
    hindquarter a.
    immediate a.
    intermediate a.
    interscapulothoracic a.
    kineplastic a.
    knee disarticulation a.
    linear a.
    major a.
    minor a.
    multiple a.
    oblique a.
    pathologic a.
    primary a.
    quadruple a.
    racket a.
    rectangular a.
    secondary a.
    subastragalar a.
    subperiosteal a.
    tarsotibial a.
    traumatic a.
amputee
AMTA
    American Massage Therapy
    Association
amulet

amyelous
amygdala
amygdalin
Amygdalis
amyloid
    beta a.
amyloidosis
amyoplasia congenita
amyostasia
amyostatic
amyosthenia
amyosthenic
amyotaxy
amyotonia congenita
amyotrophia
amyotrophic lateral sclerosis (ALS)
amyotrophy
    hemiplegic a.
    neuralgic a.
    progressive spinal a.
amyous
ANA
    antinuclear antibody
anabiotic
Anabol Naturals
anabsinthin
anadidymus
anaerobic
    a. exercise
    a. oral bacteria
    a. vaginosis
anagenesis
Anahata
anal
    a. canal
    a. fissure
    a. sphincter
    a. triangle
analeptic
analgesia
    acupuncture a. (AA)
    conduction a.
    endorphin a.
    endorphinergic a.
    endorphin-mediated
      acupuncture a.
    high-frequency low-intensity a.
    hypnotic a.
    inhalation a.
    low-frequency, high-intensity a.
    patient-controlled a. (PCA)
    spinal a.
    stress-induced a.

analgesic
    a. effect
    a. point
analgesimeter
analgetic
analysis
    amino acid a.
    behavioral a.
    bioenergetic a.
    gait a.
    hair a.
    Laban movement a.
    live enzyme a.
    mechanical a.
    motion a.
    muscle a.
    postural a.
    static a.
anamnesis
ananas
Ananase
anaphylactic shock
anaphylactoid reaction
anaphylaxis
    ocular a.
anapophysis
anascha
Ana-Sed
anastomose
anastomosing vessel
anastomosis
anastomotic branch
anatomic
    a. airway
    a. barrier
    a. position
    a. snuffbox
Anatomica
    Basle Nomina A.
anatomical
    a. landmark
    a. neck of humerus
anatomicomedical
anatomicopathologic
anatomicosurgical
anatomique
    tabatière a.

anatomist
anatomy
    applied a.
    functional a.
    general a.
    innominate a.
    neuromuscular a.
    physiologic a.
    regional a.
    rib a.
    special a.
    topographic a.
Anchusa
    A. officinalis
    A. tinctoria
ancon
anconad
anconal fossa
anconeus
    a. muscle
    musculus a.
anconitis
anconoid
androgenization
androgen metabolism
Andrographalide
androgynus
    Sauropus a.
anecdotal evidence
Anemarrhena asphodeloides
anemia
    acute hemolytic a.
    hemolytic a.
    hemorrhagic a.
    iron-deficiency a.
    local a.
    megamineral sideroblastic a.
    osteosclerotic a.
    pernicious a.
    posthemorrhagic a.
    sideroblastic a.
    spastic a.
    traumatic a.
anemic
anemone
    meadow a.

NOTES

anemone *(continued)*
   prairie a.
   A. *pulsatilla*
anencephaly
aneroid manometer
anesthesia
   acupuncture a.
   ambulatory a.
   axillary a.
   balanced a.
   basal a.
   block a.
   brachial a.
   caudal a.
   cervical a.
   circle absorption a.
   closed a.
   compression a.
   conduction a.
   dental a.
   diagnostic a.
   differential spinal a.
   a. dolorosa
   electric a.
   endotracheal a.
   epidural a.
   extradural a.
   field block a.
   general a.
   girdle a.
   high spinal a.
   hyperbaric a.
   hyperbaric spinal a.
   hypobaric spinal a.
   hypotensive a.
   hypothermic a.
   infiltration a.
   inhalation a.
   insufflation a.
   intercostal a.
   intramedullary a.
   intranasal a.
   intraoral a.
   intraosseous a.
   intraspinal a.
   intratracheal a.
   intravenous a.
   intravenous regional a.
   isobaric spinal a.
   local a.
   low spinal a.
   manipulation under a.
   medial a.

   nerve block a.
   open drop a.
   outpatient a.
   painful a.
   paracervical block a.
   paravertebral a.
   patient-controlled a. (PCA)
   peridural a.
   presacral a.
   pressure a.
   pudendal a.
   regional a.
   retrobulbar a.
   sacral a.
   saddle block a.
   segmental a.
   spinal a.
   splanchnic a.
   subarachnoid a.
   surgical a.
   tactile a.
   therapeutic a.
   to-and-fro a.
   topical a.
   total spinal a.
   traumatic a.
   visceral a.
anesthesiologist
anesthesiology
anesthetic
   epidural local a.
   flammable a.
   a. gas
   general a.
   a. index
   inhalation a.
   instillation of a.
   intravenous a.
   local a.
   primary a.
   secondary a.
   a. shock
   spinal a.
   topical a.
   a. vapor
   volatile a.
anesthetist
anesthetization
anesthetize
aneth fenouil
Anethum graveolens
aneurysm
   abdominal a.

ampullary a.
axial a.
benign bone a.
cerebral a.
compound a.
cylindroid a.
diffuse a.
ectatic a.
false a.
fusiform a.
hernial a.
mycotic a.
peripheral a.
Pott a.
saccular a.
serpentine a.
traumatic a.
true a.
aneurysmal bone cyst
angel
    a. tulip
    a. wing
Angelica
    A. *archangelica*
    A. *polymorpha*
    A. *sinensis*
angelica
    European a.
    garden a.
    a. root
    a. tree
    wild a.
angelique
angel's trumpet
anger
    inadequate a.
angiectatic
angiectopia
angiitis
angina
    a. cruris
    a. pectoris
    unstable a.
angiogenesis factor
angiohypertonia
angiohypotonia
angioneurotic edema

angioplasty
    coronary a.
    percutaneous transluminal a.
angiosclerotica
    dysbasia a.
    myasthenia a.
angiotensin
angiotensin-converting enzyme (ACE)
angle
    a. of antetorsion
    a. of anteversion
    beta a.
    carrying a.
    cephalic a.
    costal a.
    craniofacial a.
    a. of declination
    ethmoid a.
    a. of Ferguson
    Ferguson lumbosacral a.
    a. of inclination
    inferior lateral a. (ILA)
    infrasternal a.
    Louis a.
    Ludwig a.
    lumbosacral a.
    lumbosacral lordotic a.
    a. of mandible
    Mitchell lumbosacral a.
    neck-shaft a.
    ophryospinal a.
    pelvivertebral a.
    Pirogoff a.
    pubic a.
    Q a.
    quadriceps a.
    a. of retroversion
    rib a.
    slip a.
    sphenoid a.
    sternal a.
    sternoclavicular a.
    substernal a.
    a. of torsion
    Welcker a.
Angostura Bitters

NOTES

angry cat exercise
angular
    a. curvature
    a. stomatitis
angularis
    Sabbatia a.
angulation
    acute a.
    apex anterior a.
    apex posterior a.
angulus
    a. costae
    a. inferior scapulae
    a. infrasternalis
    a. lateralis scapulae
    a. mandibulae
    a. sterni
    a. superior scapulae
angustifolia
    Cassia a.
    Echinacea a.
    Lavandula a.
    Pulmonaria a.
ani
    levator a.
animal force
anion
    superoxide a.
anise
    a. fruit
    a. oil
    a. seed
anisomelia
anisosthenic
anisum
    Pimpinella a.
ankle
    a. bone
    central bone of a.
    fibular collateral ligament of a.
    a. and foot somatic dysfunction
    a. and foot tender point
    a. functional technique
    a. joint
    lateral collateral ligament of a.
    a. region
    a. tub
ankle-foot orthosis
ankylopoietic
ankylosed

ankylosing
    a. hyperostosis
    a. spondylitis
ankylosis
    artificial a.
    bony a.
    extracapsular a.
    false a.
    fibrous a.
    intracapsular a.
    spurious a.
    true a.
ankylotic
anmian
    Ex-HN 8 a. I
    Ex-HN 9 a. II
annexal
Annie
    sweet A.
annua
    Artemisia a.
annularis
    rachitis fetalis a.
annular tear
annulospiral ending
annulus fibrosis
annuum
    Capsicum a.
annuus
    Helianthus a.
anociassociation
anococcygeal
    a. body
    a. ligament
    a. nerve
anodyne imagery
anomalous development
anomaly
anonymous vein
anorectal surgery
anorexia nervosa
anosmia
anosmic
anospinal
anovulation
anovulatory
anoxia
    anoxic a.
    cerebral a.
anoxic anoxia
ANS
    autonomic nervous system

ansa
a. cervicalis
a. sacralis
a. subclavia
Vieussens a.
ansae nervorum spinalium
anserine
a. bursa
a. bursitis
answer
Nature's A.
Antabuse
antagonist
dynorphin kappa a.
endorphin a.
a. muscle
antagonistic muscle
antalgesia
antalgic gait
Antares
antebrachial
a. fascia
a. flexor retinaculum
antebrachii
chorda obliqua membranae
interosseae a.
fascia a.
margo lateralis a.
margo medialis a.
margo radialis a.
margo ulnaris a.
membrana interossea a.
antebrachium
ante cibum
antecubital space
anteflex
anteflexion
antegrade
antelope brush
anterior
a. apprehension test
a. arch
a. articular pillar
a. atlas
a. border
a. branch
a. capsule

a. caudate
a. compartment
a. component
a. convexity
a. curvature
a. direction
duplicitas a.
facies a.
a. fat pad
a. fat pad lesion
a. fibular head
fibular head a.
a. fontanelle
fossa cranii a.
a. glide
a. horn cell
a. iliac rotation
a. ilium
a. ilium functional technique
a. inferior iliac spine
a. and inferior right shoulder
girdle
a. innominate iliac rotation
a. lift therapy
linea axillaris a.
linea glutea a.
linea mediana a.
a. margin
membrana atlantooccipitalis a.
musculus sacrococcygeus a.
musculus scalenus a.
musculus serratus a.
musculus tibiofascialis a.
a. nasal aperture
a. nasal spine
a. palpation
pars a.
a. part
a. pelvic tilt
a. plane
a. posterior compression
radial head a.
regio antebrachialis a.
regio brachialis a.
regio carpalis a.
regio cervicalis a.
regio cruris a.

A

NOTES

anterior *(continued)*
   regio cubitalis a.
   regio femoris a.
   regio genus a.
   a. sacrum
   a. scalene muscle
   a. segment
   a. serratus muscle
   a. subluxation
   a. superior iliac spine (ASIS)
   a. superior iliac spine test
   a. surface
   synchondrosis intraoccipitalis a.
   a. tibial compartment syndrome
   tibialis a.
   a. tibial muscle
   a. translated sacrum
   translation a.
anterioris
   trigonum musculare regionis
     cervicalis a.
   tuberculum musculi scaleni a.
   tuberositas musculi serrati a.
   vagina tendinis musculi
     tibialis a.
anteriorly
   convex a.
   a. rotated innominate
   a. rotated right innominate
   sacroiliac bilaterally nutated a.
anterior-posterior axis
anterius
   segmentum a.
   trigonum cervicale a.
anteroexternal
anteroinferior
anterointernal
anterolateral tract (ALT)
anteromedial
anteromedian
anteroposterior (AP)
   a. axis
   a. erect lumbar spine
   a. glide
   a. movement
   a. projection
   a. rib compression
   a. translation test
anterosuperior
antetorsion
   angle of a.
anteversion
   angle of a.

anthelminthic
anthelmintic
anthocyanin
Anthoxanthum odoratum
anthranoid derivative
Anthraxiviore
Anthriscus cerefolium
anthropometer
anthropometric
anthropometry
anthroposcopy
anthroposomatology
anthroposophically extended
   medicine
anthroposophic medicine
anthroposophy
anthroquinone glycoside
antiaging drug therapy
antiaging medicine
antiallergenic
antiallergic property
AntiAllergy formula
antiandrogen
antibacterial
antibiotic
   aminoglycoside a.
   broad-spectrum a. (BSA)
antibiotic-induced diarrhea
antibiotic-resistant bacteria
antibody
   antinuclear a. (ANA)
   sperm a.
anticatarrhal
anticholinergic compound
anticipatory
   a. nausea
   a. vomiting
anticlinal
anticnemion
anticoagulant
anticonvulsive effect
anticus
   musculus scalenus a.
antidepressant
   tricyclic a.
antidiarrheal
antidiuretic
antidotal
antiedemic
antiemetic
antiestrogen
antifebrile
antifertility

antiflatulent
antifungal
antigen
    hepatitis B surface a.
    prostate-specific a. (PSA)
antigen-antibody reaction
antigenic
antigonadal
antigravity muscle
antihabituation
antihelminthic activity
antihemorrhagic
antihepatoxic
antihistamine
antihypertensive treatment
antiinflammatory
    a. agent
    a. drug
    a. effect
antilithic
antimetabolite
antimicrobial
    a. activity
    a. medication
antimony
    vegetable a.
antineoplastic
antineoplaston therapy
antinuclear
    a. antibody (ANA)
    a. antibody test
antiobesity
antioxidant
    Body Language Super A.
    cellular a.
    a. defense system
    DHEA with A.'s
    a. vitamin
antioxidative
antioxidizing agent
antiplatelet
antipodal
antipode
antipolarization biphasic pulse
antiprostatic
antipyogenic
antipyretic

antipyrine
antiretroviral drug
antirheumatic
antiseptic
    living a.
    nasal a.
    topical a.
    viable a.
antiserum
    immunoglobulin E a.
antispasmodic
antistaphylococcal
antistatin
antisterility vitamin
Anti-Stress Enzymes
antithenar
antithyroid
antithyroidal effect
antitragicus
    a. muscle
    musculus a.
antitragus
    muscle of a.
antitrope
antitropic
antitrypanosome
antituberculosis vaccine
antitumor
antitussive
antiulcerogenic
antiviral
antra (pl. of antrum)
antral
antropathy
antrum, gen. antri, pl. antra
anular
    a. ligament
    a. ligament of radius
    a. ligament of stapes
anularis
    digitus a.
anulus
    a. fibrosus disci intervertebralis
    a. fibrosus of intervertebral
    disk
    a. of fibrous sheath

NOTES

21

anxiety
    stress-induced a.
    trait a.
anxiolytic
ao
    hsia ku ts' a.
    i-mu-ts' a.
AOA
    American Osteopathic Association
aorta
    abdominal a.
    coarctation of a.
    thoracic a.
aortae
    pars thoracica a.
aortic hiatus
AP
    anteroposterior
    AP Mag
    AP projection
aparine
    Galium a.
ape hand
aperiosteal amputation
aperta
    spina bifida a.
apertura
    a. thoracis inferior
    a. thoracis superior
aperture
    anterior nasal a.
    superior thoracic a.
    thoracic a.
apex
    a. anterior angulation
    a. capitis fibulae
    a. of head of fibula
    a. ossis sacri
    a. of patella
    a. patellae
    a. posterior angulation
    a. of sacrum
aphorism
aphrodine
aphrodisiac
Aphrodyne
aphthous ulcer
apical
    a. axillary lymph node
    a. ligament of dens
apiol
Apis mellifera
apitherapy

apium
Apium graveolens
APL
    acute promyelocytic leukemia
Apley
    A. compression test
    A. scratch test
apnea
    induced a.
apneic oxygenation
apneustic center in pons
apodia
aponeurosis
    extensor a.
    a. of insertion
    a. of investment
    a. musculi bicipitis brachii
    a. of origin
    palmar a.
    a. palmaris
    plantar a.
    a. plantaris
    thoracolumbar a.
    a. of vastus muscles
aponeurositis
aponeurotic
aponeurotica
    falx a.
apophysary
apophysial, apophyseal
    a. fracture
apophysis
    basilar a.
    lenticular a.
apophysitis
    calcaneal a.
    a. tibialis
apoplexia
    hemiplegic a.
apoptosis
apparatus
    Golgi tendon a.
    a. ligamentosus colli
    a. ligamentosus weitbrechti
appearance
    Scotty dog a.
appendage
appendiceal
appendicitis
appendicular
    a. artery
    a. muscle
    a. skeleton

appendiculare
    skeleton a.
appendix
appetite stimulation
apple
    Adam's a.
    a. cider vinegar
    golden a.
    hog a.
    Indian a.
    mad a.
    marsh a.
    oak a.
    a. pectin
    a. of Peru
    a. pulp
    thorn a.
appleringie
appliance
application
    bioelectromagnetic a.
    hands-on a.
    new drug a. (NDA)
    traditional a.
applied
    a. anatomy
    a. kinesiologist
    a. kinesiology
    a. voltage
apposition
    bayonet a.
    convex-to-convex a.
appositional growth
apprehension test
approach
    Aston a.
    biofield a.
    complementary and
      alternative a. (CAA)
    hands-on a.
    mind-body a.
    mixer a.
approximate
approximation
    law of a.

apricot
    a. seed extract
    a. vine
apus
    sympus a.
Aqua-Rid
aquatica
    Mentha a.
aqueduct
aqueductus
aqueous extract
aquifolium
    Berberis a.
    Ilex a.
    Mahonia a.
Arabian myrrh
arabic
    gum a.
arabica
    Coffea a.
arabinogalactan
arachnoid
    a. granulation
    a. layer
    a. layer of meninges
    a. of spinal cord
    spinal part of a.
arachnoidea mater spinalis
arachnoiditis
Aralia racemosa
A'Ra'R A'Di
arbor
arborea
    Datura a.
arborescens
    Hydrangea a.
    lipoma a.
arborescent
arborine
arborinine
arborization
arborize
arbutin
arc
    movement a.
    reflex a.
    somatic reflex a.

NOTES

arc *(continued)*
    somatovisceral reflex a.
    visceral reflex a.
    viscerovisceral reflex a.
arcate
arch
    abdominothoracic a.
    anterior a.
    carpal a.
    coracoacromial a.
    costal a.
    fallen a.
    a. of foot
    foot a.
    Haller a.
    hemal a.
    iliopectineal a.
    lamina of vertebral a.
    Langer a.
    lateral lumbocostal a.
    lateral weightbearing a.
    medial lumbocostal a.
    medial spring a.
    metatarsal a.
    plantar a.
    plantar arterial a.
    popliteal a.
    pseudometatarsal a.
    tarsal a.
    tendinous a.
    a. of thoracic duct
    transverse a.
    unilateral fallen a.
    vertebral a.
    zygomatic a.
archangelica
    Angelica a.
architecture
    bone a.
arciform
Arctium lappa
Arctostaphylos
Arctuvan
arcual
arcuate
    a. cell
    a. ligament
    a. nucleus
    a. popliteal ligament
    a. pubic ligament
arcuation
arcus
    a. costalis

    a. costarum
    a. iliopectineus
    a. lumbocostalis lateralis
    a. lumbocostalis medialis
    a. palmaris profundus
    a. palmaris superficialis
    a. palpebralis inferior
    a. palpebralis superior
    a. pedis longitudinalis
    a. pedis longitudinalis pars lateralis
    a. pedis longitudinalis pars medialis
    a. pedis transversalis
    a. tarseus
    a. tendineus
    a. tendineus musculi solei
    a. venosus dorsalis pedis
    a. venosus palmaris profundus
    a. venosus palmaris superficialis
    a. venosus plantaris
    a. vertebra
    a. volaris profundus
    a. volaris superficialis
Ardeydystin
ardic
area
    affected a.
    diseased a.
    A. Health Education Center (AHEC)
    hypochondriac a.
    a. intercondylaris anterior tibiae
    a. intercondylaris posterior tibiae
    medial scapular a.
    pivot a.
    proximal a.
    retroorbital a.
    shawl a.
    stagnant a.
    stagnated a.
areca
    A. catechu
    a. nut
arecaidine
arecoline
Areocaps
areola, pl. **areolae**
areolar tissue
Argentine
Argentum nitricum

arginine
arguta
    Actaea a.
aristolactam
Aristolochia
    A. clematitis
    A. fangchi
    A. manshuriensis
    A. serpentaria
aristolochia
aristolochiaefolia
    Smilax a.
aristolochic acid
ark
    Noah's a.
Arkocaps
arm
    biceps muscle of a.
    deep fascia of a.
    a. drop test
    lateral surface of a.
    moment a.
    posterior region of a.
    posterior surface of a.
    swing of a.
    triceps muscle of a.
armamentarium
    manual medicine a.
armeniaca
    Prunus a.
armino
armoise
armonica
Armoracia rusticana
armpit
armrest bolster
arnica
    common a.
    A. cordifolia
    a. flower
    A. latifolia
    Mexican a.
    A. montana
    mountain a.
    a. root
    A. sororia
    A. Spray

Arnicaid
Arniflora Gel
Arnold-Chiari
    A.-C. malformation
    A.-C. syndrome
Aromamist Steam Tube
Aroma-Stream Diffuser
aromatherapy
    a. diffuser
    ousia a.
aromatica
    Eugenia a.
Aromatic Castor Oil
aromaticum
    Eugenia a.
    Syzygium a.
Aromist Personal Steam Sauna
arousal
    autonomic a.
    sympathetic a.
arrector
arrhythmia
    cardiac a.
    ventricular a.
arrhythmogenic
arrow
    green a.
arrowwood
    Indian a.
arruda
    a. brava
    a. do mato
arsenic
Arsenicum album
ART
    articulation treatment
    assisted reproductive technique
    asymmetry, range of motion
    abnormality, tissue texture
    abnormality
art
    healing a.
    martial a.
    a. therapy
artava
    sukra a.

NOTES

Artemisia
  A. absinthium
  A. annua
  A. cina
  A. dracunculus
  A. tridentata
  A. vulgaris
artemisinin
arteria
arterial dissection
arteries (*pl. of* artery)
arteriococcygeal gland
arteriola
arteriolar
arteriole
arteriovenous malformation
arteritis
  temporal a.
artery, pl. arteries
  appendicular a.
  atlantic part of vertebral a.
  atresia of vertebral a.
  axillary a.
  basilar a.
  brachial a.
  carotid a.
  celiac a.
  central sulcal a.
  cervical part of internal
    carotid a.
  cortical a.
  cremasteric a.
  digital collateral a.
  distributing a.
  femoral a.
  fibular a.
  hardening of the arteries
  humeral a.
  iliac a.
  inferior ulnar collateral a.
  intercostal a.
  internal carotid a.
  intracranial part of vertebral a.
  lowest lumbar a.
  lowest thyroid a.
  medial plantar a.
  medullary spinal a.
  mesenteric a.
  metatarsal a.
  muscular a.
  obturator a.
  peroneal a.
  popliteal a.

  prevertebral part of
    vertebral a.
  profunda brachii a.
  profunda femoris a.
  pubic branch of obturator a.
  renal a.
  rule of the a.
  spinal a.
  sternomastoid a.
  subclavian a.
  sulcus for vertebral a.
  vertebral a.
  vertebral basilar a.
artetyke
Arthease
arthragra
arthral
arthralgia
  intermittent a.
  periodic a.
  a. saturnina
arthralgic
arthritica
arthritic atrophy
arthriticum
  tuberculum a.
arthritis, pl. arthritides
  atrophic a.
  chronic absorptive a.
  chylous a.
  crystal-induced a.
  a. deformans
  degenerative a.
  filarial a.
  gonococcal a.
  gonorrheal a.
  gouty a.
  hemophilic a.
  hypertrophic a.
  infectious a.
  inflammatory a.
  juvenile a.
  a. mutilans
  neuropathic a.
  a. nodosa
  ochronotic a.
  proliferative a.
  psoriatic a.
  pyogenic a.
  rheumatoid a. (RA)
  suppurative a.
  a. tea
arthrocele

arthrocentesis
arthrochondritis
arthroclasia
arthrodesis
    triple a.
arthrodia
arthrodial
    a. articulation
    a. cartilage
    a. joint
    a. structure
arthrodynia
arthrodynic
arthrodysplasia
Arthro-Ease
arthroendoscopy
arthroereisis
arthrogenous
arthrogram
arthrography
arthrogryposis multiplex congenita
arthrokatadysis
arthrolith
arthrolithiasis
arthrologia
arthrology
arthrolysis
arthrometer
arthrometry
arthroophthalmopathy
    hereditary progressive a.
arthropathia psoriatica
arthropathology
arthropathy
    diabetic a.
    facet a.
    long-leg a.
    neuropathic a.
    static a.
    tabetic a.
arthroplasty
    gap a.
    interposition a.
arthropneumoradiography
arthropyosis
arthrorisis

Arthro-Rx
    Natural A.-R.
arthrosclerosis
arthroscope
arthroscopy
arthrosis
arthrostomy
arthrosynovitis
arthrotropic
Arth-X
Arth-X-Plus
artichoke
articular
    a. branch
    a. capsule
    a. cartilage
    a. cavity
    a. chondrocalcinosis
    a. circumference of head of radius
    a. circumference of head of ulna
    a. crepitus
    a. crescent
    a. crest
    a. disk
    a. disk of acromioclavicular joint
    a. disk of distal radioulnar joint
    a. disk of sternoclavicular joint
    a. facet
    a. facet of head of fibula
    a. facet of head of rib
    a. facet of tubercle of rib
    a. fat pad
    a. fossa of temporal bone
    a. fracture
    a. gout
    a. labrum
    a. lamella
    a. ligamentous release
    a. lip
    a. margin
    a. meniscus
    a. mobility
    a. mobility of bones

NOTES

articular *(continued)*
  a. mobility of cranial bone
  a. muscle
  a. muscle of elbow
  a. muscle of knee
  a. nerve
  a. network
  a. palpation
  a. pillar
  a. pit of head of radius
  a. process
  a. reaction
  a. receptor
  a. structure
  a. surface of acromion
  a. surface of arytenoid
    cartilage
  a. surface of mandibular fossa
    of temporal bone
  a. surface of patella
  a. vascular circle
  a. vascular network
articulare
  cavum a.
  labrum a.
  rete vasculosum a.
articularis
  capsula a.
  cartilago a.
  cavitas a.
  a. cubiti muscle
  discus a.
  facies a.
  a. genus muscle
  meniscus a.
  musculus a.
  nervus a.
articulate
articulated skeleton
articulatio
  a. acromioclavicularis
  a. atlantoaxialis lateralis
  a. atlantoaxialis mediana
  a. atlantooccipitalis
  a. bicondylaris
  a. calcaneocuboidea
  a. capitis costae
  a. carpometacarpalis pollicis
  a. cartilaginis
  a. complexa
  a. composita
  a. condylaris
  a. costotransversaria

  a. cotylica
  a. coxae
  a. cubiti
  a. cuneonavicularis
  a. ellipsoidea
  a. fibrosa
  a. genus
  a. humeri
  a. humeroradialis
  a. humeroulnaris
  a. incudomallearis
  a. lumbosacralis
  a. mediocarpalis
  a. ovoidalis
  a. plana
  a. radiocarpalis
  a. radioulnaris distalis
  a. radioulnaris proximalis
  a. sacrococcygea
  a. sacroiliaca
  a. sellaris
  a. simplex
  a. spheroidea
  a. sternoclavicularis
  a. subtalaris
  a. synovialis
  a. talocalcaneonavicularis
  a. talocruralis
  a. tarsi transversa
  a. tibiofibularis articulationes
    carpometacarpales
articulation
  acromioclavicular a.
  arthrodial a.
  atlantoaxial a.
  atlantooccipital a.
  bicondylar a.
  calcaneocuboid a.
  carpometacarpal a.
  cartilaginous a.
  compound a.
  condylar a.
  costotransverse a.
  costovertebral a.
  cuneonavicular a.
  distal radioulnar a.
  distal tibiofibular a.
  a.'s of foot
  glenohumeral a.
  a.'s of hand
  humeral a.
  humeroradial a.
  humeroulnar a.

interchondral a.
intermetatarsal a.
interphalangeal a.
intertarsal a.
metacarpophalangeal a.
metatarsophalangeal a.
occipital a.
occiput a.
parietal bone a.
peg-and-socket a.
proximal radioulnar a.
radiocarpal a.
rib a.
sacroiliac a.
a. of skull
sphenoid a.
spheroid a.
sternochondral a.
sternoclavicular a.
sternocostal a.
subtalar a.
superior tibial a.
talocalcaneal a.
talocrural a.
talonavicular a.
temporal a.
temporal bone a.
tibiofibular a.
transverse tarsal a.
a. treatment (ART)
trochoid a.
ulna-meniscal-triquetral a.
articulationes
a. cinguli membri inferioris
a. cinguli membri superioris
a. costochondrales
a. costovertebrales
a. intercarpales
a. interchondrales
a. intermetacarpales
a. intermetatarsales
a. interphalangeae manus
a. interphalangeae pedis
a. intertarseae
a. manus
a. membri inferioris liberi

a. membri superioris liberi
a. metacarpophalangeae
a. metatarsophalangeae
a. pedis
a. sternocostales
a. tarsometatarsales
articulatory
a. pop
a. procedure
a. technique
a. treatment
articulus
artifact
electrochemical potential a.
artificial
a. ankylosis
a. calculus
a. lighting
a. respiration
a. stone
a. ventilation
Artival
arvense
Equisetum a.
arytenoid
arytenoidal articular surface of cricoid
arytenoideus
asana
Asarum heterotropoides
ascalonicum
Allium a.
Ascaris lumbricoides
ascendens
cervicalis a.
musculus cervicalis a.
ascending
a. branch
hyper liver yang a.
a. myelitis
Asclepias
A. synaca
A. tuberosa
As-Comp
Ascophyllum nodosum
ascorbate

NOTES

ascorbic
a. acid
a. acid flush
aseptic necrosis
ash
bitter a.
northern prickly a.
poison a.
prickly a.
southern prickly a.
ashi point
Asian ginseng
asiatica
Centella a.
titrated extract of *Centella a.*
(TECA)
Asiatic ginseng
ASIS
anterior superior iliac spine
Aspalathus linearis
asparagine
Asparagus officinalis
aspartate
a. aminotransferase (AST)
potassium-magnesium a.
aspartic acid
aspect
posterior a.
aspen
American a.
quaking a.
aspera
lateral lip of linea a.
linea a.
medial lip of linea a.
asperae
labium laterale lineae a.
labium mediale lineae a.
Aspergillus
A. mold
A. oryzae
Asperula
A. avensis
A. odorata
asperuloside
asperum
Dracontium a.
Symphytum a.
asphodeloides
Anemarrhena a.
asphyxia
asphyxial
asphyxiant

asphyxiate
asphyxiation
aspic
aspidium oleoresin
Aspilia
aspirator
aspirin
aspirin-sensitive asthma
ASQ
Attributional Style Questionnaire
ASQ Internal Scale
ASQ Stability Scale
assafoetida
Ferula a.
assay
colorimetric redox a.
assertiveness training
assessment
biological terrain a. (BTA)
energetic a.
energy field a.
group curve a.
holistic a.
occupational therapy a.
three-dimensional a.
Ass-Hide Gelatin Decoction
assimilation
a. pelvis
a. sacrum
assist
respiratory a.
assistance
respiratory a.
assistant ingredient
assisted
a. eccentric strengthening
supine
a. reproductive technique
(ART)
assistive movement
associate
Diamond-Herpanacine A.'s
a. ingredient
association
American Chiropractic A.
(ACA)
American Heart A. (AHA)
American Holistic Health A.
(AHHA)
American Massage Therapy A.
(AMTA)
American Osteopathic A.
(AOA)

A. for Applied
  Psychophysiology and
  Biofeedback (AAPB)
Herb Trade A. (HTA)
independent practice a. (IPA)
International Chiropractic A.
  (ICA)
National Acupuncture
  Detoxification A.
National Nutritional Foods A.
  (NNFA)
New York Heart A. (NYHA)
North American Nursing
  Diagnosis A. (NANDA)
organ a.
ass's foot
AST
  aspartate aminotransferase
asterion
asternal
asthenia
asthenic
asthi
asthma
  aspirin-sensitive a.
  bronchial a.
  exercise-induced a.
  occupational a.
  a. weed
asthmaweed
  Queensland a.
Aston
  A. approach
  A. patterning
  A. therapeutics
ASTRA 8 formula
astragalar
astragalocalcanean
astragalofibular
astragaloscaphoid
astragalotibial
astragalus
  A. *gummifer*
  A. *membranaceus*
  A. 10 Plus
  a. root
astriction

astringe
astringent
  yellow a.
Astring-O-Sol
astrology
  Vedic a.
asustado
aswagandha
asymmetric
  a. chondrodystrophy
  a. motion
  a. tonic reflex
asymmetrical joint
asymmetry
  cervicothoracic a.
  congenial a.
  facet a.
  a., range of motion
    abnormality, tissue texture
    abnormality (ART)
  a., range of motion, texture
  zygapophysial joint a.
asynchronous
asystematic
atactic abasia
atavicus
  metatarsus a.
atavistic epiphysis
ataxia
  Friedreich a.
  hereditary spinal a.
  vestibulocerebellar a.
ataxiadynamia
ataxic gait
ataxy
atherogenesis
atherosclerosis
atherosclerotic lesion
athetosis
Atkinson & Barker's Gripe
  Mixture
atlamisa
atlantic part of vertebral artery
atlantis
  fovea articularis inferior a.
  fovea articularis superior a.
  fovea dentis a.

NOTES

atlantoaxial
  a. articulation
  a. cervical spine
  a. joint
  a. vertebra
atlantoepistrophic
atlantooccipital
  a. articulation
  a. joint
  a. membrane
atlantooccipitalis
  articulatio a.
atlantoodontoid
atlas
  anterior a.
  cruciate ligament of the a.
  cruciform ligament of a.
  lateral mass of a.
  longitudinal bands of cruciform
    ligament of a.
  a. motion test
  a. rotated right
  superior articular facet of a.
  transverse ligament of the a.
ATM
  Awareness Through Movement
atomizer
atonia
atonicity
atonic muscle tone
atony
atopic
  a. dermatitis
  a. eczema
Atractylis gummifer
atractylode
Atractylodes macrocephala
atrata
  Cryptotympana a.
atresia of vertebral artery
atrial
  a. fibrillation
  a. septal defect
atrioventricular
  a. block
  a. node
atrium
  intervenous tubercle of right a.
atriviridis
  Garcinia a.
Atropa belladonna
atrophica
  myotonia a.

atrophic arthritis
atrophy
  acute reflex bone a.
  arthritic a.
  facioscapulohumeral a.
  familial spinal muscular a.
  ischemic muscular a.
  juvenile muscular a.
  muscle a.
  muscular a.
  myopathic a.
  neurogenic a.
  neurotrophic a.
  peroneal muscular a.
  progressive muscular a.
  scapulohumeral a.
  spinal muscular a., type III
atropine
atropurpureus
  Euonymus a.
attachment
  ligamentous a.
  muscle-tendon a.
  muscular a.
  musculoskeletal system
    diaphragm a.
attack
  acute a.
  epileptic a.
  heart a.
  transient ischemic a. (TIA)
attention
  a. deficit disorder (ADD)
  a. deficit hyperactivity disorder
    (ADHD)
Attention! dietary supplement
attentional control
attenuate
attenuation
  posthypnotic a.
  stress a.
attitude
  observer a.
  Survey of Pain A.'s (SOPA)
attitudinal
attollens
Attributional
  A. Style Questionnaire (ASQ)
  A. Style Questionnaire Global
    Scale
attunement therapy
atypical
  a. rib

a. segment
a. thoracic vertebra
Aucklandia lappa
audioanalgesia
auditory
a. EMG feedback
a. meatus
Auerbach plexus
augmentor nerve
Auklandia
aunee
aura
brown a.
dirty green a.
gray a.
pink a.
red a.
white a.
aureus
Senecio a.
Staphylococcus a.
auricular
a. acupuncture
a. rami
auricularis
digitus a.
auriculotherapy point
Aurum metallicum
auscultation
abdominal a.
triangle of a.
Australian tea tree oil
autism
autistic parasite
autoantibody
autochthonous parasite
autoclave
autogenic
a. biofeedback
a. feedback
a. training
a. training phrase
autogenics
autohemotherapy
autoimmune
a. deficiency syndrome
a. disease

autointoxication
autolymphocyte therapy
automatic thought
autonomic
a. arousal
a. dysregulation
a. dysregulation disorder
a. ganglion
a. innervation
a. innervation pattern
a. nervous system (ANS)
a. nervous system dysfunction
a. nervous system dysregulation
a. part of peripheral nervous system
a. perception
a. reactivity
a. tone
autopod
autopodium
autosuggestion technique
autumnale
Colchicum a.
autumn crocus
Autussan "T"
auxiliary
available
motion a.
Aveeno
A. Cleansing Bar
A. Colloidal
A. Dry
A. Lotion
A. Oilated Bath
A. Regular Bath
avellanedae
Tabebuia a.
avena
A. sativa
A. Sativa Compound in Species Sedative Tea
avens
city a.
wood a.
avensis
Asperula a.

NOTES

Avogadro number
avulsion fracture
awareness
    conscious a.
    focusing of the conscious a.
    peripheral a.
    a. release technique
    A. Through Movement (ATM)
    universal a.
ax
axes (*pl. of* axis)
axial
    a. aneurysm
    a. muscle
    a. rotation
    a. section
    a. skeleton
axiale
    skeleton a.
axil
axile
axilla
    suspensory ligament of a.
axillaris
    fascia a.
    fossa a.
    plica a.
    regio a.
axillary
    a. anesthesia
    a. arch muscle
    a. artery
    a. cavity
    a. fold
    a. fold dysfunction
    a. fossa
    a. line
    a. lymph node
    a. plexus
    a. region
    a. sheath
    a. triangle
    a. vein
axion
axis, pl. **axes**
    absolute yin channel a.
    anterior-posterior a.
    anteroposterior a.
    brilliant yang channel a.
    cephalocaudal a.
    cerebrospinal a.
    cervical spine a.
    channel a.

    diagonal a.
    energy a.
    helical a.
    horizontal a.
    HPA a.
    hypothalamic-pituitary-adrenal a.
    hypothalamic-pituitary-thyroid a.
    inferior transverse a.
    innominate a.
    jue-yin a.
    jue-yin channel a.
    large yin a.
    a. ligament of malleus
    long a.
    longitudinal a.
    major yang channel a.
    major yin channel a.
    middle transverse a.
    minor yang channel a.
    minor yin channel a.
    oblique a.
    organ a.
    pituitary adrenal a.
    postural a.
    respiratory a.
    a. of rib motion
    rotation around a.
    a. of sacral motion
    sanjiao-gallbladder a.
    shao-yang a.
    shao-yang channel a.
    shao-yin a.
    shao-yin channel a.
    superior transverse a.
    tai-yang a.
    tai-yang channel a.
    tai-yin a.
    tai-yin channel a.
    thoracic a.
    thyroid a.
    translation along a.
    transverse a.
    vertebral a.
    vertical a.
    x a.
    y a.
    yang channel a.
    yang-ming a.
    yang-ming channel a.
    yin channel a.
    z a.
axoaxonic
axodendritic

axofugal
axon
axoplasmic
    a. flow
    a. transport
ayurveda, Ayur Veda, Ayurveda
    Maharishi a.
Ayurvedic medicine

Azadirachta indica
azafran
azelaic acid
azoospermia
azulene
azygos
azygous

A

NOTES

β (*var. of* beta)

B
 B cell
 B lymphocyte
B₁
 vitamin B₁
B₂
 vitamin B₂
B₃
 provitamin B₃
 vitamin B₃
B₅
 vitamin B₅
B₆
 melatonin with vitamin B₆
 vitamin B₆
B₇
 vitamin B₇
B₉
 vitamin B₉
B₁₂
 intramuscular B₁₂
 vitamin B₁₂
B₁₇
 vitamin B₁₇
ba
 b. gang
 b. gang diagnostic criteria: yin and yang, interior and exterior, deficiency and excess, cold and heat
 b. hui di huang wan
 b. ji tian
 b. wei di huang wan
 b. wei di huang wan gui zhi tang
 b. xie point
 b. zheng san
 b. zheng tang
 b. zhen san
 b. zhen tang
Babinski reflex
baccal juniper
baccata
 Taxus b.
Bachelor of Ayurvedic Medicine and Surgery (BAMS)
bachelor's button
Bach flower remedy

bacillary dysentery
bacille Calmette-Guérin (BCG, bCG)
bacilli
 acid-fast b.
 gram-negative b.
bacillus
 tubercle b.
back
 adolescent round b.
 broadest muscle of b.
 cat b.
 deep muscles of b.
 hollow b.
 muscles of b.
 b. off
 b. pain
 poker b.
 regions of b.
 retraining with sit b.
 saddle b.
 b. shu point
 sit b.
 true muscles of b.
backache
backboard splint
backbone
 two-column concept of b.
back-knee
backward
 b. bending
 b. bending test
 b. bent test
 b. curvature
 b. direction
 injury before b.
 b. torsion
backward-bending
 b.-b. dynamic film
 b.-b. vertebral motion
Bacopa Plus
bacteria
 anaerobic oral b.
 antibiotic-resistant b.
 gram-negative b.
 gram-positive b.
 symbiotic b.
bacterial
 b. abscess
 b. vaginosis

B

bactericidal
bactericide
bacteriocide
bacterium
bacteriuria
bafeng
 Ex-LE 36 b.
bafeng point
bag
 Ambu b.
 breathing b.
 nuclear b.
bai
 b. he gu jin tang
 huang b.
 b. hu tang
 b. ji
 b. shao
 b. zhen san
 b. zhu
baicalensis
 Scutellaria b.
baihui
 du 20 b.
bairnwort
baja
 patella b.
baked licorice decoction
Baker cyst
baking soda
bal
balance
 altered muscle b.
 b. and control
 dosha b.
 dynamic b.
 electrolyte b.
 energy b.
 b. and hold functional
  technique
 b. and hold procedure
 b. and hold technique
 homeostatic b.
 kinesthetic b.
 neurophysiological b.
 B. oil
 postural b.
 qi b.
 sensory motor b.
 structural b.
 sympathovagal b.
 b. testing level one
 b. testing level three

 b. testing level two
 tissue tension b.
 Vital B.
 whole energy b.
balanced
 b. anesthesia
 b. ligamentous release
 b. ligamentous tension
  technique
 b. ligamentous tension
  treatment (BLT)
 b. membranous tension
 b. tension
balancing
 craniosacral b.
 energy b.
 mouth b.
 polarity b.
 spinal b.
 zero b.
baldrianwurzel
baldrinal
ball
 b. of the foot
 b. and socket joint
balloon
 rectal b.
ballottement test
balm
 bee b.
 eye b.
 b. of Gilead
 horse b.
 Indian b.
 kamphor b.
 lemon b.
 b. mint
 mountain b.
 ox b.
 Tiger B.
balm-mint
balmony
balsam
 black b.
 Canada b.
 fir b.
 b. fir
 Friar's B.
 B. of the Holy Victorious
  Knight
 Indian b.
 Jerusalem B.
 b. of Peru

B

Peru b.
Peruvian b.
propolis b.
Thomas b.
b. of Tolu
Tolu b.
turpentine b.
Ward's B.
balsamifera
  Populus b.
balsamum
  Myroxylon b.
  Toluifera b.
  b. tolutanum
balucanat
bamboo
  b. shoot
  b. spine
BAMS
  Bachelor of Ayurvedic Medicine and
  Surgery
ban
  b. he wan
  b. xia huo po tang
band
  elastic b.
  iliotibial b.
  Maissiat b.
  moderator b.
  stress b.'s
  subcutaneous b.
bandage
  capeline b.
  circular b.
  demigauntlet b.
  elastic b.
  Esmarch b.
  figure-of-eight b.
  gauntlet b.
  immovable b.
  oblique b.
  plaster b.
  roller b.
  scarf b.
  spica b.
  spiral b.
  triangular b.

banding of muscle
bandy-leg
bane
  leopard's b.
  wolf's b.
baneberry
banji
bank
  blood b.
Bantron Tablets
bao
  b. wei di huang wan
  b. yuan wan
baohuang
  ub 53 b.
baptisia
Baptisia tinctoria
bar
  Aveeno Cleansing B.
barbadensis
  Aloe b.
Barbados aloe
barbata
  Usnea b.
barberry
  b. bark
  common b.
  European b.
  holly-leaved b.
barbotage
bardana
Bardinet ligament
bark
  barberry b.
  bayberry b.
  blackberry root b.
  buckthorn b.
  butternut b.
  cassia b.
  China b.
  cinchona b.
  cinnamon b.
  condor-vine b.
  condurango b.
  cramp b.
  eagle-vine b.
  ground cinchona b.

NOTES

bark (*continued*)
  haronga b.
  inner b.
  Jesuit's b.
  murillo b.
  oak b.
  Panama b.
  pau d'arco inner b.
  Peruvian b.
  powdered slippery elm b.
  prickly ash b.
  root b.
  sacred b.
  seven b.'s
  tanner's b.
  wahoo b.
  white willow b.
  wild cherry b.
  yoco b.
Barkow ligament
Barlean's
  B. Flax oil
  B. Vita-Flax
barley grass
Barlow test
baroreceptor reflex
Barosma betulina
barrel chest
barrier
  abnormal b.
  anatomic b.
  blood-cerebrospinal fluid b.
  b. concept
  direct b.
  elastic b.
  b. engagement
  fascial b.
  flexion b.
  indirect b.
  joint capsule b.
  joint surface b.
  ligament b.
  long muscle b.
  long restrictive b.
  b. to motion
  motion b.
  normal b.
  pain restrictive b.
  pathologic b.
  physiologic b.
  resistant b.
  restricted b.
  restricted motion b.

  restriction b.
  restrictive b.
  short muscle b.
  short restrictive b.
  skin b.
  terminal b.
Barr-Lieou syndrome
Bartholomew's tea
basad
basal
  b. anesthesia
  b. body temperature (BBT)
  b. cell carcinoma
  b. cell nevus syndrome
  b. ganglion
  b. tone
basalis
  fibrocartilago b.
base
  b. chakra
  energy b.
  b. energy center
  fracture of odontoid b.
  b. of metacarpal
  b. of metatarsal
  b. of patella
  b. of phalanx
  restricted sacral b.
  sacral b.
  b. of sacrum
  b. of stapes
  b. of support
  unleveling of b.
baseball finger
baseline hypnotic ability
basic
Basic Prenatal
basil
  common b.
  garden b.
  holy b.
  sweet b.
basilar
  b. apophysis
  b. artery
  b. axis of skull
  b. portion of occiput
  b. sinus
basilare
  os b.
basilicum
  Ocimum b.
basilicus

B

basioccipital
basiocciput
basipetal
basis
   b. ossis metacarpalis
   b. ossis metatarsalis
   b. ossis sacri
   b. patellae
   b. phalangis
basisphenoid
basivertebral
Basle Nomina Anatomica
basograph
basophil
basophile
Bassoran with Cascara
Bassora tragacanth
basswood
bastard saffron
basti
Batavia
   B. cassia
   B. cinnamon
Bates eye system
bath
   Aveeno Oilated B.
   Aveeno Regular B.
   herbal b.
   immersion b.
   medicated b.
   mud b.
   oatmeal b.
   paraffin b.
   seaweed b.
   sitz b.
   steam b.
   turpentine b.
   whirlpool b.
bathmotropic effect
Batson
   B. plexus
   B. venous plexus
battery
   skin b.
batwing deformity
baxie
   Ex-UE 28 b.

bay
   b. laurel
   b. leaf
   rose b.
   sweet b.
   b. tree
bayberry bark
bayonet
   b. apposition
   Spanish b.
BBT
   basal body temperature
BCG, bCG
   bacille Calmette-Guérin
BCIA
   Biofeedback Certification Institute
   of America
B-complex vitamin
BCP
   birth control pill
BDI
   Beck Depression Inventory
BDP pad
BEA
   below-elbow amputation
bead
   prayer b.'s
   b. vine
beading of the ribs
beaked pelvis
beam
   continuous-wave laser b.
bean
   calabar b.
   castor b.
   Dutch tonka b.
   b. juice
   kidney b.
   love b.
   navy b.
   ordeal b.
   precatory b.
   tonka b.
bearberry leaf
beargrape
bear's
   b. foot

NOTES

41

bear's *(continued)*
   b. grape
   b. paw
   b. weed
beauty
   Ageless B.
Beck
   B. Anxiety Inventory
   B. Depression Inventory (BDI)
Béclard triangle
bed
   fracture b.
   b. rest
bedsore
bedstraw
bedwetting
bee
   b. balm
   b. byproduct
   b. glue
   b. pollen
   b. propolis
   b. sting
   b. wort
beebread
beech cough drops
beefsteak plant
Bee-Gone
   Aller B.-G.
beetle
   Chinese blistering b.
beggar's button
Begin oil
behavior
   abnormal b.
   hypnotic b.
   b. modification
   pain b.
   phobic b.
   b. therapy
   type A b.
behavioral
   b. analysis
   b. medicine
   b. therapy
being therapy
beishu point
beishuxue point
bell
   lint b.'s
   B. palsy
   b. pepper
   B. respiratory nerve

belladonna
   b. alkaloid
   Atropa b.
bellerica
   Terminalia b.
Bellini ligament
belly
   b. button
   muscle b.
below-elbow amputation (BEA)
below-knee amputation (BKA)
belt
   Hackett sacroiliac cinch b.
   magnetic support b.
   sacroiliac cinch b.
Belvedere cypress
bench
   meditation b.
   monkey's b.
Bendectin
bending
   backward b.
   forward b.
   forward-to-backward b.
   b. fracture
   side b.
   b. test
benedicta
   herba b.
Benedict's herb
benedictus
   Cnicus b.
Benefin
Ben-Gay
benibana
benign
   b. bone aneurysm
   b. intracranial hypertension
   b. prostatic hyperplasia (BPH)
   b. prostatic hypertrophy (BPH)
benit
   cardon b.
benjamin
   gum b.
   stinking b.
   B. system of muscular therapy
   b. tree
bennet
   herb b.
   way b.
bent
   forward b.
benzaldehyde

benzodiazepine
benzoe
benzoic acid
benzoin
  Siam b.
  Sumatra b.
  tincture of b.
  b. tree
benzoyl peroxide
berberine salt
Berberis
  B. aquifolium
  B. vulgaris
berberry
bergamot
beriberi
  wet b.
berry
  cedar b.
  cubeb b.
  hawthorn b.
  Indian b.
  jaundice b.
  juniper b.
  levant b.
  magnolia vine b.
  partridge b.
  saw palmetto b.
  scarlet b.
  twin b.
  two-eyed b.
  wild brier b.
Bertin ligament
best
  Nature's B.
Bestatin
bet
  bouncing b.
beta, β
  b. amyloid
  b. angle
  b. blocker
  b. carotene
  b. endorphin
  b. glucan
  1,3 b. glucan

  β-glucan soluble fiber
  b. sitosterol
betaine hydrochloride
betal
  chavica b.
Betatene
betel
  b. nut
  b. nut quid
  b. palm
  b. pepper leaf
bethroot
betle
  Piper b.
betonica
  B. officinalis
  Stachys b.
betony
  Paul's b.
  wood b.
Betty
  sweet B.
betulina
  Agathosma b.
  Barosma b.
  Diosma b.
betuline
bevel change
Bevitamel
Beyond Milk Thistle
bezoar
BF&C ointment
BF&S ointment
Bhakti yoga
bhang
BHA preservative
bheda
bhringraj oil
BHT preservative
bi
  cold b.
  heat b.
  b. syndrome
bian
  b. bing
  b. zheng
  b. zheng lun zhi (BZLZ)

NOTES

biao illness
biarticular
biaxial joint
biber
Bible leaf
bicarbonate
    sodium b.
biceps
    b. brachii muscle
    b. femoris
    b. femoris muscle
    b. femoris muscle long head
    b. femoris muscle short head
    b. muscle of arm
    b. muscle of thigh
    b. reflex
Bichat ligament
bicipital
    b. fascia
    b. groove
    b. ridge
    b. tendinitis
    b. tuberosity
bicipitoradial bursa
bicondylar
    b. articulation
    b. joint
bicondylaris
    articulatio b.
bicornous
b.i.d.
    bis in die
    twice a day
bidactyly
Bidens tripartita
bi-digital O-ring test
biennis
    Oenothera b.
bierdji
    surale di b.
Bier method
Biesiadecki fossa
bifid
    b. rib
    b. thumb
    b. tip
    b. transverse process
bifida
    spina b.
Bifidobacterium bifidum
Bifido Factor
bifidum
    Bifidobacterium b.

bifidus
    Lactobacillus b.
biforate
bifurcate ligament
bifurcatio
bifurcation
big
    b. chief
    b. fever
    b. pulse
    b. qi
    b. sweating
    b. thirst
Bigelow
    B. ligament
    B. septum
    Y-ligament of B.
    B. Y-ligament
biguan
    st 31 b.
bilateral
    b. extension
    b. extension restriction
    b. lateral stretch
    b. lateral stretch technique
    b. linear cervical spine stretcl
    b. sacrum extended
    b. sacrum flexed
    b. shoulder abduction
    maneuver
bilateralism
bilaterally
    b. flexed
    b. nutated sacroiliac
bilberry
    bog b.
    b. extract
    B. Vegicap
bile
    b. acid
    b. preparation
    raw b.
biliary
    b. cholesterol
    b. colic
    b. duct
    b. dyskinesia
    b. system
biloba
    extract of *Ginkgo b.* (EGb)
    Ginkgo b.
bilobalide
bilocular joint

bimalleolar fracture
bindweed
bing
    bian b.
Bio
    B. Nutritional
    B. Rizin
    B. Star
bioactive
bioavailability
biobehavioral treatment
Bio-Bifidus
Biocarde
Bio-Cardiozyme Forte
biochanin
biochemical
    b. individuality
    b. profile
    b. substrate
biochemistry
    nutritional b.
biodynamic massage
biodynamics
bioelectric
    b. energy
    b. mechanism
    b. potential
bioelectromagnetic
    b. application
    b. medicine
bioelectromagnetism
bioelectron
bioenergetic
    b. analysis
    b. exercise
    b. field
    b. medicine
    b. synchronization technique
    b. system technique
        classification
    b. therapist
bioenergy
    b. field
    b. healing
    b. model

biofeedback
    Association for Applied
        Psychophysiology and B.
        (AAPB)
    autogenic b.
    brainwave b.
    B. Certification Institute of
        America (BCIA)
    delayed b.
    electroacupuncture b.
    electromyographic b.
    EMG b.
    b. exercise
    frontal EMG b.
    b. instrumentation
    kinesthetic b.
    b. relaxation training
    skin temperature b.
    b. therapy
    thermal b.
biofeedback-assisted relaxation
biofield
    b. approach
    b. therapeutics
bioflavonoid
BioFlex
Bioforce of America
Bioginkgo
    B. 24/6
    B. 27/7
    B. 27/7 Extra Strength
Bio-Gymnema
bioinformation system
biological
    b. energy
    b. rhythm
    b. sampling
    b. standard unit
    b. terrain assessment (BTA)
biologic feedback
biologics
biology
    molecular b.
biomagnet
biomagnetic
    b. field
    b. therapy

NOTES

biomagnetics
biomarker
biomechanical
    b. change
    b. dysfunction
    b. rehabilitation
    b. tether
biomechanics
    muscle b.
biomedicine
biomolecular element
biomolecule
bioorganism
bio-oxidative therapy
Bioperine
    DHEA with B.
biopharmacologic
biophysical methodology
Bio-PMT
biopsy
    bone marrow b.
biopsychosocial
bioreceptor feedback
biorhythm
biosafety
biosis
    intestinal b.
Biosode
biosonic repatterning
biostatics
Bio-Strath
Biota orientalis
biotaxis
Bio-Tech
biotechnology
biotherapeutic
biotin
biotoxin
biotransformation
biowater
bipalatinoid
biped stance
bipennate muscle
bipennatus
    musculus b.
biperforate
biphasic
    b. pulse
    b. stimulator
biphenyl
    polyhalogenated b.
bipolar factor

birch
    black b.
    cherry b.
    b. leaf
    b. tar oil
    white b.
    b. wood oil
bird
    b. lime
    b.-lime thistle
bird's
    b. foot
    b. nest
bird's-eye
    white b.-e.
birth
    breech b.
    b. control pill (BCP)
    b. fracture
    b. plan
    premature b.
    b. trauma
    water b.
birthing center
birthroot
birthwort
bisabolol
bisacromial
bisaxillary
biscuit
bis in die (b.i.d.)
bishop's weed
bishopswort
bisiliac
bismuth
bistoria
    Polygonum b.
bistort
    common b.
bite
    snake b.
bitrochanteric
bitter
    Angostura B.'s
    b. ash
    b. button
    b. dock
    b. fennel
    b. herb
    b. lettuce
    b. melon
    b. orange oil

B

b. root
b. wood
Bitteridina
bittersweet
European b.
b. nightshade
biventer cervicis
biventral
BKA
below-knee amputation
black
b. balsam
b. birch
b. catechu
b. choke
b. cohosh
b. cohosh syrup
b. currant seed oil
B. Draught Granules
b. drink
b. elder
b. haw
b. hellebore
b. mustard
b. nightshade
b. nightshade leaf
B. ointment
b. pepper
b. pepper essential oil
b. plum
b. poplar
b. poplar bud
b. psyllium
b. radish
b. raspberry
b. root
b. sampson
b. snakeroot
b. tang
b. tea
b. walnut
b. willow
blackberry root bark
black-eyed Susan
blackhaw
blackroot
blackstrap molasses

blackwort
bladder
b. cancer
b. innervation
b. irrigation
irritable b.
b. meridian
b. outlet obstruction
b. suspension surgery
b. wrack
bladderpod
bladderwrack
blade
b. bone
shoulder b.
blam
field b.
blanching
blanco
condurango b.
blanket
thermal space b.
blasen tang
Blastolysin
blastomycosis
blazing star
bleed
intracranial b.
bleeding
b. diathesis
gastrointestinal b.
b. gums
b. heart
intramural b.
b. needle
b. time
uterine b.
blend
SP-6 Cornsilk B.
SP-23 Eyebright B.
SP-8 Hawthorn Motherwort B.
blessed
b. thistle
b. thistle combo
b. thistle herb
Blighia sapida

NOTES

blind
b. nasotracheal intubation
b. test
blister
cutaneous b.
fracture b.
blob
may b.
block
b. anesthesia
atrioventricular b.
bone b.
depolarizing b.
diagnostic b.
diagnostic joint b.
epidural b.
field b.
IV regional b.
joint b.
nerve b.
nondepolarizing b.
phase I b.
phase II b.
sacroiliac joint b.
selective nerve b.
spinal b.
stellate b.
sympathetic b.
b. vertebra
zygapophysial joint b.
blockade
adrenergic b.
cholinergic b.
ganglionic b.
myoneural b.
sympathetic b.
blockage
cerebrospinal fluid b.
energy b.
joint b.
blocked energy
blocker
beta b.
calcium channel b.
potassium channel b.
blocking
opiate receptor b.
blond
b. plantago
b. plantago seed
blood
b. bank
b. circulation

b. circulation system
citrated autologous b.
b. count
deficiency of heart b.
deficiency of liver b.
flesh and b.
b. flow control
b. glucose
b. group
influential point of b.
b. lipid
ozone-enriched b.
b. poisoning
b. pressure (BP)
b. purification
stagnation of b.
b. stagnation
stagnation of heart b.
stasis of b.
b. sterilization
b. substitute
b. sugar
b. supply
b. type
b. urea nitrogen (BUN)
b. vessel
b. viscosity
whole b.
b. xu
blood-cerebrospinal fluid barrier
bloodless amputation
bloodletting
bloodroot
Bloodroot/Celandine Supreme
bloodstopper
blood-thinning medication
bloodwort
Canadian b.
bloom
alum b.
violet b.
winter b.
blossom
lime b.
red clover b.'s
BLT
balanced ligamentous tension
treatment
blue
b. cohosh
b. cohosh root
b. elderberry
b. flag

B

b. ginseng
b. light treatment
b. mallow
b. mauve
b. mountain tea
b. sailors
b. toe syndrome
b. vervain
b. violet
blueberry
European b.
fresh b.
blue-green alga
blunt needle
blush
b. phenomenon
b. sign
BMI
body mass index
board
Federation of Chiropractic
Licensing B.'s
boca juniros
bocco
Bochdalek gap
Bock ganglion
body
b. acupoint
b. acupuncture
anococcygeal b.
b. cavity
b. of clavicle
coccygeal b.
b. disorientation
epithelial b.
b. fluid
b. fluid metabolism
foreign b.
b. framework
glomus b.
b. habitus
b. inch
b. of ischium
B. Language Essential Green
Foods
B. Language Super Antioxidant
long axis of b.

loose b.
b. mass index (BMI)
b. mechanics
b. mechanism
melon-seed b.
b. movement
b. of nail
pacchionian b.'s
B. Polish
b. position
regions of b.
b. restructuring
b. of rib
rice b.
Sandström b.'s
sphenoid b.
b. of sternum
b. of sweat gland
Symington anococcygeal b.
b. table
b. of talus
b. therapy
b. of thigh bone
thyroid b.
b. of tibia
b. of ulna
unity of b.
b. unity
b. of vertebra
vertebral b.
body-mind
b.-m. centering
b.-m. system
body-motion electrostatic effect
BodyTable
HiLo B.
TouchAmerica B.
body-weight ratio
bodywork
Feldenkrais b.
Hakomi b.
Nationally Certified Therapeutic
Massage and B. (NCTMB)
b. practitioner
Soma b.
b. system
Trager b.

NOTES

bofareira
bog
    b. bilberry
    b. cranberry
bogbean
bogginess
boggy
    b. sensation
    b. tissue texture abnormality
boi
boil
    topical b.
bois de sassafras
bol
bola
boldine
boldo
    b. leaf
boldus
    Peumus b.
bolster
    armrest b.
    b. buddy
bolus
    intravenous b.
bombesin
bombilia
bone
    b. abscess
    adamantinoma of long b.'s
    b. age
    ankle b.
    b. architecture
    articular fossa of temporal b.
    articular mobility of b.'s
    articular mobility of cranial b.
    articular surface of mandibular
      fossa of temporal b.
    blade b.
    b. block
    b. block fusion
    body of thigh b.
    breast b.
    Breschet b.'s
    brittle b.
    B. Builder with Boron
    bundle b.
    calcaneal b.
    calcaneus b.
    calf b.
    b. canaliculus
    capitate b.
    carpal b.

cartilage b.
cavalry b.
central b.
b. chip
coccygeal b.
collar b.
contour of b.
coxal b.
cubital b.
cuboid b.
cuneiform b.
b. cyst
B. Defense
b. densitometry study
b. density
b.'s of digits
dorsal talonavicular b.
elbow b.
endochondral b.
epactal b.
episternal b.
ethmoid b.
exercise b.
external surface of frontal b.
external surface of parietal b.
facial b.
fibrous dysplasia of b.
first cuneiform b.
flank b.
flat b.
frontal b.
b. Gla protein
b. graft
greater multangular b.
hamate b.
head of thigh b.
heel b.
heterotopic b.
hip b.
hollow b.
hooked b.
iliac b.
b. infarct
b. of inferior limb
influential point of the b.
innominate b.
intermediate cuneiform b.
irregular b.
ischial b.
b. island
Krause b.
lacrimal b.
lamella of b.

lamellar b.
lateral cuneiform b.
lentiform b.
lesser multangular b.
lesser trochanter pubic b.
long b.
b. of lower limb
lunate b. ˋ
marble b.
b. marrow
b. marrow biopsy
b. marrow depression
b. marrow embolism
b. marrow suppression
b. marrow transplant
mastoid part of temporal b.
b. matrix
maxillary b.
medial cuneiform b.
membrane b.
b. metabolism
metacarpal b.'s [I–V]
metatarsal b.'s [I–V]
middle cuneiform b.
multangular b.
nasal b.
navicular b.
neck of thigh b.
nonlamellar b.
occiput b.
b. pain
paired skull b.
palatine b.
parietal b.
pelvic b.
perichondral b.
peroneal b.
petrous b.
ping-pong b.
pipe b.
Pirie b.
pisiform b.
pneumatic b.
postsphenoid b.
presphenoid b.
pubic b.
replacement b.

b. resorption
reticulated b.
rider's b.
sacred b.
b. scan
scaphoid b.
b. sclerosis
second cuneiform b.
semilunar b.
sesamoid b.
shin b.
short b.
somatic dysfunction of
  cuboid b.
somatic dysfunction of
  tarsal b.
sphenoid b.
styloid process of temporal b.
styloid process of third
  metacarpal b.
superior branch of the
  pubic b.
b. of superior limb
B. Support
suprasternal b.
sutural b.
tail b.
tarsal b.
temporal b.
thigh b.
third cuneiform b.
three-cornered b.
trapezium b.
trapezoid b.
triangular b.
triquetrum b.
tubercle of scaphoid b.
tubercle of trapezium b.
tuberosity of cuboid b.
tuberosity of fifth metatarsal b.
  [V]
tuberosity of first metatarsal b.
  [I]
tuberosity of navicular b.
unciform b.
unpaired skull b.
b. of upper limb

NOTES

bone *(continued)*
   Vesalius b.
   b. wax
   wedge b.
   b. window
   wormian b.
   woven b.
   zygomatic margin of greater
     wing of sphenoid b.
Bonefos
bonelet
bonemeal
bones
boneset
bonesetter
   lightning b.
bonesetting
Bonjean
   Elixir B.
bonnet
   Hydro B.
Bonnie Prudden myotherapy
Bontanifuge
bony
   b. ankylosis
   b. crepitus
   b. lock
borage
   common b.
   b. leaf
   b. powder
   b. seed
   b. seed oil
Borago officinalis
border
   anterior b.
   free b.
   inferior b.
   interosseous b.
   lateral b.
   medial b.
   superior b.
   ventral b.
borderline personality
boretree
Bori
   Shanti B.
Born Again's DHEA Eyelift Serum
boron
   Bone Builder with B.
boss
boswellic acid
Boswelya-Plus

botanical
   b. essential oil
   b. hallucinogen
   b. medicine
   b. supplement
botanomedicine
botany
botfly maggot
bottle brush
botulinic acid
bough
   golden b.
bouncing bet
Bountiful Harvest tea
bouquet
   Riolan b.
Bourbon vanilla
Bourgery ligament
boutonnière deformity
bovina
   facies b.
bovine
   b. cartilage
   b. colostrum
   b. donor cell
bowel
   B. Build
   b. cleansing
   irritable b.
bowl
   rubber spa b.
bow-leg, bowleg
bowman's
   b. reflex
   b. root
box
   fracture b.
   b. holly
   light b.
   mountain b.
   steam b.
   view b.
boxberry
boxer's fracture
boxthorn seed
boy's love
BP
   blood pressure
BPC 1973
BPH
   benign prostatic hyperplasia
   benign prostatic hypertrophy

brace
   cast b.
bracelet
brachia (*pl. of* brachium)
brachial
   b. anesthesia
   b. artery
   b. fascia
   b. gland
   b. lymph node
   b. muscle
   b. nerve entrapment
   b. neuritis
   b. plexus
   b. plexus neuropathy
   b. pulse
brachialgia
   cervical b.
   b. statica paresthetica
brachialis
   b. muscle
   musculus b.
   pars infraclavicularis plexus b.
   pars supraclavicularis plexus b.
brachii
   aponeurosis musculi bicipitis b.
   caput breve musculi bicipitis b.
   caput laterale musculi tricipitis b.
   caput longum musculi bicipitis b.
   caput longum musculi tricipitis b.
   caput mediale musculi tricipitis b.
   fascia b.
   musculus biceps b.
   musculus triceps b.
   short head of biceps b.
brachiocephalic vein
brachiocrural
brachiocubital
brachioradialis
   b. muscle

   musculus b.
   b. reflex
brachium, pl. **brachia**
brachybasia
brachybasocamptodactyly
brachybasophalangia
brachycnemic
brachydactylia
brachydactylic
brachydactyly
brachykerkic
brachymelia
brachymesophalangia
brachymetacarpalia
brachymetacarpia
brachymetapody
brachymetatarsia
brachymorphic
brachypellic
brachyphalangia
brachypodous
brachyskelic
brachysyndactyly
brachytelephalangia
brachytype
bracken
   sweet b.
bracteatum
   Onosma b.
bradyarrhythmia
bradycardia
   sinus b.
bradykinesia, bradycinesia
bradykinetic
bradykinin
brain
   coiling of b.
   b. death
   fourth ventricle of b.
   B. Gum
   b. lesion
   b. lipid
   mobility of b.
   b. nutrient
   b. wave
   b. wave activity
brain-injury associated cephalgia

B

NOTES

brainstem pathway
brainwave biofeedback
brake
    knotty b.
    sweet b.
bramble of Mount Ida
bran
    oat b.
    Quaker Oat B.
    rice b.
branch
    acetabular b.
    anastomotic b.
    anterior b.
    articular b.
    ascending b.
    deep b.
    deltoid b.
    descending b.
    dorsal b.
    inferior b.
    joint b.
    lateral cutaneous b.
    left b.
    medial b.
    meningeal b.
    muscular b.
    perforating b.
    peroneal communicating b.
    posterior b.
    qi b.
    superficial b.
    superior b.
    ventral b.
branching
brandy mint
Brassica
    B. alba
    B. juncea
    B. nigra
brauche
brava
    arruda b.
    pareira b.
Brazilian
    B. cocoa
    B. ginseng
    B. Herbal Tea
Brazil nut
breach of taboo
breakdown
    cartilage b.

breakstone
    parsley b.
breast
    b. bone
    chicken b.
    funnel b.
    pigeon b.
    suspensory ligaments of b.
breath
    abdominal b.
    deepening of b.
    exhalation b.
    focusing of b.
    b. of life
    b. suspension
Breath-Aid
breath-directed inner healing
Breathe Ease
breathing
    b. bag
    coarse b.
    b. consciously
    diaphragmatic b.
    b. exercise
    b. exercise-oriented qigong
    b. qigong
    b. reflex
    shallow b.
    slow b.
    b. technique
breathwork
    holotropic b.
    integrative b.
    radiance b.
breech
    b. birth
    b. delivery
Breeze Free
bregma
Breschet
    B. bones
    B. vein
bretylium tosylate
breve
    caput b.
    os b.
breves
    musculi levatores costarum b.
brevicollis
brevifolia
    Taxus b.
    Yucca b.

brevis
 adductor b.
 caput profundum musculi
  flexoris pollicis b.
 caput superficiale musculi
  flexoris pollicis b.
 deep head of flexor pollicis b.
 extensor carpi radialis b.
  (ECRB)
 extensor digitorum b. (EDB)
 musculus abductor pollicis b.
 musculus adductor b.
 musculus extensor carpi
  radialis b.
 musculus extensor digitorum b.
 musculus extensor hallucis b.
 musculus extensor pollicis b.
 musculus fibularis b.
 musculus flexor digitorum b.
 musculus flexor hallucis b.
 musculus flexor pollicis b.
 musculus palmaris b.
 musculus peroneus b.
 musculus supinator radii b.
 superficial head of flexor
  pollicis b.
brew
 Congming Anti-HIV herbal b.
brewer's yeast
bridal myrtle
bridewort
bridge
 Wheatstone b.
brief
 B. Screen for Depression
 B. Social Phobia Scale (BSPS)
brier fruit
Brigham tea
bright
 see b.
brightness
 yang b.
brilliant yang channel axis
brim
Brinase
brinton root
brisement

Bristol diet therapy
British
 B. Indian lemongrass
 B. myrrh
 B. oak
brittle
 b. bone
 b. diabetes
 b. nails
broadest muscle of back
broad fascia
broadleaf plantain
broad-spectrum antibiotic (BSA)
Brodie
 B. bursa
 B. ligament
bromelain
bromocriptine
Bronc-Ease
bronchial
 b. asthma
 b. hyperresponsiveness
bronchiolitis
 acute b.
 b. obliterans
bronchitis
 chronic b.
bronchoconstriction
bronchodilating
bronchodilation
bronchospasm
Broncrin
Bronhillor Natural Source Cough
 Candies & Throat Disks
broom
 butcher's b.
 Dyer's b.
 old woman's b.
 Scotch b.
 sweet b.
 b. top
broomrape
broth
 potato b.
brown
 b. alga
 b. aura

B

NOTES

brown *(continued)*
    b. mustard
    b. oak
    b. rice
    b. tumor
Brucella
bruisewort
brunella
brush
    antelope b.
    bottle b.
brushing
    skin b.
bruxism
Bryonia
    B. agaricus
    B. alba
bryony root
bryostatin
BSA
    broad-spectrum antibiotic
BSPS
    Brief Social Phobia Scale
BTA
    biological terrain assessment
    BTA S-2000
    BTA S-2000 biofeedback
      system
bu
    gu sui b.
    b. gu zi
    kun b.
    b. method
    shi zi bai b.
    b. yang huang wu tang
    b. zhong yi qi tang
buccinator muscle
buccopharyngeus
    musculus b.
buchu leaf
buckbean
bucket-handle
    b.-h. motion of rib
    b.-h. rib motion
    b.-h. tear
buckhorn
buckle
buckthorn
    alder b.
    b. bark
    Californian b.
    common b.

    European b.
    purging b.
buckwheat pollen
Bucky
    B. diaphragm
    upright B.
bud
    black poplar b.
    calendula b.
    periosteal b.
    poplar b.
Buddhist meditation
Buddhi yoga
buddy
    bolster b.
buffalo neck
Bufo bufo gargarizans
bugbane
bugle
    common b.
    water b.
bugleweed
bugloss
    common b.
bugwort
build
    Bowel B.
builder
    deep chi b.
buildup
    excessive energy b.
bulb
    b. compression
    garlic b.
bulbar
bulbi
bulbocapnine
bulbospinal
bulbus
bulgaricus
    Lactobacillus b.
bulge
    b. of muscle
    b. test
bulimia
bulk
    Laxacil B.
    b. laxative
bulla, pl. bullae
bullsfoot
bump
    b. and hollow
    b. and hollow contour

BUN
  blood urea nitrogen
bundle
  b. bone
  neurovascular b.
bunion
Bunnel-Littler test
bunny's ears
bupleuri radix
Bupleurum chinese
bur
  great b.
  thorny b.
burden
burdock
  edible b.
  great b.
  b. root
burner
  lower b.
  middle b.
  triple b.
  upper b.
burnet
  lesser b.
  salad b.
burning
  b. mugwort
  b. quality
  skin b.
burning-bush
burn plant
Burns
  B. ligament
  B. space
Burow solution
burr marigold
bursa, pl. **bursae**
  Achilles b.
  adventitious b.
  anserine b.
  bicipitoradial b.
  Brodie b.
  coracobrachial b.
  deep infrapatellar b.
  gluteofemoral b.
  gluteus medius bursae

gluteus minimus b.
iliac b.
iliopectineal b.
intermuscular gluteal b.
ischial b.
radial b.
rider's b.
subacromial b.
subfascial prepatellar b.
synovial b.
bursal
  b. abscess
  b. synovitis
bursa-pastoris
  Capsella b.-p.
bursitis
  Achilles tendon b.
  anserine b.
  calcific b.
  infrapatellar b.
  ischial b.
  ischiogluteal b.
  olecranon b.
  pes anserinus b.
  prepatellar b.
  b. of shoulder
  subacromial b.
  subdeltoid b.
  trochanteric b.
bursolith
bursopathy
bursotomy
burst
bursting heart
bursula
bush
  creosote b.
  oleander b.
  pepperridge b.
  strawberry b.
  trumpet b.
butcher's
  b. broom
  b. broom extract 4:1
  b. broom root
butter
  clarified b.

B

NOTES

butter *(continued)*
   cocoa b.
   snake b.
butterbur root extract
butterfly
   b. fragment
   b. vertebra
   b. weed
butternut bark
buttocks
button
   bachelor's b.
   beggar's b.

   belly b.
   bitter b.
   cockle b.
   golden b.
   mescal b.
   peyote b.
   yellow b.
buttress plate
byproduct
   bee b.
BZLZ
   bian zheng lun zhi

C
centesimal dilution
C fiber
CAA
complementary and alternative
approach
cabbage
meadow c.
c. palm
pole-cat c.
skunk c.
cacao
Theobroma c.
c. tree
cachexia
cactus
large-flowered c.
sweet-scented c.
vanilla c.
cactus-hawthorn compound
cacumen
cacuminal
CAD
coronary artery disease
cadmium
C. sulfate
C. sulfuricum D3
C. sulfuricum D3 drops
cafe
caffeic
c. acid
c. acid phenethyl ester (CAPE)
caffeine
cage
thoracic c.
cake catechu
Cal
Fem C.
calabar bean
calabarica
faba c.
calamine lotion
Calamintha montana
calamus
Acorus c.
calcanea
regio c.
calcaneal
c. apophysitis
c. articular surface of talus

c. bone
c. gait
c. heel spur
c. motion
c. process of cuboid
c. region
c. sulcus
c. tendon
c. tuber
c. tubercle
c. tuberosity
c. valgus deformity
c. varus deformity
calcaneoapophysitis
calcaneoastragaloid
calcaneocavus
calcaneocuboid
c. articulation
c. joint
c. joint dysfunction
c. ligament
calcaneocuboidea
articulatio c.
calcaneodynia
calcaneofibular ligament
calcaneonavicular ligament
calcaneoscaphoid
calcaneotibial ligament
calcaneovalgocavus
calcaneovalgus
talipes c.
calcaneovarus
talipes c.
calcaneum
rete c.
calcaneus, pl. calcanei
c. bone
cuboidal articular surface of c.
interosseous groove of c.
middle talar articular surface
of c.
peroneal trochlea of c.
posterior talar articular surface
of c.
sulcus calcanei
talipes c.
tendo c.
trochlea fibularis calcanei
tuber calcanei
tuberculum calcanei

calcar
   c. femorale
   c. pedis
calcarea
   C. carbonica
   peritendinitis c.
   C. phosphorica
calcarine
calceoulus
   Cypripedium c.
calces (*pl. of* calx)
calciferol
calcification
   metastatic c.
calcific bursitis
calcinosis
   c. intervertebralis
   renal c.
   tumoral c.
calciokinesis
calciokinetic
calcis
   os c.
   tuber c.
calcitonin gene-related peptide
calcium
   c. alginate
   c. carbonate
   c. channel blocker
   chelated c.
   c. citrate
   c. hydroxide
   c. lysinate
   c. oxalate
   c. oxalate renal stone
   c. oxalate urolithiasis
   c. pyrophosphate deposition
     disease
calcodynia
calculus
   artificial c.
Caldani ligament
calendula
   c. bud
   C. officinalis
   c. petal
calf
   c. bone
   football c.
   gnome's c.
   triceps muscle of c.
calf-bone

calf's nose point
California
   C. Personality Inventory (CPI)
   C. poppy
   C. rape
   C. yew
Californian buckthorn
californica
   Eschscholzia c.
californicum
   Eriodictyon c.
caliper
   c. motion
   c. motion of rib
   c. rib motion
calisya
   Cinchona c.
Callahan technique
Callanetics therapy
callus
   central c.
   definitive c.
   ensheathing c.
   medullary c.
   permanent c.
   provisional c.
   temporary c.
calm
   C. Child
   C.'s Forte Homeopathic
     Formula
   C.'s Forte Sleep Aid
Calmacin
Calmette-Guérin
   bacille C.-G. (BCG, bCG)
Calmo
Calms
caloric intake
calorie
   ratio of saturated fat and
     cholesterol to c.'s
calumba
calx, *pl.* calces
calyceal
CAM
   complementary and alternative
     medicine
cambium
cambogia
   Garcinia c.
camellia
Camellia sinensis

camera
    gamma c.
    scintillation c.
camomile (*var. of* chamomile)
cAMP
    cyclic 3′,5′ adenosine
    monophosphate
Campbell ligament
campeche
Camper chiasm
camphor
    laurel c.
    c. of the poor
    c. tree
camphora
    Cinnamomum c.
camptocormia
camptodactyly, camplodactyly
camptomelia
camptomelic
    c. dwarfism
    c. syndrome
camptothecin tree
Campylobacter jejuni
Canada
    C. balsam
    C. snakeroot
    C. tea
canadense
    Menispermum c.
    Teucrium c.
canadensis
    Collinsonia c.
    Hydrastis c.
    Sambucus c.
    Sanguinaria c.
Canadian bloodwort
canadine
canal
    adductor c.
    anal c.
    carpal c.
    cervical c.
    cervicoaxillary c.
    costoclavicular c.
    Dupuytren c.
    external anal c.

    femoral c.
    c. of Guyon
    Hoyer c.
    Hunter c.
    intervertebral c.
    nutrient c.
    obturator c.
    sacral c.
    spinal c.
    subsartorial c.
    Sucquet c.
    Sucquet-Hoyer c.
    tarsal c.
    van Horne c.
    vertebral c.
canales (*pl. of* canalis)
canalicular
canaliculi
canaliculus
    bone c.
canalis, pl. canales
    c. adductorius
    c. carpi
    c. centralis medullae spinalis
    c. condylaris
    c. femoralis
    c. musculotubarius
    c. nutricius
    c. obturatorius
    c. sacralis
    c. vertebralis
Cananga odorata
Cancell
cancellous tissue
cancer
    bladder c.
    colon c.
    colorectal c.
    gastrointestinal c.
    c. jalap
    metastatic breast c.
    oral c.
    c. root
cancerroot
candicans
    Populus var. balsamifera c.

C

NOTES

candida
    C. albicans
    c. infection
candidiasis
candidissima
    Packera c.
Candistroy
candle
    citronella c.
    Our Lord's c.
candleberry
candleflower
candlenut
candlewick
cang zhu
canina
    Rosa c.
canister
canker sore
cankerwort
cannabinoid
Cannabis
    C. afghanica
    C. indica
    C. sativa
cannabis
cannula, pl. cannulae
    thin disposable c.
Canscora decussata
cantharides
cantharidin
cantharis
Cantharis vesicatoria
canthaxanthin
Cantrol
cao
    c. ma huang
    xia ku c.
    zhi gan c.
caoutchouc pelvis
cap
    Castor Oil C.'s
    friar's c.
    Hain Pumpkin Seed Oil C.'s
    Sanhelio's Circu C.'s
    soldier's c.
capacitance
    skin c.
capacity
    functional c.
    hypnotic c.
CAPE
    caffeic acid phenethyl ester

cape
    C. aloe
    C. periwinkle
capeline bandage
capensis
    Matricaria c.
caper plant
capillary
    c. circulation
    c. density
    c. fracture
    c. network
    c. pressure
capim-cidrao
capita
capitata
    Lactuca c.
capitate bone
capitatum
    os c.
capitellum
capitis
    musculus longissimus c.
    musculus longus c.
    musculus semispinalis c.
    musculus spinalis c.
    musculus splenius c.
    musculus transversalis c.
capitopedal
capitula
capitular joint
capitulum
    c. humeri
    c. of humerus
    c. motion
Capparis spinosa
Capralin
Caprinex
capri ulnaris
caprylic acid
Caprystatin
capsaicin
    c. cream
    topical c.
capsella
Capsella bursa-pastoris
capsicastrum
    Solanum c.
Capsicum
    C. annum
    C. frutescens
capsicum
Capsin

Cap-Stun
capsula
  c. articularis
  c. fibrosa
capsular
  c. compression theory
  c. ligament
  c. portion of sacroiliac joint
capsulation
capsule
  aloe vera inner leaf c.
  anterior c.
  articular c.
  devil's claw c.
  dong quai c.
  fibrous c.
  fibrous articular c.
  garlic c.
  hypericum extract c.
  joint c.
  linden c.
  lobelia c.
  Morinda citrifolia c.
  nettles c.
  octacosanol c.
  uva ursi c.
capsulitis
  adhesive c.
  c. of shoulder
capsuloplasty
caput
  c. breve
  c. breve musculi bicipitis
   brachii
  c. breve musculi bicipitis
   femoris
  c. costae
  c. femoris
  c. fibulae
  c. humerale
  c. humerale musculi flexoris
   carpi ulnaris
  c. humerale musculi pronatoris
   teretis
  c. humeri
  c. laterale
  c. laterale musculi gastrocnemii

  c. laterale musculi tricipitis
   brachii
  c. longum
  c. longum musculi bicipitis
   brachii
  c. longum musculi bicipitis
   femoris
  c. longum musculi tricipitis
   brachii
  c. mallei
  c. mediale
  c. mediale musculi
   gastrocnemii
  c. mediale musculi tricipitis
   brachii
  c. obliquum
  c. obliquum musculi adductoris
   hallucis
  c. obliquum musculi adductoris
   pollicis
  c. ossis femoris
  c. ossis metacarpalis
  c. ossis metatarsalis
  c. profundum musculi flexoris
   pollicis brevis
  c. radii
  c. superficiale musculi flexoris
   pollicis brevis
  c. transversum musculi
   adductoris hallucis
  c. transversum musculi
   adductoris pollicis
  c. ulnare
  c. ulnare musculi flexoris carpi
   ulnaris
  c. ulnare musculi pronatoris
   teretis
  c. zygomaticum quadrati labii
   superioris
Capzasin
carageenan
carang
  layor c.
caraway
carb
  kali c.
carbamazepine

NOTES

carbenoxolone
carbohydrate
    complex c.
    c. intolerance
carbohydrate-rich food
carbon
    c. dioxide exchange
    c. tetrachloride
    c. tetrachloride-induced
        hepatotoxicity
carbonaceous activated water
    (CAW)
carbonate
    calcium c.
carbonica
    Calcarea c.
carbuncle
carcinogenesis
carcinoma
    basal cell c.
    colorectal c.
    squamous cell c.
carcinomatosis
    leptomeningeal c.
carcinomatous
    c. myelopathy
    c. myopathy
    c. neuropathy
carcinosin
cardamom
    Malabar c.
cardamomum
    Elettaria c.
cardamons
cardiac
    c. arrhythmia
    c. glycoside
    c. infarction
    c. insufficiency
    c. mechanoreceptor
    c. neurosis
    c. plexus
    c. tamponade
    c. tonic
cardiaca
    Leonurus c.
cardinal
    c. flower
    c. plane
cardioglycoside
    digitalis c.
cardiomyopathy
    dilated c.

cardiopathy
    toxin-induced c.
cardioprotective
cardiopulmonary resuscitation
cardiothoracic ratio
cardiotonic
cardiovascular
    c. disease
    c. disorder
Cardiplant
Carditone
cardon benit
cardopatiae
    radix c.
cardo santo
cardunculus
    Cynara c.
Carduus marianus
care
    Allergy C.
    complementary health c.
    comprehensive c.
    conventional c.
    integrated c. (IC)
    integrative health c.
    supportive c.
Carex hirtha
cari
    oleum c.
caribe
    ruibarbo c.
Carica papaya
caries
    dental c.
carina
carinatum
    pectus c.
caring-healing modalities
Carleton University Responsiveness
    to Suggestion Scale
Carlina vulgaris
carline thistle
Carmen
    Agua del C.
carmichaeli
    Aconitum c.
Carmichaeli Tea Pills
carminative
carne de vibora
carnitine
carnivora
carnosic acid

carnosus
  panniculus c.
caro quadrata sylvii
carosella
carotene
  beta c.
  Multigenics Without Beta C.
carotenoid
  c. complex
  orange c.
caroticoclinoid ligament
carotid
  c. artery
  c. artery dissection
  c. artery palpation
  c. ganglion
  c. nerve
carotidynia
Caro-xan
carp
  grass c.
carpal
  c. arch
  c. articular surface of radius
  c. bone
  c. canal
  c. groove
  c. joint
  c. tunnel
  c. tunnel syndrome (CTS)
carpenter's
  c. herb
  c. square
Carpenter syndrome
carpi
  canalis c.
  ossa c.
  sulcus c.
carpocarpal
carpometacarpal
  c. articulation
  c. joint
  c. joint of thumb
  c. ligaments dorsal and palmar
carpometacarpales
  articulatio tibiofibularis
  articulationes c.

carpopedal
carpus curvus
carrageen
carriage
  head c.
carrisyn
carrot
  oil of c.
  wild c.
carrying angle
Carthamus tinctorius
Carticin
Cartilade
cartilage
  arthrodial c.
  articular c.
  articular surface of
    arytenoid c.
  c. bone
  bovine c.
  c. breakdown
  connecting c.
  cornua of thyroid c.
  costal c.
  cricoid c.
  cuneiform c.
  diarthrodial c.
  elastic c.
  falciform c.
  fibrous c.
  floating c.
  GNC Liquid Shark C.
  hyaline c.
  hypsiloid c.
  Informed Nutrition Shark C.
  interosseous c.
  intervertebral c.
  intraarticular c.
  intrathyroid c.
  investing c.
  c. knife
  loose c.
  c. matrix
  Morgagni c.
  Natural Brand Shark C.
  oblique line of thyroid c.
  parachordal c.

NOTES

cartilage *(continued)*
  permanent c.
  posterior process of septal c.
  Reichert c.
  semilunar c.
  shark c.
  slipping rib c.
  sternal c.
  supraarytenoid c.
  tarsal c.
  temporary c.
  triangular c.
  triquetrous c.
  triticeal c.
  uniting c.
  Weitbrecht c.
  Wrisberg c.
  xiphoid c.
  Y c.
cartilaginea
  junctura c.
cartilagines (*pl. of* cartilago)
cartilaginis
  articulatio c.
cartilaginous
  c. articulation
  c. joint
  c. part of skeletal system
  c. septum
cartilago, pl. cartilagines
  c. articularis
  c. costalis
  c. thyroidea
  c. triticea
cart track plant
Carum carvi
caruncle
caruncula
carvacrol
carvi
  Carum c.
  oleum c.
caryophylli
  oleum c.
caryophyllum
cas
cascara
  Bassoran with C.
  Kondremul with C.
  c. sagrada
case
  long-term c.

c. study
therapy-resistant c.
casein
caseous osteitis
Cas-Evac
caseweed
cassava
Casser perforated muscle
cassia
  C. acutifolia
  C. angustifolia
  c. bark
  Batavia c.
  Cinnamomum c.
  Padang c.
  Saigon c.
  C. senna
cassine
  Ilex c.
cast
  c. brace
  halo c.
castor
  c. bean
  c. oil
  C. Oil Caps
  c. oil pack
  c. oil plant
Castoria
  Fletcher's C.
cat
  c. back
  c. back exercise
catabolism
catalase
catalepsy
catalysis
catalyst altered water (CAW)
cataract
  poikiloderma atrophicans
    and c.
cataria
  Nepeta c.
catarrh
Catarrh Mixture
catastrophize
catchweed
catechin
catecholamine
  c. O-methyl transferase
    (COMT)
  reactive c.

catechu
Acacia c.
Areca c.
black c.
cake c.
category
point c.
traditional diagnostic c.
catgut
chromic c.
Catha edulis
Catharanthus roseus
catharsis
cathartic
saline c.
cathartica
Rhamnus c.
catheter
catlin
catmint
catnip
c. and fennel extract
c. herb
c. mist
c. tea
c. tea enema
cat's
c. claw
C. Claw Defense Complex
c. claw inner bark extract
c. foot
c. play
catshair
catwort
cauda
c. equina
c. equina syndrome
caudad
c. to cranial
translation c.
caudal
c. anesthesia
c. direction
c. ligament
c. retinaculum
caudale
retinaculum c.

caudate
anterior c.
caudocephalad
caught
c. in exhalation
c. in inhalation
Caulophyllum
C. robustum
C. thalictroides
causal factor
causalgia
causality
causam
tolle c.
cause
identifiable c.
necessary c.
root c.
sufficient c.
cauterant
cauterization
cautery
cava (*pl. of* cavum)
caval
cavalry bone
cave
Meckel c.
cavernosum
corpus c.
cavitas
c. articularis
c. medullaris
c. pelvis
c. thoracis
cavitation
c. phenomenon
c. pop
c. pop sound
cavity
articular c.
axillary c.
body c.
cotyloid c.
greater peritoneal c.
huiyin c.
idiopathic bone c.
lesser peritoneal c.

C

NOTES

cavity *(continued)*
    medullary c.
    peritoneal c.
    c. of pharynx
    pleural c.
    thoracic c.
cavum, pl. **cava**
    c. articulare
    foramen of vena cava
    manus cava
    c. medullare
    c. pelvis
    c. peritonei
    c. thoracis
cavus
    pes c.
    talipes c.
CAW
    carbonaceous activated water
    catalyst altered water
cayenne
    c. ginger
    c. pepper
CBC
    complete blood count
CBT
    cognitive behavior therapy
CCE
    Council on Chiropractic Education
CCK
    cholecystokinin
CC Pollen
CCTET
    contact, control, test, evaluate,
      treatment
C-cysteine
    N-acetyl C.-c.
cedar
    c. berry
    Eastern white c.
    false white c.
    oil of c.
    yellow c.
Cefkava
celandine
    common c.
    garden c.
    greater c.
    lesser c.
    c. poppy
    c. tops and root
Celebrate oil
celendine extract

celery
    c. seed
    c. seed oil
    wild c.
celiac
    c. artery
    c. disease
    c. ganglion
    c. plexus reflex
    c. rickets
    c. sprue
cell
    ALT c.
    anterior horn c.
    arcuate c.
    B c.
    bovine donor c.
    daughter c.
    dried c.
    endorphinergic c.
    fresh c.
    C. Guard
    helper T c.
    Langhans c.'s
    Langhans-type giant c.'s
    c. membrane composition
    mother c.
    motor c.
    natural killer c.
    NK c.
    osteochondrogenic c.
    osteogenic c.
    osteoprogenitor c.
    physaliphorous c.
    plasma c.
    red blood c.
    stem c.
    STT c.
    suppressor c.
    T c.
    tendon c.
    c. therapy
    c. treatment
    Virchow c.
cella
Cellasene
Cellguard Co-Q10 Nac
cell-mediated immunity
cellula
cellular
    c. antioxidant
    c. element
    c. immune response

c. memory
c. metabolism
c. milieu
c. proliferation
c. repatterning technique
c. spill
c. therapy
c. toxin
cellule
cellulite
cellulose
    oxidized c.
cellulosic acid
Cel-Ray
    Dr. Brown's C.-R.
cement
    c. disease
    c. line
Centaurea cyanus
centaury
    common c.
    European c.
    lesser c.
    minor c.
Centella asiatica
center
    Area Health Education C. (AHEC)
    base energy c.
    birthing c.
    chondrification c.
    crown energy c.
    diaphysial c.
    energy c.
    heart energy c.
    Kerckring c.
    main energy c.
    major energy c.
    minor energy c.
    ossification c.
    c. of ossification
    c. of rotation
centering
    body-mind c.
centesimal dilution (C)
centra

central
    c. amputation
    c. axillary lymph node
    c. bone
    c. bone of ankle
    c. callus
    c. canal of spinal cord
    c. canal stenosis
    c. disk herniation
    c. nervous system (CNS)
    c. nervous system inherent mobility
    c. neurohumoral mechanism
    c. osteitis
    c. palmar space
    c. spinal stenosis
    c. stimulation
    c. sulcal artery
    c. tendon
centrale
    os c.
centrally acting stimulant
Centranthus ruber
centrifugal
centrofacial lentiginosis
centrum of a vertebra
cepa
    Allium c.
Cephaelis ipecacuanha
cephalad pubic dysfunction
cephalgia
    brain-injury associated c.
cephalic
    c. angle
    translation c.
cephalocaudal axis
cephalopharyngeus
    musculus c.
cephalorrhachidian
cephalothoracic
cephalward
ceratocricoid
cerclage
cerea
    flexibilitas c.
    c. flexibilitas

NOTES

69

cereal
>fortified c.

cerebelli
>falx c.
>tentorium c.

cerebellum
>subacute degeneration of c.

cerebral
>c. aneurysm
>c. anoxia
>c. arteriovenous malformation
>c. cortex
>c. death
>c. hemorrhage
>c. infarction
>c. insufficiency
>c. insufficiency syndrome
>c. insult
>c. palsy
>c. spinal fluid fluctuation
>c. thrombosis
>c. vein
>c. ventricle

cerebri
>falx c.
>tentorium c.

cerebrospinal
>c. axis
>c. fluid (CSF)
>c. fluid blockage
>c. fluid fluctuation
>c. fluid pulse wave
>c. system

cerebrum
>fourth ventricle of c.

cerefolium
>*Anthriscus c.*

ceremonial procedure
ceremony
>spirit-calling c.
>sweat-lodge c.

cereus
>*C. grandiflorus*
>night-blooming c.

cerifera
>*Myrica c.*

certification
>guild c.
>holistic nurse c. (HNC)

certified
>guild c.
>holistic nurse c. (HNC)

cerulea
>*Sambucus c.*

cervical
>c. anesthesia
>c. articulatory technique
>c. brachialgia
>c. canal
>c. cranial syndrome
>c. degeneration
>c. degeneration of
>   intervertebral disk
>c. disk
>c. dysplasia
>c. enlargement
>c. enlargement of spinal cord
>c. facet
>c. flexion test
>c. flexor muscle
>c. fusion syndrome
>c. gland
>c. iliocostal muscle
>c. interspinal muscle
>c. isometric exercise
>c. longissimus muscle
>c. loop
>c. and lumbar lordoses
>c. lymph node
>c. mobilization
>c. myelogram
>c. nerves [C1–C8]
>c. orthosis
>c. part of esophagus
>c. part of internal carotid
>   artery
>c. part of spinal cord
>c. part of thoracic duct
>c. plexus
>c. rib
>c. roll
>c. root
>c. rotation
>c. rotator muscle
>c. scoliosis
>c. segment articular pillar
>c. segments of spinal cord
>   [C1–C8]
>c. spine
>c. spine axis
>c. spine diagnosis
>c. spine functional technique
>c. spine motion testing
>c. spine muscle energy
>   technique

c. spine myofascial technique
c. splanchnic nerves
c. spondylitis
c. spondylosis
c. syndrome
c. tender point
c. triangle
c. vertebra
c. vertebrae [C1–C7]
c. vertigo
cervicale
trigonum c.
cervicales
regiones c.
vertebrae c. [C1–C7]
cervicalis
ansa c.
c. ascendens
costa c.
descendens c.
fascia c.
lamina superficialis fasciae c.
cervicalium
tuberculum anterius
vertebrarum c.
tuberculum posterius
vertebrarum c.
cervices (*pl. of* cervix)
cervicis
biventer c.
musculi intertransversarii
anteriores c.
musculi intertransversarii
posteriores c.
musculi rotatores c.
musculus iliocostalis c.
musculus interspinalis c.
musculus longissimus c.
musculus semispinalis c.
musculus spinalis c.
musculus splenius c.
musculus transversalis c.
cervicoaxillary canal
cervicobrachial syndrome
cervicocephalic syndrome
cervicocranial syndrome
cervicofacial

cervicothoracic
c. articulatory technique
c. asymmetry
c. ganglion
c. orthosis
c. transition
cervix, pl. **cervices**
c. uteri
Cervus nippon
cessation
smoking c.
Cetraria
C. islandica
Ceylon cinnamon
CFS
chronic fatigue syndrome
CGI
Clinical Global Improvement
CGI scale
Chaenomeles japonica
chai hu su gan tang
chair
EasyChair massage c.
chakra
c. acupuncture
c. acupuncture treatment
base c.
crown c.
fifth c.
first c.
fourth c.
heart c.
integrating c.
lower c.
main c.
opening of the c.
c. point
polarity c.
c. region
second c.
seventh c.
sixth c.
solar plexus c.
c. system
third c.
throat c.
upper c.

C

NOTES

chamaedrys
  Teucrium c.
Chamaelirium luteum
Chamaemelum nobile
chamazulene
chamber
  Hyper-Oxy portable
  hyperbaric c.
chamomile, camomile
  Classic C.
  common c.
  English c.
  c. flower
  German c.
  C. Grande
  Hungarian c.
  organic c.
  Roman c.
  sweet false c.
  c. tea
  true c.
  wild c.
chamomilla
  Matricaria c.
Chamomilla recutita
Champion's Choice
change
  adaptive c.
  bevel c.
  biomechanical c.
  dysfunctional cellular c.
  homeostatic c.
  immunological c.
  Life C.
  lumbar tissue texture c.'s
  neuroreflexive c.
  C. oil
  osseous c.
  palpatory c.
  reflex c.
  rhythmic c.
  thoracic tissue texture c.'s
  tissue texture c.'s
  trophic c.'s
Change-O-Life
changqiang
  du 1 c.
changras
channel
  acupuncture c.
  c. axis
  cold stagnation in the liver c.

cold stagnation in the
  lower c.
corresponding c.
coupled c.
c. course
course of c.'s
cycles of c.'s
du mai c. (du)
eight psychic c.'s
energy c.
extraordinary c.
gallbladder c. (gb)
heart c. (he)
irregular c.
kidney c. (ki)
kidney-heart c.
large intestine c. (li)
liver c. (liv)
lung c. (lu)
lymphatic c.
main c.
marvelous c.
pair of c.'s
pericardial c.
pericardium c. (pe)
propagated sensation along
  the c. (PSC)
ren c.
ren mai c. (ren)
sanjiao c. (sj)
shao yin c.
small intestine c. (si)
small intestine-bladder c.
spleen c. (sp)
stomach c. (st)
tai yang c.
triple burner c.
triple heater c.
triple warmer c.
urinary bladder c. (ub)
yang c.
yin c.
channel-structural level
chan su
ch'an su leaf
chant
chanting
chaparral
Chapman
  C. reflex
  C. reflex point

character
c., onset, location, duration, exacerbation, remission (COLDER)
psychogenic c.
yang c.
characteristic
pulse c.
charantia
Momordica c.
charcoal
activated c.
c. hemoperfusion
c. tablet
charge
coulomb of c.
charley horse
Charlie
creeping C.
charlock
chart
symptom c.
Chassaignac space
chassediable
chaste
agneau c.
c. tree
c. tree fruit
chasteberry
chaulmogra, chaulmoogra
c. oil
chavica betal
chaw
CHD
coronary heart disease
che
zi he c.
chebula
Terminalia c.
check
Sinus C.
checkerberry
two-eyed c.
checklist
Everyday Problem C. (EPCL)
Hopkins Symptom C. (HSCL)

checkup
energy c.
cheeseflower
cheeseweed
cheilitis
cheirarthritis
cheiropodalgia
cheirospasm
chelate
chelated
c. calcium
c. mineral
chelation
c. chemical
energy c.
c. therapist
c. therapy
Chelidonium majus
Chelone glabra
chemical
chelation c.
c. sampling
chemoimmunotherapy
chemonucleolysis
chemopreventative
chemoprevention
chemoprotective
chemotaxis
chemotherapy
Revici guided c.
chengfu
ub 36 c.
chengqi
st 1 c.
Chenopodium ambrosoides
chenopodium oil
cherry
c. birch
choke c.
maraschino c.
rum c.
wild c.
cherubism
chervil
cow c.
garden c.

C

NOTES

73

chervil *(continued)*
    salad c.
    sweet c.
chest
    alar c.
    barrel c.
    flat c.
    foveated c.
    c. index
    keeled c.
    phthinoid c.
    c. physical therapy
    pterygoid c.
    c. qi
    regions of c.
    c. wall
    c. wall motion
chestnut
    horse c.
chewable
    Multigenics C.
Cheweez
chewing
    abnormal c.
Cheyne-Stokes respiration
CHF
    congestive heart failure
chi, ch'i
    c. circulation
    consolidated c.
    c. cuang zi
    deep c.
    c. disturbance
    extended c.
    extrinsic c.
    c. flow
    c. gong
    c. imbalance
    internal c.
    intrinsic c.
    c. kung
    c. movement
    Nature's C.
    c. nei tsang
    c. reservoir
    shan c.
    sick c.
    stored c.
    tai c.
chiang huo
chiao
chiasm
    Camper c.

chiasma tendinum
chiasmatic
chicken breast
chickpea
chickweed
    star c.
Chicorium intybus
chicory
chief
    big c.
chien
    chih c.
child
    Calm C.
childbirth
childhood fall
chili pepper
Chimaphilia umbellata
chin
    c. ch'iao mai
    c. dao
China
    C. bark
    C. Gold
    C. root
China-wood oil
chinensis
    Coptis c.
    Cuscuta c.
    Lycium c.
    Schisandra c.
    Simmondsia c.
chinese
    C. blistering beetle
    Bupleurum c.
    C. cinnamon
    C. classification
    C. cornbind
    C. cucumber
    C. dietary therapy
    C. doctor
    C. ephedra
    C. gelatin
    C. ginger
    C. ginseng
    C. herbalist
    C. herbal medicine
    C. jujube
    C. kidney system
    C. licorice
    C. medicine
    C. motherwort
    C. nutrition

C. organ
C. parsley
C. rhubarb
C. syndrome
C. taoism
C. toad
ching qi tang
chinwood
Chionanthus virginicus
chip
    bone c.
chirarthritis
chiropodalgia
chiropodist
chiropody
chiropractic
    c. adjustment
    doctor of c. (DC)
    c. manipulation
    c. medicine
    National College of C.
    network c.
    c. radiology
    rational c.
    straight c.
    c. subluxation
    subluxation-based c.
    World Federation of C. (WFC)
chiropractor
chiropraxy
chirospasm
chitosamine
chitrak
chize
    lu 5 c.
Chlorella
chloride
    ethyl c.
Chlorofresh
chlorogenic acid
chlorophyll
    Papaya Enzyme with C.
chlorophyllin
chlorosis
chocolate flower

choice
    Champion's C.
    Physician's C.
choke
    black c.
    c. cherry
cholagogic
cholangitis
cholecalciferol
cholecystitis
cholecystokinin (CCK)
cholelithiasis
choleretic
choleric temper
cholesterol
    biliary c.
    c. gallstone
    high c.
    LDL c.
    c. metabolite
    serum c.
Cholestin
choline
cholinergic blockade
Cholosum N
chondral
chondralgia
chondralloplasia
chondrification center
chondritis
chondroblast
chondroblastoma
chondrocalcinosis
    articular c.
chondroclast
chondrocostal
chondrocyte
chondrodynia
chondrodystrophy
    asymmetric c.
    hereditary deforming c.
    hypoplastic fetal c.
chondroectodermal
chondrogenesis
chondroglossus
chondroid tissue

C

NOTES

chondroitin
  c.-4-sulfate
  c.-6-sulfate
  c.-C
  c. sulfate
  c. sulfate A
chondrology
chondrolysis
chondroma
  juxtacortical c.
  periosteal c.
chondromalacia patellae
chondromatosis
  synovial c.
chondromatous
chondromere
chondromyxoma
chondroosseous
chondroosteodystrophy
chondropathy
chondrophyte
chondroplasty
chondroporosis
chondrosarcoma
chondroskeleton
chondrosternal
chondrotrophic
chondroxiphoid ligament
chondrus
  C. crispus
  c. extract
chong
  c. mai
  c. xian san
chongras
Chopart joint
chop nut
choppy pulse
chorda, pl. **chordae**
  c. magna
  c. obliqua membranae
    interosseae antebrachii
  chordae tendineae
chordal
chordoma
chorea
  Huntington c.
christe herbe
Christi
  palma C.
Christian Science
Christmas
  C. factor

  C. flower
  C. rose
Christopher
  stinking C.
chromatography
  gas c. (GC)
  high-performance liquid c.
  (HPLC)
  thin-layer c. (TLC)
chromatotherapy
chromic catgut
chromium picolinate
chromosomal
chromosome
chromotherapy
chronic
  c. absorptive arthritis
  c. allograft rejection
  c. back pain
  c. bronchitis
  c. condition
  c. conjunctivitis
  c. dysfunction
  c. facial nerve paralysis
  c. fatigue syndrome (CFS)
  c. headache
  c. hemorrhagic villous
    synovitis
  c. hepatitis
  c. inflammation
  c. muscle tension
  c. musculoskeletal pain
  c. obstructive pulmonary
    disease (COPD)
  c. pain
  c. pain condition
  c. pelvic pain (CPP)
  c. postural deficit
  c. recurrent anteriorly nutated
    sacroiliac dysfunction
  c. rheumatism
  c. somatic dysfunction
  c. stagnation
  c. type
  c. urticaria
chronically
  c. recurrent low back pain
  c. recurring back pain
chronobiology
chronobiotic
chronophotograph
Chronoset
chronotherapy

chronotropic effect
Chrysanthemum
  C. morifolium
  C. vulgare
chua ka massage
chuan, ch'uan
  tai chi c., tai ji c., tai ji quan
    c. yang
chuang gui er chen tang
chuanxiong
  Ligusticum c.
chung
  jen c.
church-flower
church steeple
chyle cistern
chyli
  cisterna c.
chylous arthritis
Chymodiactin
chymopapain
chymotrypsin
cibum
  ante c.
Cicaderma
cicatricial
cicatrix, pl. cicatrices
cicatrizant
cicatrization
cicely
  smooth c.
  sweet c.
Cichorium intybus
Cicuta
  C. douglasii
  C. maculata
cigar
  indirect moxibustion with
    moxa c.
  moxa c.
  moxibustion with moxa c.
cigarette
  herbal c.
  lettuce-leaf c.
cilantro
cimetidine
Cimexon

Cimicifuga
  C. dahurica
  C. foetida
  C. heracleifolia
  C. racemosa
cina
  Artemisia c.
cinae
  semen c.
cinchona
  c. bark
  C. calisya
  C. Homeopathic
  C. ledgeriana
  red c.
  C. succirubra
  yellow c.
cinchonism
cinefluorography
cinefluoroscopy
cinematic amputation
cineplastic amputation
cineplastics
cineradiography
cineraria
  Senecio c.
Cineraria maritima
cinerariifolium
  Tanacetum c.
cineroentgenography
cingulum
  c. membri inferioris
  c. membri superioris
cinnamomea
  Rosa c.
Cinnamomum
  C. camphora
  C. cassia
  C. verum
  C. zeylanicum
cinnamon
  c. bark
  Batavia c.
  Ceylon c.
  Chinese c.
  false c.
  Panang c.

C

NOTES

cinnamon *(continued)*
   Saigon c.
   c. wood
cinquefoil
circadian
   c. pacemaker
   c. pattern of onset of
     myocardial infarction
   c. rhythm
   c. rhythm sleep disorder
   c. sequence
   c. shift
circle
   c. absorption anesthesia
   articular vascular c.
   goddess c.
   hermeneutic c.
circuit
   oscillatory c.
circular
   c. amputation
   c. bandage
   c. sinus
circulation
   blood c.
   capillary c.
   chi c.
   collateral c.
   compensatory c.
   dural c.
   energy c.
   greater c.
   lymph c.
   microcosmic orbit c.
   peripheral c.
   perivascular interstitial fluid c.
   qi c.
   systemic c.
   water qi c.
circulatory
   c. effect
   c. function
   c. system
circulus articularis vasculosus
circumarticular
circumaxillary
circumbulbar
circumduction
circumference
circumferentia
   c. articularis capitis radii
   c. articularis capitis ulna

circumferential
   c. fibrocartilage
   c. lamella
circumflex
circumscribed
circumscripta
   osteitis fibrosa c.
circus
   c. movement
   c. performer
Cirflo
cirrhosis
   micronodular c.
cis-linoleic acid
cistern
   chyle c.
   lumbar c.
   Pecquet c.
cisterna chyli
cisternal
citral
citrate
   calcium c.
   tamoxifen c.
citrated autologous blood
citratus
   Cymbopogon c.
citrifolia
   Morinda c.
citrin
citriodora
   Lippia c.
citronella
   c. candle
   oil of c.
citrulline
citrus
Citrus reticulata
city avens
Civinini process
clarified butter
clary
   c. oil
   c. sage
clasp-knife reflex
class
   New York Heart Association
     functional c.
classic
   c. acupuncture
   c. acupuncture point
   C. Chamomile

classical
    c. acupuncture
    c. homeopathy
    c. migraine
classification
    bioenergetic system
      technique c.
    Chinese c.
    energy balance technique c.
    Nursing Interventions C. (NIC)
claudication
    intermittent c.
    neurogenic c.
claudicatory
clavatum
    Lycopodium c.
Claviceps purpurea
clavicle
    acromial articular facies of c.
    acromial articular surface of c.
    acromial end of c.
    acromial extremity of c.
    body of c.
    conoid tubercle of c.
    c. muscle energy technique
    sternal articular surface of c.
    sternal end of c.
    sternal extremity of c.
clavicula
claviculae
    corpus c.
    extremitas acromialis c.
    extremitas sternalis c.
clavicular
    c. facet
    c. head of pectoralis major
      muscle
    c. notch of sternum
    c. part of pectoralis major
      muscle
clavicularis
    incisura c.
claviculus
clavipectoral fascia
clavipectoralis
    fascia c.

claw
    cat's c.
    devil's c.
    c. toe
clawfoot, claw foot
clawhand, claw hand
clay shoveler's fracture
clean
    c. air tea
    c. needle technique (CNT)
cleanse
    Aerobic Bulk C. (ABC)
    A.M./P.M. Ultimate C.
cleanser
    Red Clover C.
cleansing
    bowel c.
    colon c.
    c. enema
    c. fast
    c. therapy
clearance
    mucociliary c.
clear eye
clearing
    homeopathic c.
ClearLungs
cleavage line
cleavers
Cleen
    Hemo C.
cleft
    c. hand
    c. point
    c. spine
cleidal
cleidocostal
cleidocranial
    c. dysostosis
    c. dysplasia
cleidoepitrochlearis
    musculus c.
cleidomastoideus
    musculus c.
clematitis
    Aristolochia c.

C

NOTES

click
    joint c.
clidal
clidocostal
clidocranial
clignetiae
    Vitis c.
climacteric
clinic
    acupuncture c.
clinical
    C. Global Improvement (CGI)
    C. Global Improvement scale
    c. herbalist
    c. hypnosis
    c. hypnotherapy
    c. nutrition
    c. phobia
    c. sensitivity
    c. trial
clinicopathologic
clinocephaly
clinodactyly
clip
    ear c.
clive
clock
    pelvic c.
clodronate
closed
    c. anesthesia
    c. dislocation
    c. facet
    c. fracture
    c. reduction of fracture
    c. surgery
closed-head injury
Clostridium ramosum
clotbur
clote
    fox's c.
clotrimazole
clotting factor
clove
    dog c.'s
    oil of c.'s
    c. oil
    c. pepper
    c. root
    c. stem
    c. tea
clover
    cow c.

    dried sweet c.
    meadow c.
    purple c.
    red c.
    wild c.
    winter c.
cloverleaf skull syndrome
club
    Hercule's c.
clubbing
    finger c.
clubfoot, club foot
clubhand, club hand
    radial c.
    ulnar c.
cluster
    affinity c.
Clutton joint
clycitein
CMP
    complementary medical practice
CMV
    cytomegalovirus
cnemial
cnemis
C1–C8 nerves
Cnicus benedictus
Cnidium monnieri
CNME
    Council on Naturopathic Medical
      Education
CNS
    central nervous system
      CNS plasticity
CNT
    clean needle technique
coagula
coagulable
coagulans
    Withania c.
coagulant
coagulation
coagulopathy
    disseminated intravascular c.
      (DIC)
coakum
coapt
coaptation splint
coarctation of aorta
coarse breathing
coat
    muscular c.
cobalamin

Cobb
    C. measurements in scoliosis
    C. method of scoliosis curve
       measurement
coca
    Erythroxylum c.
    c. leaf
cocaine addiction
cocainization
cocashweed
cocci (*pl. of* coccus)
coccobacillary
coccobacillus
coccoid
Cocculus
    C. indicus
    C. palmatus
cocculus
coccus, pl. **cocci**
coccyalgia
coccydynia
coccygalgia
coccygea, pl. **coccygeae**
    foveola c.
    vertebrae coccygeae [Co1–Co4]
coccygeal
    c. body
    c. bone
    c. cornu
    c. dimple
    c. foveola
    c. ganglion
    c. gland
    c. joint
    c. nerve [Co]
    c. nerve plexus
    c. part of spinal cord
    c. plexus
    c. segment of spinal cord
      [Co]
    c. vertebrae [Co1–Co4]
    c. whorl
coccygealia
    cornua c.
coccygeus muscle

coccygis
    musculus extensor c.
    os c.
coccygodynia
coccyodynia
coccyx
cochin lemongrass
cochlear nerve
Cochlospermum
    C. gossypium
cocklebur
cockle button
cock's crow diarrhea
cocktail
    Myers c.
    c. party syndrome
    c. syndrome
cock-up-hat
cocoa
    Brazilian c.
    c. butter
cocos
    C. nucifera
    Poria c.
    Sclerotium Poriae c.
14C-octacosanol
codeine
codfish vertebra
Codman triangle
Codonopsis pilosula
coelom
Coenzyme B complex
coenzyme Q10 (CoQ_{10})
cofactor
Coffea arabica
coffee
    c. enema
    c. retention enema
    robusta c.
    Santos c.
cognition
    critical analytic c.
cognitive
    c. avoidance technique
    c. behavioral stress
      management
    c. behavior therapy (CBT)

C

NOTES

cognitive *(continued)*
    c. function
    c. learning
    c. perceptual motor evaluation
    c. restructuring
    c. therapy
Cognitive-Somatic Anxiety
    Questionnaire
cohosh
    black c.
    blue c.
    white c.
coiling
    c. of brain
    c. motion
Coix lachryma jobi
Cola
    C. acuminata
    C. nitida
cola
    c. seed
    c. tree
colchicine
Colchicum autumnale
cold
    c. bi
    common c.
    c. disturbance
    interior c.
    c. laser therapy
    pathogenic c.
    c. sore
    c. stagnation in the liver
      channel
    c. stagnation in the lower
      channel
    c. symptom
    c. therapy
cold-based hydrotherapy
Cold-Eeze
COLDER
    character, onset, location, duration,
      exacerbation, remission
    condition, onset, location, duration,
      exacerbation, remission
coldness symptom
Cold-Plus
cold-pressed olive oil
coleus
    wild c.
colewort
Coley toxin

coli
    diverticulosis c.
    Escherichia c.
    melanosis c.
colic
    biliary c.
    renal c.
    c. root
colicroot
colitis
    ulcerative c.
colla (*pl. of* collum)
collagen fiber
collagenosis
collagen-vascular disease
collapse
collapsed energy
collar
    c. bone
    herbal flea-repellent pet c.
collar-button abscess
collards
collateral
    c. circulation
    c. ganglion
    c. ligament
    c. ligament of knee
    c. system
    c. vessel
collaterale
    vas c.
colle du japon
Colles fascia
colli
    apparatus ligamentosus c.
    musculi c.
    musculus longus c.
    musculus semispinalis c.
    musculus spinalis c.
    musculus splenius c.
    trigonum c.
colliculus
collina
    Achillea c.
Collinson
    Tincture C.
Collinsonia canadensis
collodion
    flexible c.
    hemostatic c.
    styptic c.
collodium

colloid
psyllium c.
styptic c.
thyroid c.
colloidal
Aveeno C.
C. Energy Formula
c. silver
c. silver protein
collum, pl. **colla**
c. anatomicum humeri
c. chirurgicum humeri
c. costae
c. femoris
c. fibulae
c. humeri
c. mallei
c. ossis femoris
c. radii
c. scapulae
c. tali
colocynth fruit
Coloklysis-7
colon
c. cancer
c. cleansing
c. hydrotherapy
iliac c.
mucosa of c.
c. therapist
c. therapy
colonic
c. adenoma
high c.
c. hygienist
c. irrigation
c. practitioner
color
c. affinity
c. healing
red c.
c. therapy
colorado
lapacho c.
colorectal
c. adenoma

c. cancer
c. carcinoma
colored-light therapy
colorimetric redox assay
coloring
food c.
colostrum
bovine c.
coltsfoot
false c.
sweet c.
Western c.
columbo root
columella
column
intermediolateral cell c.
lateral c.
posterior c.
spinal c.
superincumbent vertebral c.
vertebral c.
columna vertebralis
columnella
coma
comatose patient
comb flower
combination
Vikonon C.
combined
c. method
c. method joint mobilization
c. sclerosis
c. technique
c. vertebral and rib
dysfunction
combo
blessed thistle c.
ginger peppermint c.
red clover c.
comfort
position of c.
Women's C.
comfrey
middle c.
c. ointment
c. root
spotted c.

NOTES

C

83

commensalism
commensal parasite
comminuted fracture
comminution
Commiphora
    C. abyssinica
    C. madagascariensis
    C. molmol
    C. mukul
    C. myrrha
commissura
commissural
commissure
common
    c. arnica
    c. barberry
    c. basil
    c. bistort
    c. borage
    c. buckthorn
    c. bugle
    c. bugloss
    c. celandine
    c. centaury
    c. chamomile
    c. cold
    c. compensatory pattern
    c. cotton
    c. daisy
    c. elder
    c. fennel
    c. figwort
    c. flexor sheath of hand
    c. horehound
    c. indigo
    c. juniper
    c. marjoram
    c. mold
    c. myrtle
    c. nettle
    c. oak
    c. parsley
    c. peroneal tendon sheath
    c. plantain
    c. quince
    c. rue
    c. sundew
    c. tansy
    c. tendinous ring of
      extraocular muscles
    c. thyme
commun
communal healing

commune
    integumentum c.
communicans
communicantes
    white rami c.
communication
    holistic c.
    intercellular c.
communis
    musculus extensor digitorum c.
    Ricinus c.
    vagina communis tendinum
      musculorum fibularium c.
    vagina tendinum musculorum
      fibularium c.
compact
compages thoracis
companion vein
compartment
    anterior c.
    fascial c.
    c. syndrome
compartmentalization
compartmentalize
compass plant
compensate
compensated posture
compensation
    postural c.
    structural c.
compensatory
    c. circulation
    c. fascial pattern
    c. hypermobility
    c. pattern
competitive inhibition
complaint
    gastrointestinal c.
complementary
    c. and alternative approach
      (CAA)
    c. and alternative medicine
      (CAM)
    c. health care
    c. medical practice (CMP)
    c. therapy
complete
    c. blood count (CBC)
    c. disinfectant
    C. oil
complex
    Advanced Carotenoid C.
    c. carbohydrate

carotenoid c.
Cat's Claw Defense C.
Coenzymate B c.
c. fracture
ginseng c.
glucosamine c.
guaiacum c.
Herbal Diuretic C.
Kidney-Liver C. #406
Lung C. #407
osteopathic lesion c.
panax c.
pareira c.
c. polysaccharide
Pulsatilla Med C.
c. regional pain syndrome
  (CRPS)
Sinus and Catarrh C.
verbascum c.
viburnum c.
complexa
articulatio c.
complexus
musculus c.
compliance
complication
neurological c.
postoperative c.
vascular c.
component
anterior c.
exhalation restriction, bucket-
  handle c.
exhalation restriction, pump-
  handle c.
involuntary c.
lesioned c.
posterior c.
somatic c.
voluntary c.
composita
articulatio c.
composite joint
composition
cell membrane c.
compound
c. aneurysm

anticholinergic c.
c. articulation
c. benzoin tincture
cactus-hawthorn c.
conchae c.
c. dislocation
endorphin c.
c. fracture
goldenrod-horsetail c.
c. joint
lungwort c.
organic c.
tocopherol c.
wild cherry bark c.
willow-meadowsweet c.
comprehensive care
compress
eyebright c.
goldenseal c.
mullein c.
compressible-rigid
compression
c. anesthesia
anterior posterior c.
anteroposterior rib c.
bulb c.
c. of fourth ventricle
lateral rib c.
c. plate
c. plating
pubic symphysis c.
rib c.
sphenobasilar c.
suboccipital c.
c. syndrome
c. test
traumatic c.
compressive
c. force
c. stress
compulsive strangury
Computabs
Lobidram C.
computed tomography (CT)
COMT
catecholamine O-methyl transferase
Concentrace trace mineral drops

NOTES

concentrate
    licorice ATC c.
    mixed tocopherol c.
    senna c.
concentrated
    C. Caraway Water
    C. Dill Water BPC 1973
concentration
    focal point of c.
    mineral c.
    One-A-Day Memory and C.
concentrative meditation
concentric
    c. contraction
    c. isotonic contraction
    c. isotonic muscle contraction
    c. lamella
    c. muscle contraction
concept
    barrier c.
    cranial c.
    ease-bind c.
    holistic c.
    myofascial tight-loose c.
    c. therapy technique
    tight-loose c.
    traditional Chinese c.
conception
    c. meridian
    c. vessel
conceptional vessel (cv)
conchae compound
concoction
concomitant
concussion
    spinal c.
    spinal cord c.
concussor
condensans
    osteopathia c.
condensing osteitis
condition
    acutely painful c.
    chronic c.
    chronic pain c.
    deficiency c.
    deficiency-type c.
    energy c.
    excess c.
    excess-type c.
    exhaustion c.
    exterior c.
    fear c.

    irreversible c.
    c., onset, location, duration, exacerbation, remission (COLDER)
    pain c.
    precancerous c.
    psychosomatic c.
    rheumatological c.
    shi c.
    shi-type c.
    type O c.
    visceral c.
    xu c.
    yang c.
    yang-type c.
    yin c.
conditioned
    c. healing
    c. reflex
conditioning
    aerobic c.
    operant c.
    verbal c.
condor-vine bark
conduction
    c. analgesia
    c. anesthesia
    perivascular sympathetic fiber c.
    c. velocity
conduit
Conduran
condurango
    c. bark
    c. blanco
    Gonolobus c.
    Marsdenia c.
condylar
    c. articulation
    c. decompression
    c. glide
    c. joint
    c. portion
    c. portion of occiput
condylaris
    articulatio c.
    canalis c.
    fossa c.
condylarthrosis
condyle
    c. cord
    c. of humerus
    lateral c.

lateral femoral c.
mandible c.
medial c.
medial femoral c.
occipital c.
condylion
condyloid process of mandible
condyloma
Condylox
condylus
c. humeri
c. lateralis
c. lateralis femoris
c. lateralis tibiae
c. medialis
c. medialis femoris
c. medialis tibiae
cone
moxa c.
coneflower
c. extract
narrow-leaved purple c.
purple c.
purple Kansas c.
conexus intertendineus
confluent
c. point
c. point of dai mai
c. point of yinwei
congenial asymmetry
congenita
amyoplasia c.
amyotonia c.
arthrogryposis multiplex c.
myatonia c.
congenital
c. abnormality
c. alteration
c. atonic pseudoparalysis
c. disorder
c. hip dysplasia
c. hypothyroidism
c. neural-tube defect
c. sternal foramen
c. torticollis
congenitale
poikiloderma c.

congestion
intracranial c.
liver qi c.
sinus c.
toxic c.
venous c.
congestive heart failure (CHF)
Congming Anti-HIV herbal brew
conical receptor
Conium maculatum
conjoined tendon
conjoint tendon
conjugated linoleic acid
conjugation
conjunctivitis
allergic c.
chronic c.
conjunctivus
tendo c.
connecting
c. cartilage
c. point
connection
energetic c.
luo c.
mind-body c.
myofascial c.
connective
c. tissue
c. tissue disease
c. tissue system
connexus intertendinei musculi extensoris digitorum
conoid
c. ligament
c. process
c. tubercle of clavicle
conscious awareness
consciously
breathing c.
consciousness
cosmic c.
force of c.
nonordinary state of c.
pure c.
consecutive amputation
consensual

C

NOTES

consolidant
Consolida regalis
consolidated chi
consolidation technique
consortium
    Faith and Health C. (FHC)
constancy lily
constant rest position
constipation
    spastic c.
constituent
constitution
constitutional weakness
constriction
constrictive pericarditis
constrictor
construct
consuelda menor
consultation
    dietetic c.
consumption moss
consumptive's weed
contact
    c. allergen
    c., control, test, evaluate, treatment (CCTET)
    c. dermatitis
    c. eczema
    four-point c.
    c. point
    c. urticaria
contained disk herniation
container
    quartz-glass c.
contaminant
contaminate
contamination
contemplation
contiguous
continuity
    amputation in c.
    c. of fascia
    myofascial c.
continuous passive motion
continuous-wave laser beam
continuum movement technique
contour
    c. of bone
    bump and hollow c.
    finite skin c.
    serrated sutural c.
contracted muscle

contractility
    muscle c.
    c. of muscle
    myocardial c.
contraction
    concentric c.
    concentric isotonic c.
    concentric isotonic muscle c.
    concentric muscle c.
    eccentric c.
    eccentric isotonic c.
    eccentric isotonic muscle c.
    eccentric muscle c.
    idiomuscular c.
    c. intensity
    isolytic c.
    isolytic muscle c.
    isometric c.
    isometric muscle c.
    isotonic c.
    isotonic muscle c.
    muscle c.
    muscular c.
    myotatic c.
    patient-active muscle c.
    postural c.
    static c.
    static muscle c.
    tetanic c.
    tetanic spastic c.
    tonic c.
    uterine c.
contraction-relaxation
contracture
    c. deformity
    Dupuytren c.
    functional c.
    gangliform c.
    muscle c.
contractured muscle
contrafissura
contraindication
contralateral
    c. dorsolateral funiculus
    c. partner
    c. side
control
    attentional c.
    balance and c.
    blood flow c.
    diffuse noxious inhibitory c. (DNIC)
    c. experiment

fluoroscopic c.
c. group
motor c.
neuroendocrine c.
pain c.
pelvic c.
voluntary c.
controlled
c. fasting
c. joint position
c. substance
C. Substance Act (CSA)
c. trial
contusion
conus medullaris
Convallaria majalis
conventional
c. acupuncture
c. care
c. TENS
c. therapy
c. tomography
convex
c. anteriorly
c. posteriorly
c.-to-convex apposition
convexity
anterior c.
Convolvulus
C. pluricaulis
C. scammonia
convulsion
cookware
iron c.
cooling agent
cool tankard
cool-warm
Cooper
C. ligament
suspensory ligaments of C.
cooperation
intensive c.
muscle c.
respiratory c.
coordinate system
coordinating effect

coordination
hand-eye c.
muscular c.
COPD
chronic obstructive pulmonary
disease
cope
copper deficiency
coprophil, coprophile
Coptis chinensis
copula
CoQ$_{10}$
coenzyme Q10
coracoacromial
c. arch
c. ligament
coracobrachial
c. bursa
c. muscle
coracobrachialis
c. muscle
musculus c.
coracoclavicular ligament
coracohumeral ligament
coracoid
c. process
c. tuberosity
coracoidea
tuberositas c.
coralberry
cord
arachnoid of spinal c.
central canal of spinal c.
cervical enlargement of
spinal c.
cervical part of spinal c.
coccygeal part of spinal c.
coccygeal segment of spinal c.
[Co]
condyle c.
dura mater of spinal c.
glioma of the spinal c.
inherent mobility of brain and
spinal c.
c. lesion
c. level
lumbar part of spinal c.

C

NOTES

cord *(continued)*
    lumbosacral enlargement of
      spinal c.
    Rexed layers of spinal c.
    sacral part of spinal c.
    spinal c.
    subacute combined degeneration
      of the spinal c.
    tendinous c.'s
    tethered c.
    c. tumor
    Weitbrecht c.
cordata
    Aleurites c.
    Tilia c.
    Tilia c.
cordifolia
    Arnica c.
cordis
    lacertus c.
Cordyceps sinensis
CordyMax Cs-4
core
    c. body temperature
    inner c.
    c. value
corelease
coreolis
    c. effect
    c. force
coriander
Coriander sativum
corkwood tree
corn
    crow c.
    c. germ
    c. poppy
    c. rose
    c. silk
cornbind
    Chinese c.
cornea, pl. corneae
corneal
Cornell Medical Index
cornflower
cornsilk buchu formula
cornstarch
cornu, gen. cornus, pl. cornua
    coccygeal c.
    cornua coccygealia
    c. inferius cartilaginis
      thyroideae
    sacral c.

    c. sacrale
    c. superius cartilaginis
      thyroideae
    cornua of thyroid cartilage
cornual
Cornus officinalus
corona
coronad
coronal
    c. plane
    c. suture
coronale
coronalis
coronaria
coronary
    c. angioplasty
    c. artery disease (CAD)
    c. heart disease (CHD)
    c. ligament of knee
    c. node
    c. plane
    c. plane postural
      decompensation
    c. thrombosis
    c. vessel
coronoid fossa of humerus
corpora (*pl. of* corpus)
corporeal
corpse
corpus, gen. corporis, pl. corpora
    c. adiposum
    c. adiposum infrapatellare
    c. cavernosum
    c. claviculae
    c. costae
    c. femoris
    c. fibulae
    c. humeri
    c. ossis femoris
    c. ossis ilii
    c. ossis ischii
    c. ossis metacarpalis
    c. ossis pubis
    c. radii
    regiones corporis
    c. sterni
    c. tali
    c. tibiae
    c. ulna
    c. vertebra
corpuscle
    Meissner c.

pacinian c.
Ruffini c.
corpuscula
corpusculum
corrective force
correlate
psychological c.
correlation
inverse c.
negative c.
positive c.
correspondence
somatic-tropic c.
corresponding
c. channel
c. organ
corrigent
corrugator
corset
lumbar c.
cortex, pl. **cortices**
cerebral c.
premotor c.
c. quercus
cortical
c. adrenal hormone
c. arteries
c. osteitis
c. pathway
corticobulbar pathway
corticospinal pathway
corticosteroid
corticotropin-releasing
c.-r. factor (CRF)
c.-r. hormone
cortisol secretion
corydalis
Corydalis yanhusuo
Corynanthe yohimbe
Corynebacterium diphtheriae
corynine
Cosamin
cosamine
cosmic consciousness
costa, gen. and pl. **costae**
angulus costae
articulatio capitis costae

caput costae
c. cervicalis
collum costae
corpus costae
crista capitis costae
crista colli costae
costae fluctuantes [XI–XII]
costae fluitantes
musculus levator costae
costae spuriae [VII–XII]
sulcus costae
tuberculum costae
costae verae [I–VII]
costal
c. angle
c. arch
c. articulatory technique
c. cartilage
c. diaphragm
c. facet
c. groove
c. notch
c. pit of transverse process
c. process
c. surface
c. surface of scapula
c. tuberosity
costale
os c.
costales
incisurae c.
costalis
arcus c.
cartilago c.
tuberositas c.
costarum
arcus c.
levatores c.
musculi levatores c.
costicartilage
costiform
costmary
costocentral
costocervical arterial trunk
costochondral
c. joint

C

NOTES

costochondral *(continued)*
   c. junction
   c. region
costochondrales
   articulationes c.
costoclavicular
   c. canal
   c. ligament
   c. line
   c. test
costocoracoid
costoinferior
costoscapular
costoscapularis
costosternal
   c. joint
   c. joint of first rib
costosuperior
costotransversaria
   articulatio c.
costotransversarium
   foramen c.
costotransverse
   c. articulation
   c. foramen
   c. joint
   c. ligament
costovertebral
   c. articulation
   c. joint
   c. ligament
costovertebrales
   articulationes c.
costoxiphoid ligament
costus root
cotrimoxazole
cotton
   American upland c.
   common c.
   styptic c.
   upland c.
   wild c.
cottonseed oil
cottonweed
cotunnii
   liquor c.
cotyle
cotylica
   articulatio c.
cotyloid
   c. cavity
   c. joint

   c. ligament
   c. notch
couchgrass, couch grass
cough
   c. activation
   c. root
   whooping c.
coughweed
coughwort
coulomb of charge
coumarin
council
   Alternative Medicine Program
     Advisory C. (AMPAC)
   American Botanical C. (ABC)
   C. on Chiropractic Education
     (CCE)
   C. on Naturopathic Medical
     Education (CNME)
counseling
   health enhancement c.
   lifestyle c.
counselor
   spiritual care c.
count
   blood c.
   complete blood c. (CBC)
   eosinophil c.
counter
   over the c. (OTC)
counteract
counterextension
counterforce
counterirritant effect
counternutation
   sacral c.
counternutational movement
counterstrain
   knee c.
   strain and c.
   c. technique
countertraction
coupled
   c. channel
   c. motion
   c. motion of spine
   c. movement
   c. sidebending
course
   channel c.
   c. of channels
   c. down
   c. up

covering
cow
    c. chervil
    c. clover
    c. face
cowcumber (*var. of* cucumber)
cowherd
cowl muscle
cowslip
    American c.
    Jerusalem c.
cow's milk
coxa
    c. adducta
    c. magna
    c. plana
    c. valga
    c. vara
    c. vara luxans
coxae
    articulatio c.
    malum c.
    musculus triceps c.
    os c.
    retinaculum capsulae
      articularis c.
coxal bone
coxale
    punctum c.
coxalgia
coxarthritis
coxarthrosis
Cox flexion/extension technique
coxitic scoliosis
coxodynia
coxofemoral
coxotuberculosis
CPA
    cumulative phase advancement
CPI
    California Personality Inventory
CPP
    chronic pelvic pain
crab's eye
cramp
    c. bark

menstrual c.
muscular c.
Crampton line
cramp-type pain
crampweed
cranberry
    bog c.
    high c.
    c. juice
    mountain c.
    C. Power
    small c.
    c. whole fruit
cranesbill
    American c.
    spotted c.
    stinking c.
    wild c.
cranial
    c. bone articular mobility
    c. bone embryology
    caudad to c.
    c. concept
    c. diagnosis
    c. manipulation
    c. mechanics
    c. meninges
    c. motion
    c. nerve
    c. nerve entrapment
    c. nerve neuropathy
    c. nerves II–XII
    c. osteopathy
    c. pivot
    c. rhythmic impulse (CRI)
    c. rhythmic impulse amplitude
    c. rhythmic impulse rate
    c. rhythmic impulse rhythm
    c. rhythm impulse (CRI)
    c. somatic dysfunction
    c. strain
    c. suture
    c. technique
    c. therapy
    c. torsion

C

NOTES

craniocarpotarsal
  c. dysplasia
  c. dystrophy
craniocervical junction
craniocleidodysostosis
craniodidymus
cranioelectrical stimulation
craniofacial
  c. angle
  c. dysostosis
  c. somatic dysfunction
craniolacunia
cranio-occipital junction
craniopagus
  c. occipitalis
  c. parasiticus
craniopathy
cranioplasty
  nonoperative c.
craniorrhachischisis
craniosacral
  c. activity
  c. balancing
  c. diagnosis
  c. extension
  c. flexion
  c. manual medicine
  c. massage
  c. mechanism
  c. reciprocal tension membrane
  c. system
  c. technique
  c. therapist
  c. therapy
  c. treatment (CST)
  c. vault (CV)
  c. vault four (CV4)
  c. vault four procedure
  c. vault technique
  c. vault technique, fourth variation
  c. V technique
cranioschisis
craniospinal sensory ganglion
craniostenosis
craniosynostosis
craniotomy
cranium
  osseous c.
crank test
Cran Relief
Cran-Tastic

crataegus
  c. extract
  C. laevigata
  C. monogyna
craterization
cream
  capsaicin c.
  GH3 c.
  Joint and Muscle Relief C.
  L-lysine c.
  tea tree oil c.
  Witch Hazel C.
crease
  digital c.
  digital flexion c.
  elbow c.
  flexion c.
  palmar c.
  patellar c.
  wrist c.
creatine monohydrate
creep
  fascial c.
creeping Charlie
cremasteric
  c. artery
  c. reflex
crena
creosote bush
crepitans
  tenalgia c.
  tenosynovitis c.
crepitant
crepitation
crepitus
  articular c.
  bony c.
crescent
  articular c.
crescentic
cress
  garden c.
crest
  articular c.
  deltoid c.
  external lip of iliac c.
  c. of greater tubercle
  c. of head of rib
  iliac c.
  intermediate line of iliac c.
  intermediate sacral c.
  internal lip of iliac c.
  interosseous c.

intertrochanteric c.
lateral epicondylar c.
lateral supracondylar c.
c. of lesser tubercle
medial epicondylar c.
medial supracondylar c.
median sacral c.
c.'s of nail matrix
c. of neck of rib
obturator c.
occipital c.
sacral c.
c. of scapular spine
supraventricular c.
terminal c.
tibial c.
trochanteric c.
tubercle of iliac c.
unleveling of iliac c.
cretinism
crewel
CRF
corticotropin-releasing factor
CRI
cranial rhythmic impulse
cranial rhythm impulse
CRI amplitude
CRI rate
CRI rhythm
CRI still point
cribriform fascia
cribrosa
fascia c.
cricoid
arytenoidal articular surface
of c.
c. cartilage
cricopharyngeal sphincter muscle
cricothyroidei
pars recta musculi c.
crippled
crispum
Petroselinum c.
crispus
Chondrus c.
Rumex c.
crista, pl. **cristae**

c. capitis costae
c. colli costae
cristae cutis
c. galli
c. iliaca
c. intertrochanterica
c. medialis fibulae
c. musculi supinatoris ulna
c. obturatoria
c. sacralis
c. sacralis intermedia
c. sacralis lateralis
c. sacralis mediana
c. supracondylaris lateralis
c. supracondylaris medialis
c. supraventricularis
c. terminalis
c. tuberculi majoris
c. tuberculi minoris
criteria
ba gang diagnostic c.: yin
and yang, interior and
exterior, deficiency and
excess, cold and heat
diagnostic c.
outcome c.
critical
c. analytic cognition
c. zone of shoulder
crocetin
crochet
main en c.
crocin
crocinic acid
crocus
autumn c.
Crocus sativus
Crohn disease
crossed
c. extensor reflex
c. straight leg raising
c. system
c. tract
crossed-hand thrust technique
cross-fiber friction massage
cross-matching
crossover trial

C

NOTES

cross-patterning of gait
cross-pattern pep walking
cross-section
cross-tolerance
cross-tolerant
crosswort
Crotalaria
croton
    c. oil
    C. tiglium
    c. tincture
crowberry
crow corn
crowfoot
crown
    c. chakra
    c. energy center
    c. of head
crow-soap
CRPS
    complex regional pain syndrome
cruces (*pl. of* crux)
cruciate
    c. eminence
    c. ligament
    c. ligament of the atlas
    c. ligament of leg
    c. ligaments of knee
    c. muscle
cruciatus
    musculus c.
cruciferous vegetable
cruciform
    c. eminence
    c. ligament of atlas
cruor
crura (*pl. of* crus)
crural
    c. diaphragm
    c. fascia
    c. ring
crureus
cruris
    angina c.
    fascia c.
    membrana interossea c.
    musculus biceps flexor c.
crus, pl. **crura**
    lateral c.
    c. laterale
    medial c.
    c. mediale

crush syndrome
crutch palsy
Cruveilhier
    C. joint
    C. ligament
crux, pl. **cruces**
cryoanesthesia
cryotherapy
crypt
    synovial c.
crypta, pl. **cryptae**
cryptenamine
Cryptococcus neoformans
cryptopodia
Cryptotympana atrata
cry reflex
crystal
    c. healing
    red beet c.
crystal-induced arthritis
crystalline
    c. free-form amino acid
    c. niacin
Cs-4
    CordyMax Cs-4
CSA
    Controlled Substance Act
CSF
    cerebrospinal fluid
CST
    craniosacral treatment
CT
    computed tomography
    CT myelogram
CTR Support
CTS
    carpal tunnel syndrome
C-type compensated structural
    scoliosis
cubeb berry
cubital
    c. bone
    c. fossa
    c. joint
    c. lymph node
    c. tunnel syndrome
cubitalis
    fossa c.
cubiti
    articulatio c.
    musculus articularis c.
    rete articulare c.

cubitus
  c. valgus
  c. varus
cuboid
  c. bone
  calcaneal process of c.
  c. pronated medial tubercle
  c. pronation
cuboidal articular surface of calcaneus
cuboidei
  tuberositas ossis c.
cuboideonavicular
  c. joint
  c. ligament
cuboideum
  os c.
cuckoo's meate
cuckoo sorrow
cucullaris muscle
cucumber, cowcumber
  Chinese c.
  sea c.
  squirting c.
  wild c.
  zombie's c.
Cucurbita
  C. maxima
  C. moschata
  C. pepo
cudweed
  marsh c.
cuff
  musculotendinous c.
cuirass respirator
cul-de-sac
  Gruber c.-d.-s.
Culver's
  C. physic
  C. root
cumaru
cumin
  sweet c.
cumin-coriander-fennel tea
Cuminum cymium
cumulative
  c. action

  c. effect
  c. phase advancement (CPA)
  c. trauma disorder
cun
  horizontal c.
  lateral c.
  c. measurement
  c. position
cuneate nucleus
cuneiform
  c. bone
  c. bone dysfunction
  c. cartilage
  depression of c.
  medial c.
cuneiforme
  tuberculum c.
cuneocuboid
  c. joint
  c. ligament
cuneometatarsal joint
cuneonavicular
  c. articulation
  c. joint
  c. ligament
cuneonavicularis
  articulatio c.
cuneoscaphoid
cunometer
cup
  Diogenes c.
  fairy c.
  c. of palm
cupana
  Paullinia c.
cupola
cupping
cupula, pl. **cupulae**
Curaco aloe
curanderismo
curare
curarization
Curcuma
  C. domestica
  C. longa
  C. xanthorrhiza
curcumin

C

NOTES

curer
curious meridian
curl
    neck flexion c.
    reverse torso c.
    torso c.
    c. up
curled dock
curling up
curl-up
    retraining with c.-u.
curly dock
current
    c. density
    electrical c.
    high-voltage pulsed c.
    c. intensity
    interferential c.
    low-frequency pulsed c.
    low-intensity direct c.
    microampere c.
    peak c.
    resultant c. (I)
current/voltage intensity
curvatura
curvature
    angular c.
    anterior c.
    backward c.
    lateral c.
    posterior c.
    spinal c.
curve
    active length-tension c.
    dose-response c.
    force-velocity c.
    lateral pelvic tilt functional c.
    lordotic c.
    muscle c.
    passive length-tension c.
    pelvic tilt functional c.
    phase-response c. (PRC)
    receiver operating
      characteristic c.
    sagittal c.
    sidebending rotational c.
    spinal c.
    stress-strain c.
    tension c.
    vertebral column c.
curvus
    carpus c.
Cuscuta chinensis

Cushing
    C. disease
    C. syndrome
cushion
    Samadhi c.
cusp
cuspidata
    Taxus c.
cuspis
cutanea-organ reflex point
cutaneomucosal
cutaneous
    c. blister
    c. eruption
    c. erythema
    c. innervation
    c. mechanoreceptor
    c. muscle
    c. nervous system
    c. sensation
    c. soft tissue
    c. threshold
    c. vasodilatation
cutaneus
    musculus c.
cutch
cuticle
cuticula
cutis
    cristae c.
CV
    craniosacral vault
      CV technique
CV4
    craniosacral vault four
      CV4 procedure
      CV4 technique
cv
    conceptional vessel
C1–C7 vertebrae
Cyamopsis tetragonoloba
cyanosis
cyanus
    Centaurea c.
cyclarthrodial
cyclarthrosis
cycle
    c.'s of channels
    23-day c.
    28-day c.
    33-day c.
    walk c.
    walking c.

cyclic 3′,5′ adenosine
  monophosphate (cAMP)
cyclosporin A, cyclosporine
Cydonia
  C. japonica
  C. lagenaria
  C. vulgaris
cylinder
cylindroid aneurysm
cymatics
cymatic therapy
Cymbopogon
  C. citratus
  C. flexuosus
cymium
  Cuminum c.
Cynara cardunculus
cynocephaly
Cynoglossum officinale
cyparissias
  Euphorbia c.
Cyperus rotundus
cypress
  Belvedere c.
Cypripedium calceoulus
Cyriax manipulation
cyristicin
cyst
  aneurysmal bone c.
  Baker c.
  bone c.
  myxoid c.
  osseous hydatid c.
  popliteal c.
  simple bone c.

  solitary bone c.
  synovial c.
  traumatic bone c.
  unicameral bone c.
cystein
  S-allyl c.
  S-ethyl c.
  S-propyl c.
cysteine
cystica
  osteitis fibrosa c.
  osteitis tuberculosa multiplex c.
  spina bifida c.
cystic fibrosis
cystine
cystis, pl. cystides
cystitis
  interstitial c.
  radiation-induced interstitial c.
Cystone
cystous
cytisine
Cytisus scoparius
cytochrome P$_{450}$
cytokine
cytologic
  c. examination
  c. specimen
cytomegalovirus (CMV)
  human c.
Cytopure
cytosis
cytotoxicity
cytotoxic T-cell
Cytozyme-F

C

NOTES

D
direct treatment
D3
Cadmium sulfuricum D.
da
d. bu yin wan
d. bu yin wen
d. cheng qi
d. cheng qi tang
d. ching qi tang
d. chi san
d. ding feng zhu
d. ling point
d. qing ye
d. suan
dabao
sp 21 d.
d'accoucheur
main d.
dachangshu
d. point
ub 25 d.
dactyl
dactylalgia
dactylocampsis
dactylocampsodynia
dactylodynia
dactylogryposis
dactylomegaly
dactylus
dadun
liv 1 d.
daffodil
daffydown-dilly
dagga
dagger flower
daheng
sp 15 d.
Dahuang Liujingao
dahurica
Cimicifuga d.
daidzein
daily
D. Detox I
D. Detox II
D. Hassles Scale
D. Stress Inventory
Wellness Multiple Max D.
daimai
gb 26 d.

dai mai
daisy
common d.
ewe d.
midsummer d.
mountain d.
Dakin solution
daling
pe 7 d.
dalmatian
Dalrymple
D. pump
D. technique
D. treatment
damage
free radical d.
ligamentous d.
damiana
d. leaf
Mexican d.
d. root
damp
d. cold in the spleen
d. disturbance
d. heat
d. heat in the liver and
gallbladder
d. heat in the spleen
pathogenic d.
dan
d. gui xhao yao tang
huo lou xiao ling d.
d. shen
d. yu tan rao
danazol
dance
Sun D.
d. therapist
d. therapy
dancing
d. mushroom
square d.
dandelion
d. extract
d. greens
d. root
dandruff
danewort
dang
d. gui

D

dang *(continued)*
    d. gui si ni tang
    d. shen
dangerous point
danger thought
danshu
    ub 19 d.
Dantian reservoir
dao
    chin d.
d'arco
    pau d.
dark female force
darshanam
d'Arsonval galvanometer
dartos fascia
das
dashu
    ub 11 d.
da-suan
Datura
    D. arborea
    D. ferox
    D. metel
    D. sanguinea
    D. stramonium
Daubenton line
daughter cell
day
    four times a d. (q.i.d.)
    three times a d. (t.i.d.)
    twice a d. (b.i.d.)
daying
    st 5 d.
day's eye
Dayto Himbin
dazhong
    ki 4 d.
dazhui
    du 14 d.
DC
    doctor of chiropractic
DDS-Acidophilus
de
    D. Kleyn test
    d. qi
    d. qi needling sensation
    d. qi sensation
    d. Quervain disease
    d. Quervain tenosynovitis
dead arm syndrome
deadly nightshade

death
    brain d.
    cerebral d.
    sudden cardiac d. (SCD)
    voodoo d.
debility
debridement
    wound d.
debris
    particulate wear d.
    toxic d.
debulking
    tumor d.
decandra
    Phytolacca decandra
declination
    angle of d.
    pelvic d.
    sacral base d.
decoction
    Ass-Hide Gelatin D.
    baked licorice d.
    d. enema
    Four Gentlemen D.
    herbal d.
    Minor Construct the
      Middle D.
    Polyporus D.
    Regulate the Middle D.
    Rock on Tai Mountain D.
    White Tiger D.
decompensated posture
decompensation
    coronary plane postural d.
    horizontal plane postural d.
    postural d.
    sagittal plane postural d.
decompression
    condylar d.
    spinal d.
decongest
decongestant
decongestion
decontamination
decreased mobility
decubitus
    d. film
    d. ulcer
decussata
    Canscora d.
deep
    d. branch
    d. cervical fascia

d. chi
d. chi builder
d. fascia
d. fascia of arm
d. fascia of forearm
d. fascia of leg
d. fascia of neck
d. fascia of thigh
d. flexor muscle of finger
d. head of flexor pollicis brevis
d. infrapatellar bursa
d. lamina
d. lateral cervical lymph node
d. layer
d. muscles of back
d. neck flexor
d. needling
d. nerve sensation
d. parasympathetic response
d. part of flexor retinaculum
d. part of masseter muscle
d. posterior sacrococcygeal ligament
d. pressure
d. relaxation
d. tendon reflex
d. tissue massage technique
d. tissue sculpting
d. touch
d. transverse metacarpal ligament
d. transverse metatarsal ligament
d. transverse perineal muscle

deepening of breath
deepithelialized rectus abdominis muscle
deep-level looseness
deep-water ocean fish
deer
    musk d.
deerberry
deernut
defacilitation
defect
    atrial septal d.

congenital neural-tube d.
fibrous cortical d.
metaphysial fibrous cortical d.
neural tube d.
septal d.
defense
    Bone D.
    d. mechanism
    Pepper D.
    Urban Air D.
defensive qi
deferens
    vas d.
deficiency
    d. condition
    copper d.
    d. disturbance
    folate d.
    d. of the gallbladder and stagnation of phlegm
    G6PD d.
    d. of heart blood
    d. of heart qi
    d. of heart yang
    d. of heart yin
    insulin d.
    jing d.
    d. of kidney jing
    d. of kidney qi
    d. of kidney yang
    kidney yang d.
    d. of kidney yin
    d. of liver blood
    liver yin d.
    d. of liver yin
    d. lung
    d. of lung qi
    d. of lung yin
    magnesium d.
    middle jiao d.
    primary carnitine d.
    proximal femoral focal d.
    secondary d.
    spleen d.
    d. of spleen qi
    d. of spleen yang
    d. of the stomach yin

D

NOTES

deficiency *(continued)*
    d. symptom
    d. syndrome
    thiamine d.
    vision d.
    visual d.
    vitamin B_{12} d.
    yang d.
    yin d.
    zhong d.
deficiency-induced disturbance
deficiency-type
    d.-t. condition
    d.-t. disharmony
    d.-t. disturbance
deficient
    d. energy
    G6PD d.
    d. organ
    d. wound healing
    yin d.
deficit
    chronic postural d.
    neurologic d.
    photocurrent d.
definition
    segmental d.
definitive callus
deformans
    arthritis d.
    dystonia musculorum d.
    hyperostosis corticalis d.
    osteitis d.
    osteochondrodystrophia d.
    spondylitis d.
deformation
    elastic d.
    plastic d.
deformity
    batwing d.
    boutonnière d.
    calcaneal valgus d.
    calcaneal varus d.
    contracture d.
    Erlenmeyer flask d.
    gunstock d.
    lobster-claw d.
    reduction d.
    silver-fork d.
    swan neck d.
    torsional d.
    valgus d.
    varus d.

degeneration
    cervical d.
    fascicular d.
    gray d.
    macular d.
    retrograde d.
degenerative
    d. arthritis
    d. disk disease
    d. joint disease
    d. vessel disease
degloving injury
deglycyrrhizinated licorice (DGL)
dehydroepiandrosterone (DHEA)
    d. sulfate (DHEA-S)
dehydrogenase
    glucose-6-phosphate d. (G6PD, G-6-PD)
dehydrotestosterone (DHT)
deionized water
delayed
    d. biofeedback
    developmentally d.
delicate organ
delight
    queen's d.
delirium
delivery
    breech d.
    vaginal d.
delta mesoscapulae
delta-9-tetrahydrocannabinol (THC)
deltoid
    d. branch
    d. crest
    d. eminence
    d. impression
    d. ligament
    d. muscle
    d. region
    d. tuberosity of humerus
deltoidea
    regio d.
deltoideopectoral
    d. triangle
    d. trigone
deltoideopectorale
    trigonum d.
deltoideus
    musculus d.
demand cardiac pacemaker

dementia
    Alzheimer d.
    multi-infarct d.
Demerol
demifacet
demigauntlet bandage
demineralization
demineralized water
demipenniform
Demosvelte-N
demulcent
Dendrobrium Monilforme Night
  Sight Pills
denervate
denervation
denitrogenation
dens
    apical ligament of d.
    facet of atlas for d.
    posterior articular surface of d.
dense
    d. connective tissue
    d. dispersed
    d. fascia
density
    bone d.
    capillary d.
    current d.
dental
    d. anesthesia
    d. caries
    d. equilibration
    d. hygiene
    d. hypnosis
    d. kinesiology
    d. phobia
    d. socket
dentate fracture
dentifrice
Dent-Zel-Ite Toothache Relief Drops
Denucé ligament
denudation
deossification
deoxyribonucleic acid (DNA)
depersonalization syndrome
depigmentation

depletion
    energy d.
depolarizing block
deposition
deprenyl
depression
    bone marrow d.
    Brief Screen for D.
    d. of cuneiform
    Hamilton Rating Scale for D.
    mental d.
    situational d.
    stress-induced d.
depressive disorder
depth of needle insertion
depurative
deputy ingredient
derangement
    intervertebral d.
    minor intervertebral d.
derivative
    anthranoid d.
    shark d.
Dermaide Aloe
Derma-Klear
dermal
    d. papillae
    d. sinus
Dermamed
dermatica
    zona d.
dermatitis
    allergic contact d.
    atopic d.
    contact d.
    exfoliative d.
    poison plant d.
    seborrheic d.
    toxicodendron d.
dermatomal
    d. level
    d. pattern
dermatome
    lower extremity d.
    lumbar d.
    d. mapping
    thoracic d.

D

NOTES

dermatomyositis
dermis
    papillae d.
dermopathy
    kava d.
    pellagroid d.
dermoskeleton
derotation
descendens cervicalis
descending
    d. brainstem pathway
    d. branch
    d. cortical pathway
    d. neural pathway
    d. serotonin-DLT inhibitory
        system
descriptive myology
descurrens
    Libocedrus d.
desensitization
    allergy d.
    systematic d.
    d. technique
desert
    lily of the d.
    d. tea
desiccated liver
desiccation
    pyramidal d.
desmitis
desmocranium
desmology
desmoplasia
detector
    electrical resistance d.
detorsion
    law of d.
detox
    D. Blend Bulk Herbs
    Daily D. I
    Daily D. II
    D. Pak
detoxification
    acupuncture d.
    d. enzyme
    heat stress d.
    liver d.
    d. procedure
    d. therapy
detoxify
Detoxygen

detrusor
    d. muscle
    d. pressure
deva
development
    anomalous d.
developmental hip dysplasia
developmentally delayed
deviation
    posterior postural d.
    radial d.
    radial-ulnar d.
    ulnar d.
device
    diode laser d.
    electroacupuncture d.
    electromagnetic microcurrent d.
    foot orthotic d.
    Libbe lower bowel
        evacuation d.
    Metrecom d.
    MicroStim 100 TENS d.
    muscle and neurological
        stimulation electrotherapy d.
    orthotic d.
    pneumatic d.
    probe d.
    restraining orthopedic d.
    TENS d.
devil's
    d. claw
    d. claw capsule
    d. claw secondary root
    D. Claw Vegicaps
    d. fuge
    d. plague
    d. scourge
    d. shrub
    d. trumpet
devil's-apple
devil's-bit
devil weed
dewberry
    swamp d.
dewcup
dew plant
dexter
    ductus thoracicus d.
dextrad
dextri
    tuberculum intervenosum
        atrii d.
d-gamma tocopherol

DGL
deglycyrrhizinated licorice
DGLA
dihomogammalinolenic acid
d-glucosamine
DHA
docosahexaenoic acid
Neuromins DHA
dhatu agni
DHEA
dehydroepiandrosterone
DHEA Men's Formula
DHEA therapy
DHEA with Antioxidants
DHEA with Bioperine
DHEA-S
dehydroepiandrosterone sulfate
DHGA
dihomogammalinolenic acid
DHT
dehydrotestosterone
diabetes
adult-onset d.
brittle d.
diabetic
d. arthropathy
d. neuropathy
D. Nutrition RX
diaclasis
Diacure
diadochokinesia, diadochocinesia
diadochokinetic
diagnosis (dx)
cervical spine d.
cranial d.
craniosacral d.
false-negative d.
false-positive d.
hand d.
holistic nursing d.
palpatory d.
pathologic d.
pulse d.
remote d.
segmental d.
structural d.
tongue d.

traditional Chinese d.
traditional pulse d.
Western d.
diagnostic
d. anesthesia
d. block
d. criteria
d. identification
d. injection
d. joint block
d. mode
d. palpation
d. procedure
d. reading
d. sensitivity
d. specificity
D. and Statistical Manual of
Mental Disorders, Fourth
Edition (DSM-IV)
d. triad
diagnostician
diagonal
d. axis
d. conjugate diameter
d. hip sink
d. section
dialectic
d. opposite
d. pattern
dialogue
d. technique
therapeutic imagery and d.
dialysis
renal d.
diameter
diagonal conjugate d.
external conjugate d.
d. obliqua
oblique d.
d. transversa
transverse d.
Diamond-Herpanacine Associates
diane
pas d.
diaphoresis
diaphoretic

NOTES

diaphragm
  Bucky d.
  costal d.
  crural d.
  d. embryology
  d. innervation
  myofascial technique for
    pelvic d.
  pelvic d.
  posterior d.
  release of d.
  respiratory d.
  d. sellae
  sternal part of d.
  thoracoabdominal d.
  three d.'s
  urogenital d.
diaphragma sellae
diaphragmatic
  d. breathing
  d. release
diaphragmatis
  pars sternalis d.
  trigonum lumbocostale d.
diaphysial, diaphyseal
  d. center
  d. dysplasia
diaphysis
diaplasis
diaplastic
Diapulse
Diarcalm
Dia-Relief
Diarid
diarrhea
  antibiotic-induced d.
  cock's crow d.
  osmotic d.
  secretory d.
  toxigenic d.
diarthric
diarthrodial
  d. cartilage
  d. joint
diarthrosis
diarticular
diary
  headache d.
  symptom d.
diastema
diastematocrania

diastolic
  d. blood pressure
  d. hypertension
diastrophic dwarfism
diathesis
  bleeding d.
  hemorrhagic d.
dibenzofuran
DIC
  disseminated intravascular
    coagulopathy
dicang
  st 4 d.
dichromate
  potassium d.
  sodium d.
  d. toxicity
diclofenac
Dictamnus albus
didactylism
die
  bis in d. (b.i.d.)
  mother's d.
  quater in d. (q.i.d.)
  ter in d. (t.i.d.)
diet
  elimination d.
  exclusion d.
  Feingold d.
  food elimination d.
  Gerson d.
  gluten-free vegan d.
  MacDougall d.
  macrobiotic d.
  Moerman anticancer d.
  natural foods d.
  Pritikin d.
  rotation d.
  d. therapy
  vegan d.
  whole-food d.
  Zen macrobiotic d.
dietary
  d. advice
  d. manipulation
  d. supplement
dietetic consultation
Di Ferrante syndrome
differential spinal anesthesia
differentiate
differentiation
difficult movement

diffuse
  d. aneurysm
  d. esophageal spasm
  d. idiopathic skeletal
    hyperostosis
  d. noxious inhibitory control
    (DNIC)
  d. pain
  d. symptom
diffuser
  Aroma-Stream D.
  aromatherapy d.
  Ultra Scent D.
diffusible stimulant
digastric muscle
Digesta-Lac
digestion
digestive enzyme
Digestozym
digit
  bones of d.'s
  ventral surface of d.
digital
  d. collateral artery
  d. crease
  d. flexion crease
  d. fossa
  d. furrow
  d. joint
digitalis
  d. cardioglycoside
  d. glycoside
Digitalis purpurea
digitation
digiti
  musculus extensor minimi d.
  musculus opponens minimi d.
digitorum
  connexus intertendinei musculi
    extensoris d.
  intertendinous connections of
    extensor d.
  d. longus muscle
  musculus extensor d.
  musculus extensor brevis d.
  musculus extensor longus d.

  musculus flexor brevis d.
  musculus flexor longus d.
  ossa d.
digitus
  d. anularis
  d. auricularis
  d. manus
  d. manus medius
  d. manus minimus
  d. manus primus
  d. manus quintus [V]
  d. manus secundus [II]
  d. manus tertius [III]
  d. pedis
  d. valgus
  d. varus
digoxin
dihe
**dihomogammalinolenic acid (DGLA,
  DHGA)**
dihydrochloride
  L-lysine d.
diji
dilatator
dilated cardiomyopathy
dilator
dill seed
dillweed
diltiazem
dilution
  centesimal d. (C)
  potentization by d.
  serial-agitated d. (SAD)
dimba
dimelia
dimenhydrinate
dimension
dimethyl
  d. fumarate
  d. sulfide (DMS)
  d. sulfoxide (DMSO)
dimethylaminoethanol
N,N-**dimethylglycine (DMG)**
  DMG
dimple
  coccygeal d.

D

NOTES

dingchuan
    Ex-B 17 d.
dinitrochlorobenzene (DNCB)
dinucleotide
    nicotinamide adenine d.
    (NADH)
diode laser device
Diogenes cup
diogenis
    poculum d.
dioica
    Urtica d.
Dionaea muscipula
diorthosis
Dioscorea
    D. floribunda
    D. opposita
    D. paniculata
    D. villosa
diosgenin
Diosma betulina
diosmin
dioxide
    inorganic germanium d.
Dioxychlor
diphenylhydantoin
diphtheriae
    Corynebacterium d.
diploë
diploica
    vena d.
diploic vein
diplomyelia
diploneural
diplopodia
dipodia
dipping
    snuff d.
diprosopus
dipsogen
Dipteryx odorata
dipus
    sympus d.
dipygus
DIR
    direct treatment
direct
    d. action technique
    d. barrier
    d. cranial molding technique
    d. energy
    d. hit
    d. infrared radiation

d. method
d. method joint mobilization
d. method technique
d. motion technique
d. osteopathic manipulative
    technique
d. suggestion
d. technique
d. treatment (D, DIR)
directed healing
direction
    anterior d.
    backward d.
    caudal d.
    downward d.
    lateral d.
    medial d.
    posterior d.
    proximal d.
    ventral d.
dirty
    d. green aura
    d. half dozen
disappearing bone disease
disarticulated
disarticulation
disc (*var. of* disk)
disci (*pl. of* discus)
disciform
discitis
discogenic
    d. pain syndrome
    d. radiculopathy
discogram
discography
discoid
discomfort
    gastrointestinal d.
discontinuation test
discopathy
    traumatic cervical d.
discrepancy
    leg length d.
discrimination
discus, pl. disci
    d. articularis
    d. articularis acromioclavicularis
    d. articularis radioulnaris
        distalis
    d. articularis sternoclavicularis
    d. interpubicus
    d. intervertebralis

disease
  Addison d.
  Alzheimer d.
  autoimmune d.
  calcium pyrophosphate
    deposition d.
  cardiovascular d.
  celiac d.
  cement d.
  chronic obstructive
    pulmonary d. (COPD)
  collagen-vascular d.
  connective tissue d.
  coronary artery d. (CAD)
  coronary heart d. (CHD)
  Crohn d.
  Cushing d.
  degenerative disk d.
  degenerative joint d.
  degenerative vessel d.
  de Quervain d.
  disappearing bone d.
  disk d.
  diverticular d.
  fibrocystic breast d.
  fishskin d.
  genetotrophic d.
  Hodgkin d.
  hypokinetic d.
  inflammatory bowel d. (IBD)
  inflammatory joint d.
  ischemic heart d.
  Jüngling d.
  Kashin-Bek d.
  Legg-Calvé-Perthes d.
  marble bone d.
  metabolic bone d.
  metastatic bone d.
  neoplastic d.
  neurological d.
  Newcastle d.
  Ollier d.
  organic d.
  Osgood-Schlatter d.
  Paget d.
  Parkinson d.
  pearl-worker's d.

  peptic ulcer d.
  peripheral arterial occlusive d.
    (PAOD)
  peripheral occlusive arterial d.
    (POAD)
  peripheral vascular d.
  primary inflammatory d.
  primary joint d.
  primary malignant bone d.
  quiet hip d.
  Raynaud d.
  rheumatoid d.
  secondary inflammatory d.
  senile hip d.
  sexually transmitted d. (STD)
  shao yang d.
  sickle cell d.
  Trevor d.
  tryptophan-associated
    eosinophilic connective
    tissue d.
  zygapophysial joint
    degenerative d.
diseased
  d. area
  d. region
disengagement technique
dishabituation
disharmony
  deficiency-type d.
  pattern of d.
  d. of yin and yang
dish face
disimpaction
disinfectant
  complete d.
  incomplete d.
disk, disc
  acromioclavicular d.
  anulus fibrosus of
    intervertebral d.
  articular d.
  Bronhillor Natural Source
    Cough Candies &
    Throat D.'s
  cervical d.

D

NOTES

disk *(continued)*
 cervical degeneration of
  intervertebral d.
 d. disease
 herniated d.
 herniated intervertebral d.
 d. herniation
 interpubic d.
 intervertebral d.
 lumbar d.
 Merkel d.
 d. pathology
 protruded d.
 radioulnar d.
 ruptured d.
 sacrococcygeal d.
 d. sequestration
 d. space
 sternoclavicular d.
 d. syndrome
 thoracic d.
diskitis
diskogram
diskography
dislocate
dislocatio erecta
dislocation
 d. of articular processes
 closed d.
 compound d.
 fracture d.
 d. fracture
 hip d.
 open d.
 perilunar d.
 shoulder d.
 simple d.
dismember
dismutase
 superoxide d. (SOD)
disodium
 edetate d.
disorder
 acute d.
 attention deficit d. (ADD)
 attention deficit
  hyperactivity d. (ADHD)
 autonomic dysregulation d.
 cardiovascular d.
 circadian rhythm sleep d.
 congenital d.
 cumulative trauma d.
 depressive d.

 Diagnostic and Statistical
  Manual of Mental D.'s,
  Fourth Edition (DSM-IV)
 dissociative d.
 endocrine d.
 enterometabolic d.
 equilibrium d.
 eye d.
 functional d.
 gastroenterological d.
 genetic d.
 gynecological d.
 hip joint d.
 immune dysregulation d.
 locomotor d.
 menstrual d.
 muscle d.
 neurological d.
 neuromuscular d.
 obsessive-compulsive d. (OCD)
 panic d.
 posttraumatic stress d. (PTSD)
 premenstrual dysphoric d.
 psychosomatic d.
 psychosomatic heart d.
 repetitive strain d.
 repetitive stress d.
 respiratory d.
 schizoaffective d.
 seasonal affective d. (SAD)
 d. of the sense organs
 simple d.
 skin d.
 stress d.
 swallowing d.
 thyroid d.
 unilateral d.
 urological d.
disorientation
 body d.
dispersed
 dense d.
dispersing method
dispersion
disposable
 d. acupuncture needle
 d. needle
disposition
 planetary d.
disproportionate dwarfism
disregulation
dissecans
 osteochondritis d.

dissection
    arterial d.
    carotid artery d.
    vertebral artery d.
disseminata
    osteitis fibrosa d.
disseminated intravascular coagulopathy (DIC)
dissociation
dissociative disorder
dissymmetry
distachya
    Ephedra d.
distad
distal
    d. ba xie point
    d. interphalangeal joint
    d. nonsegmental needling
    d. point
    d. radioulnar articulation
    d. radioulnar joint
    d. radioulnar joint dysfunction
    d. tibiofibular articulation
    d. tibiofibular joint
    d. tibiofibular joint dysfunction
distalis
    articulatio radioulnaris d.
    discus articularis radioulnaris d.
distant healing
distention
    abdominal d.
    gaseous d.
    rectal d.
    d. of visceral peritoneum
distinct meridian
distortion
distraction
    joint d.
    mental d.
    d. osteogenesis
distributing artery
distribution
    energy d.
    median nerve d.
    myotomal d.
    segmental d.
    weight d.

disturbance
    chi d.
    cold d.
    damp d.
    deficiency d.
    deficiency-induced d.
    deficiency-type d.
    energy d.
    energy field d.
    excess d.
    excess-type d.
    functional d.
    han d.
    heat d.
    heat-type d.
    internal d.
    li d.
    liver d.
    pathogenic internal wind d.
    phlegm d.
    re d.
    shi d.
    sleep d.
    xu d.
    xu-type d.
    yin-type d.
disulfram
diterpene ester
Diuplex
diuresis
diuretic
Diurite
Diurnal
diurnal therapy
divaricata
    Larrea d.
    Ledebouriella d.
diversified technique
diversilobum
    Toxicodendron d.
diverticular disease
diverticulitis
diverticulosis coli
diverticulum
    Nuck d.
Divinal-Bohnen

D

NOTES

divination
    medical d.
divine will
division
    posterior primary d.
divot
dizziness
DL-carnitine
DL-phenylalanine
DLT
    dorsolateral tract
DMG (*N,N*-dimethylglycine)
    N,N-dimethylglycine
    Aangamik DMG
DMS
    dimethyl sulfide
DMSO
    dimethyl sulfoxide
DNA
    deoxyribonucleic acid
    rapid amplification of
        polymorphic DNA (RAPD)
DNCB
    dinitrochlorobenzene
DNIC
    diffuse noxious inhibitory control
DO
    doctor of osteopathy
do
    jin shin d.
dock
    bitter d.
    curled d.
    curly d.
    elf d.
    narrow d.
    patience d.
    sour d.
    velvet d.
    yellow d.
docosahexaenoic acid (DHA)
docosenoic acid
doctor
    Chinese d.
    d. of chiropractic (DC)
    naturopathic d. (ND, NMD)
    d. of Oriental medicine
        (DOM)
    d. of osteopathy (DO)
    witch d.
doctrine of similars
dodecandra
    Phytolacca d.

DOE
    dyspnea on exertion
dog
    d. cloves
    d. grass
    d. rose fruit
    d. standard
dogwood
    Jamaican d.
    poison d.
    West Indian d.
doing therapy
dolendi
    locus d.
dolichocephalic
dolichocephaly
dolichopellic
doll
    wax d.
dolloff
doll's eye
dolomite
Dolorac
dolorimeter
dolorosa
    anesthesia d.
dolorosus
    hallux d.
DOM
    doctor of Oriental medicine
domestica
    Curcuma d.
dominant
    d. eye
    d. eye test
    right-eye d.
dong
    gan feng nei d.
    d. quai
    d. quai capsule
    d. quai fluid extract
dopa decarboxylase inhibitor
dopamine
Doppler study
dorsa (*pl. of* dorsum)
dorsabdominal
dorsad
dorsal
    d. branch
    d. calcaneocuboid ligament
    d. carpal ligament
    d. carpal network
    d. carpometacarpal ligament

d. cuboideonavicular ligament
d. cuneocuboid ligament
d. cuneonavicular ligament
d. fascia of foot
d. fascia of hand
d. forearm
d. hood
d. horn
d. interossei interosseous
  muscles of foot
d. interossei interosseous
  muscles of hand
d. interosseous muscle
d. mesentery of esophagus
d. metacarpal ligament
d. metatarsal ligament
d. muscle
d. to plantar glide
d. radiocarpal ligament
d. root
d. root ganglion
d. sacrococcygeal muscle
d. sacrococcygeus muscle
d. sacroiliac ligament
d. spine
d. surface
d. surface of digit of foot
d. surface of digit of hand
d. surface of sacrum
d. surface of scapula
d. talonavicular bone
d. tilt
d. tubercle of radius
d. vertebra
dorsale
  rete carpale d.
dorsales
  regiones d.
dorsalgia
dorsalis
  facies d.
  musculus sacrococcygeus d.
  spina d.
dorsi
  latissimus d.
  musculi d.
  musculus iliocostalis d.

musculus latissimus d.
musculus longissimus d.
musculus semispinalis d.
musculus spinalis d.
dorsiflexed
  talus d.
dorsiflexion
  restricted d.
dorsiscapular
dorsispinal
dorsocephalad
dorsodynia
dorsolateral
  d. pathway
  d. tract (DLT)
dorsolumbar
dorsoventrad
dorsum, pl. **dorsa**
  d. of foot
  d. of hand
  d. manus
  d. pedis
  d. scapulae
  d. sellae
dosage
  soft tissue procedure d.
dose
  effective d.
  lethal d.
  minimal lethal d.
  supraphysiologic d.
dose-response curve
dosha
  d. balance
  d. imbalance
  kapha d.
  pitta d.
  vata d.
double
  d. flap amputation
  d. fracture
double-blind
  d.-b. study
double-webbed needle
douche
  acidophilus d.
  yogurt d.

D

NOTES

doughy tissue texture abnormality
douglasii
   Cicuta d.
doulua
dove's foot
dowel graft
down
   course d.
   D. syndrome
downward
   d. direction
   injury above d.
dowsing
doxylamine
dozen
   dirty half d.
D-phenylalanine
Dr.
   Dr. Brown's Cel-Ray
   Dr. John R. Christopher
    Formula
Dracontium
   D. asperum
   D. foetidum
dracunculus
   Artemisia d.
drag
   skin d.
dragon
   d. flower
   green d.
   gum d.
dragonhead needle
dragon's mugwort
drainage
   Galbreath mandibular d.
   infusion-aspiration d.
   lymphatic d.
   mandibular d.
   nasal d.
   d. pathway
   rectal lymphatic d.
   venous d.
   venous sinus d.
draining method
Dramamine
drawer
   d. sign
   d. test
   d. test of knee
drawing
   mandala d.
   pain d.

dream
   Rice D.
drelip
dressing
   fixed d.
   gauze d.
   transparent d.
dribbling
   urinary d.
dried
   d. cell
   d. flower
   d. herb
   d. medicinal
   d. rattlesnake meat
   d. sweet clover
   d. venom
drink
   black d.
   green d.
drip
   intravenous d.
drip-suck irrigation
dromotropic
drop (gt)
   d. arm test
   d. finger
   d. foot
   d. test of hip
drop-off sign
drops (gtt)
   beech cough d.
   Cadmium sulfuricum D3 d.
   Concentrace trace mineral d.
   Dent-Zel-Ite Toothache
    Relief D.
   Traumeel oral d.
dropwort
drosera
dross
   hive d.
drug
   addictive d.
   antiinflammatory d.
   antiretroviral d.
   d. interaction
   investigational new d. (IND)
   nonsteroidal antiinflammatory d.
    (NSAID)
   orphan d.
   psychotropic d.
   schedule I d.
drug-herb interaction

drug-induced
   d.-i. hepatitis
   d.-i. hypertension
dry
   d. amputation
   Aveeno D.
   d. energy
   d. heat
   d. mouth
   d. needling
   d. pasta
   d. socket
   d. stool
   d. synovitis
dry-kuei
Dryopteris filix-mas
DSM-IV
   Diagnostic and Statistical Manual of
   Mental Disorders, Fourth Edition
du
   du mai channel
   d. 20 baihui
   d. 1 changqiang
   d. 14 dazhui
   d. 16 fengfu
   d. huo ji sheng wan
   d. 6 jizhong
   d. jung
   d. 4 mingmen
   d. 17 naohu
   d. 26 renzhong
   d. 11 shendao
   d. 24 shenting
   d. 25 suliao
   d. 13 taodao
   d. 15 yamen
   d. 2 yaoshu
   d. 3 yaoyangguan
duan
   xu d.
dubi
   st 35 d.
Ducase
duct
   abdominal part of thoracic d.

arch of thoracic d.
biliary d.
cervical part of thoracic d.
hemithoracic d.
Pecquet d.
subclavian d.
thoracic d.
ductal
duction
   resistive d.
ductular
ductule
ductulus
ductus
   d. hemithoracicus
   d. thoracicus
   d. thoracicus dexter
dulcamara
   Solanum d.
dull pain
d'ulmaire
   fleur d.
dulse
dung
   mai men d.
duodenal ulcer
duodenum
duplicitas
   d. anterior
   d. posterior
Dupré muscle
Dupuytren
   D. canal
   D. contracture
   D. fascia
dura
   external layer of d.
   d. layer
   d. layer of meninges
   d. mater
   d. mater mobility
   d. mater of spinal cord
   d. mater spinalis
dural
   d. blood flow

NOTES

dural *(continued)*
 d. circulation
 d. innervation
 d. layer
 d. membrane
 d. restriction
 d. venous sinus
duralumin
duration
 pulse d.
dushu
 ub 16 d.
Dutch
 D. myrtle
 D. rush
 D. tonka bean
dwarf
 d. elder
 d. palm
dwarfism
 camptomelic d.
 diastrophic d.
 disproportionate d.
 proportionate d.
dx
 diagnosis
D-xylose test
dye
 Indian d.
dyer's
 D. broom
 d. madder
 d. saffron
dynamic
 d. balance
 d. exercise
 d. friction
 d. functional principle
 d. functional procedure
 d. functional technique
 d. mechanoreceptor
 d. motion
 d. phasic muscle
 d. posture
 d. potential
 d. reciprocal tension
 d. splint
 d. study
 symptom d.
 d. tension
dynamical
 d. energy
 d. energy system

dynamics
dynamism
dynamogenesis
dynamograph
dynamometer
dynamoscope
dynamoscopy
Dynatronics
 D. Model 1650
 D. Model 1620 laser
dynorphin kappa antagonist
dysarthrosis
dysbasia
 d. angiosclerotica
 d. lordotica progressiva
dyscephalia
dyscephaly
dyschondroplasia with hemangiomas
dyschondrosteosis
dysdiadochokinesia
dysentery
 amebic d.
 bacillary d.
dysergia
dyserythropoiesis
dysfibrinogenemia
dysfunction
 acromioclavicular joint d.
 acute somatic d.
 ankle and foot somatic d.
 autonomic nervous system d.
 axillary fold d.
 biomechanical d.
 calcaneocuboid joint d.
 cephalad pubic d.
 chronic d.
 chronic recurrent anteriorly
  nutated sacroiliac d.
 chronic somatic d.
 combined vertebral and rib d.
 cranial somatic d.
 craniofacial somatic d.
 cuneiform bone d.
 distal radioulnar joint d.
 distal tibiofibular joint d.
 elbow somatic d.
 ERS d.
 extended, rotated, sidebent d.
 external torsion d.
 fascial d.
 fibular head d.
 fibular somatic d.
 flexed, rotated, sidebent d.

FRS d.
group d.
hand somatic d.
hepatocellular d.
hip d.
hip joint d.
hip somatic d.
iliosacral d.
iliosacral joint d.
iliosacral rotational d.
iliosacral somatic d.
inferior pubic d.
innominate shear d.
joint d.
knee joint d.
knee somatic d.
left superior innominate
   shear d.
low back d.
lower extremity d.
lumbar spine flexed, rotated,
   sidebent d.
lumbar spine FRS d.
lumbar spine somatic d.
manubrioglodiolar sternal d.
metabolic d.
metatarsal bone d.
muscular d.
navicular bone d.
neurologic d.
neutral d.
nonneutral d.
pelvic floor d.
pelvic girdle d.
pelvic somatic d.
proximal tibiofibular joint d.
psoas muscle d.
pubic d.
pubic symphysis d.
radius d.
respiratory rib d.
rib d.
rib cage d.
rib cage somatic d.
rib torsional d.
right inferior innominate
   shear d.

sacral base d.
sacral somatic d.
sacroiliac d.
sacroiliac articulation d.
sacroiliac joint d.
sacroiliac somatic d.
sacrum restriction d.
secondary somatic d.
segmental d.
shoulder girdle d.
shoulder somatic d.
single vertebral motion
   segment d.
skeletal d.
soft-tissue d.
somatic d.
sphenobasilar junction d.
structural rib d.
subacute d.
superior pubic d.
symphysis pubis d.
talocalcaneal d.
talotibial joint d.
temporomandibular joint d.
T1-4 group d.
T3-6 group d.
torsional d.
type I somatic d.
type II somatic d.
upper rib cage d.
vasomotor d.
vertebral d.
vertebral motion d.
vertebral somatic d.
visceral d.
viscerosomatic reflex d.
viscerosomatic somatic d.
wrist somatic d.
zygapophysial joint d.

dysfunctional
   d. cellular change
   d. segment
dysglycemia
dyskinesia
   biliary d.
   d. intermittens
   tardive d.

D

NOTES

dysmenorrhea
  primary d.
dysosteogenesis
dysostosis
  cleidocranial d.
  craniofacial d.
  mandibuloacral d.
  mandibulofacial d.
  metaphysial d.
  d. multiplex
dysphoric mood
dysplasia
  cervical d.
  cleidocranial d.
  congenital hip d.
  craniocarpotarsal d.
  developmental hip d.
  diaphysial d.
  d. epiphysealis multiplex
  d. epiphysialis hemimelia
  d. epiphysialis punctata
  faciodigitogenital d.
  mandibulofacial d.
  metaphysial d.
  monostotic fibrous d.
  multiple epiphyseal d.
  oculoauriculovertebral d.
  oculovertebral d.
  polyostotic fibrous d.
  skeletal d.
  spondyloepiphyseal d.
dysplastic spondylolisthesis
dyspnea
  d. on exertion (DOE)
  paroxysmal nocturnal d. (PND)

dysraphism
  spinal d.
dysregulation
  autonomic d.
  autonomic nervous system d.
  immune d.
dysspondylism
dysstasia
dysstatic
dyssynergia
dystelephalangy
dystonia
  d. lenticularis
  d. musculorum deformans
  torsion d.
dystrophia myotonica
dystrophica
  myotonia d.
dystrophy
  adult pseudohypertrophic
    muscular d.
  craniocarpotarsal d.
  facioscapulohumeral
    muscular d.
  limb-girdle muscular d.
  muscular d. (MD)
  myotonic d.
  pelvofemoral muscular d.
  reflex sympathetic d. (RSD)
  thoracic-pelvic-phalangeal d.
dysuria
dzao
  shan d.

e
e jiao
e zhu

E$_1$
prostaglandin E$_1$ (PGE$_1$)

E$_2$
prostaglandin E$_2$ (PGE$_2$)

E406

E413

EA
electroacupuncture
EA intensity

eagle-vine bark

ear
e. acupuncture
bunny's e.'s
e. clip
electronic e.
e. heart point
e. kidney point
level of e.
e. liver point
e. magnet
mouse e.
e. point
e. seed
e. shenmen point
e. sympathicus point

earache

earth
e. element
phases: metal, water, wood, fire, and e.
e. salts
e. smoke

earthbank

EarthClay

ease
e. and bind concept in motion
e. and bind phenomenon
Breathe E.
point of maximum e.
range of e.

ease-bind
e.-b. concept
e.-b. functional technique

east
E. Indian lemon grass
E. Indian root

Easter
E. flower
E. ledge
E. mangiant
E. rose

eastern
E. acupuncture
E. medicine
E. poison oak
E. white cedar

easy
e. movement
e. normal (EN)
e. normal left (ENL)
e. normal right (ENR)

EasyChair massage chair

Eaton-Lambert syndrome

EAV
electroacupuncture according to Voll

ebimar

ebulus
Sambucus e.

eburnation

EBV
Epstein-Barr virus

eccentric
e. amputation
e. contraction
e. isotonic contraction
e. isotonic muscle contraction
e. muscle contraction

eccentrochondroplasia

ecchondroma

ecchondrosis

ECG
electrocardiogram

echinacea
E. angustifolia
e. care liquid
e. fresh freeze-dried
E. Glycerite
E. Herbal Comfort Lozenges
e. mother tincture
E. pallida
E. purpurea
e. tea

Echium

echter lavendel

Echtrosept-GT

eclampsia

E

121

eclectic manipulation
Ecologica
ecology
    human e.
    pediatric e.
ECRB
    extensor carpi radialis brevis
    ECRB muscle
ECRL
    extensor carpi radialis longus
    ECRL muscle
ecstasy
    liquid e.
    natural e.
ectad
ectal
ectatic aneurysm
ectocervical
ectomorphic body type
ectosteal
ectrocheiry
Ecuadorian sarsaparilla
eczema
    allergic e.
    allergic contact e.
    atopic e.
    contact e.
EDA
    electrodermal activity
EDB
    extensor digitorum brevis
    EDB muscle
edema
    angioneurotic e.
    peripheral e.
    pulmonary e.
    Quincke e.
edetate
    e. disodium
edetic acid
edible burdock
edodes
    Lentinus e.
EDR
    electrodermal response
EDRF
    endothelium-derived relaxing factor
EDTA
    ethylenediaminetetraacetic acid
education
    Council on Chiropractic E.
    (CCE)

    Council on Naturopathic
    Medical E. (CNME)
    movement e.
edulis
    Catha e.
EEG
    electroencephalogram
    electroencephalograph
    EEG feedback
    theta EEG
    EEG theta wave feedback
EFA
    essential fatty acid
Efamol
effect
    additive e.
    analgesic e.
    anticonvulsive e.
    antiinflammatory e.
    antithyroidal e.
    bathmotropic e.
    body-motion electrostatic e.
    chronotropic e.
    circulatory e.
    coordinating e.
    coreolis e.
    counterirritant e.
    cumulative e.
    Fenn e.
    frequency/intensity e.
    ganglionic-blocking e.
    Haldane e.
    harmonizing e.
    homeostatic e.
    immune-enhancing e.
    local e.
    mentally relaxing e.
    neurological e.
    neurovascular side e.
    nocebo e.
    nonsegmental e.
    Orbeli e.
    parasympathetic e.
    placebo e.
    psychic e.
    psychological e.
    raphe serotonin e.
    relaxing e.
    sedative e.
    segmental e.
    side e.
    somatic e.
    spasmolytic e.

specific e.
stereospecific e.
synergistic e.
therapeutic e.
tonic e.
tonifying e.
effective
   e. dose
   e. refractory period
efferent
   e. fiber
   e. fibers of vagus nerve
   e. nerve
   e. vessel
Effer-Syllium
effleurage massage technique
effusion
   e. knee joint test
   malignant e.
EGB 761
EGb
   extract of *Ginkgo biloba*
egg lecithin
Egoscue method
ego strengthening
egrelti
   erkek e.
Egyptian's herb
Egyptian thorn
Ehlers-Danlos syndrome
eicherinde
eicosapentaenoic acid (EPA)
eight
   e. influential points
   E. Precious Herbs
   e. psychic channels
EKG
   electrocardiogram
elacy
elaiopathia
elastic
   e. band
   e. bandage
   e. barrier
   e. cartilage
   e. deformation

   e. fiber
   e. people
elasticity
   muscle e.
   e. of muscle
elastin
elata
   Gastrodia e.
Elaut triangle
Elavil
elbow
   articular muscle of e.
   e. bone
   e. crease
   golfer's e.
   interosseous bursa of e.
   intratendinous bursa of e.
   e. joint
   lateral ligament of e.
   Little Leaguer's e.
   lymph nodes of e.
   medial collateral ligament of e.
   miner's e.
   e. motion testing
   e. muscle energy technique
   nursemaid's e.
   point of e.
   posterior region of e.
   posterior surface of e.
   e. region
   restricted e.
   e. somatic dysfunction
   e. tender point
   tennis e.
   tip of e.
   transverse ligament of e.
   triangle of e.
elbowed
elder
   black e.
   common e.
   dwarf e.
   European e.
   e. flower
   e. leaf
   poison e.

E

NOTES

elder *(continued)*
    red-fruited e.
    sweet e.
elderberry
    blue e.
    hockle e.
    e. powder
    red e.
Eldisine
elecampane
electric
    e. anesthesia
    e. irritability
    e. pulse
electrical
    e. current
    e. field
    e. formula
    e. resistance detector
    e. stimulation
    e. stimulation therapy
    e. tonification
electricity
    low-level e.
    pulse of e.
    static e.
electroacupuncture (EA)
    e. according to Voll (EAV)
    e. biofeedback
    e. device
electroanalgesia
electroanesthesia
electrocardiogram (ECG, EKG)
electrochemical potential artifact
electrocontractility
electrode
    grounding pad e.
    e. pad
    e. patch
    e. resistance
electrodermal
    e. activity (EDA)
    e. response (EDR)
    e. skin resistance
electrode-to-skin interface
electrodiagnosis
electrodiagnostic study
electroencephalogram (EEG)
electroencephalogram-driven
    stimulation
electroencephalograph (EEG)
electrogalvanism
electrolysis

electrolyte balance
electromagnetic (EM)
    e. bioinformation system
    e. energy
    e. energy field
    e. energy treatment
    e. field (EMF)
    e. microcurrent device
    e. radiation (EMR)
    e. signal
    e. system
    e. therapy
electromagnetism
electromassage
electromyogram (EMG)
electromyograph feedback
electromyographic (EMG)
    e. biofeedback
electromyography (EMG)
electronarcosis
electronic ear
electrooculogram (EOG)
electroparacentesis
electrophoresis
electrophysiologic
electrophysiology
electrospinogram
electrospinography
electrostatic
electrostimulate
electrostimulation
electrotherapy
    interferential e.
electrotonification
electuary
element
    biomolecular e.
    cellular e.
    earth e.
    entrapment of neural e.
    fire e.
    lymphatic e.
    metal e.
    mother e.
    neural e.
    son e.
    trace e.
    vascular e.
    water e.
    wood e.
elemental zinc
elementary reproductive force
eleopathy

elephant's gall
Elettaria cardamomum
Eleutherococcus senticosus
elevata
    scapula e.
elevation
    rest, ice, compression, e.
    (RICE)
    rest, ice, heat, e.
    e. stretch
elevator
    e. muscle of rib
    e. muscle of scapula
    periosteal e.
elfdock, elf dock
    e. root
elfwort
eliminate
elimination diet
elixir
    E. Bonjean
    Kernosan E.
    E. Spark
ellipsoidal joint
ellipsoidea
    articulatio e.
elliptical amputation
elm
    American e.
    Indian e.
    moose e.
    red e.
    slippery e.
    sweet e.
EM
    electromagnetic
    extraordinary meridian
emaciation
emanate
emblica
    Phyllanthus e.
embolism
    bone marrow e.
embolus
    pulmonary e.
embrace
    Steam E.

embryologist
embryology
    cranial bone e.
    diaphragm e.
emedullate
E-mergen-C
emergence
emergency
    acute e.
    e. treatment
Emerge oil
emesis
emetic
EMF
    electromagnetic field
EMG
    electromyogram
    electromyographic
    electromyography
    EMG biofeedback
    surface EMG
eminence
    cruciate e.
    cruciform e.
    deltoid e.
    hypothenar e.
    iliopectineal e.
    iliopubic e.
    intercondylar e.
    e. of scapha
    thenar e.
    thyroid e.
eminentia
    e. carpi radialis
    e. carpi ulnaris
    e. hypothenaris
    e. iliopubica
    e. intercondylaris
    e. intercondyloidea
    e. scaphae
    e. thenaris
emission
    nocturnal e.
emmenagogue
emollient
emotion
    seven e.'s

E

NOTES

emotional
  e. expression
  e. factor
  e. imbalance
  e. stressor
  e. toxin
emphysema
  pulmonary e.
empiric
empirical principle
empowerment
emptiness pattern
empty
  e. end feel
  e. pulse
empyemic scoliosis
EMR
  electromagnetic radiation
EMS
  eosinophilia-myalgia syndrome
emulsion
  Fleet Castor Oil E.
Emulsoil
EN
  easy normal
enabling objective
enarthrodial joint
enarthrosis
encephalitis
encephalomyelitis
encephalopathy
  epileptic e.
  hypertensive e.
  uremic e.
enchanter's herb
enchondral
enchondromatosis
Encialina
encina
enclosed source energy
end
  e. feel
  e. feel sensation
endemic hypertrophy
ending
  annulospiral e.
  free nerve e.
endive
  garden e.
  green e.
  wild e.
endocarditis
  subacute bacterial e.

endocervical
endochondral
  e. bone
  e. ossification
endocrine
  e. disorder
  e. status
  e. system
endocrinotherapy
  endogenous e.
endocytosis
endodermal sinus tumor
endogenous
  e. endocrinotherapy
  e. toxicity
endolymphatic sac
endometriosis
endonasal acupuncture
endorphin
  e. analgesia
  e. antagonist
  beta e.
  e. compound
  e. mechanism
  e. molecule
  e. peptide
  e. release
endorphin-dependent system
endorphinergic
  e. analgesia
  e. cell
  e. link
**endorphin-mediated acupuncture
  analgesia**
endoskeleton
endothelial myeloma
**endothelium-derived relaxing factor
  (EDRF)**
endotracheal
  e. anesthesia
  e. intubation
endurance
  e. exercise
  Target E.
enema
  catnip tea e.
  cleansing e.
  coffee e.
  coffee retention e.
  decoction e.
  oil e.
  purgative e.

retention e.
therapeutic e.
Eneractin
energetic
    e. assessment
    e. connection
    e. flow
    e. imbalance
    e. therapy
    e. treatment
energetics
    acupuncture e.
Energizer
energy
    active e.
    e. axis
    e. balance
    e. balance technique
      classification
    e. balancing
    e. base
    bioelectric e.
    biological e.
    e. blockage
    blocked e.
    e. center
    e. channel
    e. checkup
    e. chelation
    e. circulation
    e. circulation network
    e. circulation plate
    collapsed e.
    e. condition
    deficient e.
    e. depletion
    direct e.
    e. distribution
    e. disturbance
    dry e.
    dynamical e.
    electromagnetic e.
    enclosed source e.
    even e.
    e. examination
    excessive e.
    excess of vital e.

    e. exercise
    e. expenditure
    e. field
    e. field assessment
    e. field disturbance
    healing e.
    heart e.
    hot e.
    e. imbalance
    indirect e.
    e. integration
    kidney e.
    kinetic e.
    latent e.
    e. leakage
    e. medicine
    e. meridian
    meridian e.
    metabolic e.
    muscle e. (ME)
    organ e.
    e. pattern
    piercing e.
    e. of position
    potential e.
    qi e.
    e. reservoir
    scattered e.
    sea of vital e.
    sick e.
    solidified e.
    somatic e.
    stagnated e.
    subtle e.
    e. therapy
    total e.
    vital e.
    wet e.
    e. work
    yang e.
    yin-yang e.
energy-field therapeutic
energy-functional level
energy-moving needle
energy-producing organ
engage

NOTES

E

engagement
  barrier e.
engelwurzel
English
  E. chamomile
  E. lavender
  E. oak
  E. plantain
  E. sarsaparilla
  E. violet
Enhance
Enhanced Glucosamine sulfate
enhancement
  immune e.
enhancer
enkephalin
ENL
  easy normal left
enlargement
  cervical e.
  lumbosacral e.
  prostate e.
ENR
  easy normal right
Enrg-V
ensheathing callus
ensiform process
ensisternum
entad
ental
Entelev Formula JS 114
enteral
enterica
  Salmonella e.
enteric-coated
  e.-c. fish oil
  e.-c. squill
enteric nervous system
enteroabsorbent
enteroclysis
enterocolitis
  necrotizing e.
Enterodyne
enterometabolic disorder
Entero-Sanol
enthesitis
enthesopathic
enthesopathy
enthnobotany
entire plant
entoectad
entrainment
  frequency-pulling e.

entrap
entrapment
  brachial nerve e.
  cranial nerve e.
  femoral nerve e.
  iliohypogastric nerve e.
  intercostal nerve e.
  median nerve e.
  nerve e.
  nerve plexus e.
  neural e.
  e. of neural element
  e. neuropathy
  neurovascular e.
  peroneal nerve e.
  radial nerve e.
  trigeminal nerve e.
  ulnar nerve e.
Entrin
entropy
enucleation
enuresis
  nocturnal e.
envelope
environment
  therapeutic e.
  withdrawal from the e.
environmental
  e. medicine
  e. toxin
envoy ingredient
enzymatic therapy
enzyme
  angiotensin-converting e. (ACE)
  Anti-Stress E.'s
  detoxification e.
  digestive e.
  glutamine synthetase e.
  e. monoamine oxidase
  pancreatic e.
  papaya e.
  proteolytic e.
  e. therapy
EOG
  electrooculogram
E'Ola Products
eosinophil, eosinophile
  e. count
eosinophilia
eosinophilia-myalgia syndrome (EMS)
EPA
  eicosapentaenoic acid

epactal bone
eparterial
epaxial
EPCL
  Everyday Problem Checklist
ependyma
ephedra
  Chinese e.
  E. distachya
  E. gerardiana
  E. helvetica
  Mongolian e.
  E. nevadensis
  E. Plus
  E. sinica
ephedrae
  herba e.
ephedrine
Epices
  Quatre E.
epicondylalgia externa
epicondyle
  lateral e.
epicondyli (*pl. of* epicondylus)
epicondylian
epicondylic
epicondylitis
  lateral humeral e.
epicondylus, pl. epicondyli
  e. lateralis humeri
  e. lateralis ossis femoris
  e. medialis humeri
  e. medialis ossis femoris
epicoracoid
epicranial muscle
epicranius
  e. muscle
  musculus e.
epidemiology
epidermal ridge
epidermidis
  Staphylococcus e.
epidermis
epididymis
epidural
  e. anesthesia
  e. block

  e. local anesthetic
  e. steroid
  e. stimulation
epigastrium
epilepsy
  grand mal e.
epileptic
  e. attack
  e. encephalopathy
  e. fit
Epimedium grandiflorum
epimysiotomy
epinephrine
epipharynx
epiphysial
  e. aseptic necrosis
  e. fracture
  e. line
  e. plate
epiphysialis
  linea e.
epiphysiodesis
epiphysiolysis
epiphysiopathy
epiphysis
  atavistic e.
  pressure e.
  slipped capital femoral e.
  stippled e.
  traction e.
episiotomy
  mediolateral e.
episode
  traumatic e.
episodic inhibition of respiration
epispinal
episternal bone
episternum
epistropheus
epitarsus
epithelial body
epithelioserosa
  zona e.
epithelium
epithesis
epitonin
epitrochlea

E

NOTES

129

epitrochlear
epitrochleoanconeus
  musculus e.
EPO
  evening primrose oil
Epogam
Epsom salts
Epstein-Barr
  E.-B. viral infection
  E.-B. virus (EBV)
equiaxial
equilibration
  dental e.
  e. treatment
equilibrium disorder
equimolar
equina
  cauda e.
equine gait
equinovalgus
  pes e.
  talipes e.
equinovarus
  pes e.
  talipes e.
equinus
  talipes e.
Equisetum
  E. arvense
  E. palustre
er
  e. chan tang
  e. chen tang
Erechtites hieracifolia
erecta
  dislocatio e.
  luxatio e.
erect film
erector
  e. muscle of spine
  e. spinae
  e. spinae mass
  e. spinae muscle
erectum
  Trillium e.
erg
ergocalciferol
ergodynamograph
ergoesthesiograph
ergograph
  Mosso e.
ergometer
ergonomic

ergonomics
ergostat
ergot
ergotherapy
erh-ch'a
Erichsen test
Eriobotrya japonica
Eriodictyon
  E. californicum
  E. glutinosum
eriodictyon
erkek egrelti
Erlenmeyer flask deformity
ermen
  sj 21 e.
error
  interobserver e.
  intraobserver e.
ERS
  extended, rotated, sidebent
    ERS dysfunction
    ERS position
    ERS vertebral
ERSL
  extended, rotated, sidebent left
ERSR
  extended, rotated, sidebent right
erucic acid
eruption
  cutaneous e.
  skin e.
eryngo
erythema
  cutaneous e.
  e. test
erythematosus
  lupus e.
  systemic lupus e. (SLE)
erythematous lesion
erythrocyte
  e. copper level
  e. magnesium level
erythrostachys
  Amaranthus hybridus var. e.
Erythroxylum coca
Escherichia coli
Eschscholzia californica
escine
esculenta
  Manihot e.
E-Sel
esere nut

Esmarch
  E. bandage
  E. tourniquet
esodic nerve
esophageal
  e. hiatus
  e. opening
esophagi
  pars cervicalis e.
  pars thoracica e.
esophagitis
esophagus
  cervical part of e.
  e. dorsal mesentery
  dorsal mesentery of e.
  mesentery of e.
esoteric healing
espiritismo
espresso
ESRRL
  extension, sidebent right, rotated left
essence
  flower e.
  kidney e.
  life e.
  mother e.
  original e.
  Peerless Composition E.
essential
  e. fatty acid (EFA)
  e. hypertension
  e. oil
Essiac
  E. formula
  E. tea
ester
  caffeic acid phenethyl e.
    (CAPE)
  diterpene e.
  fumaric acid e.
  stanol e.
esthesioneurocytoma
Estramonio
estrogen
  phenolic e.
Estroven
ethanol

ethanolamine
ethanolic
  e. extract
  e. solution
ether
  xylostyptic e.
ethics
  holistic e.
ethmoid
  e. angle
  e. bone
  perpendicular plate of e.
  e. sinus
ethnobotany
  Native American e.
ethnocentrism
ethnomedicine
ethnopharmacology
ethyl chloride
**ethylenediaminetetraacetic acid
  (EDTA)**
etiology
  multicausal e.
etoposide
Eucalyptamint
eucalyptus
  E. globulus
  e. leaf vapor
  oil of e.
  e. oil
  e. oil in vaporizer
Eucommia ulmoides
Euflat 1
Eugalan Forte
Eugenia (*See also Syzygium*)
  E. aromatica
  E. aromaticum
  E. jambolana
  E. paniculata
Euonymus atropurpureus
eupatoria
  Agrimonia e.
Eupatorium
  E. perfoliatum
  E. purpureum
  E. rugosum

E

NOTES

Euphorbia
E. *cyparissias*
E. *hirta*
E. *longana*
E. *poinsettia*
E. *pulcherrima*
euphoria
euphoric agent
Euphrasia
E. *officinalis*
E. *stricta*
eupraxia
eupsychia
eurhythmy
europaeus
Lycopus e.
European
E. angelica
E. barberry
E. bittersweet
E. blueberry
E. buckthorn
E. centaury
E. elder
E. linden
E. mandrake
E. massage
E. mullein
E. pennyroyal
E. pestroot
E. spindle tree
E. squill
E. vervain
E. white hellebore
eustachian tube
eutonic
evaluation
cognitive perceptual motor e.
musculoskeletal system e.
nutritional e.
psychological e.
urodynamic e.
even
e. energy
e. method of needling
evening
e. primrose
e. primrose oil (EPO)
event
sensory e.
event-related brain potential

everlasting
life e.
march e.
Every Body's Protein Powder
everyday
E. Life Questionnaire
E. Problem Checklist (EPCL)
evidence
anecdotal e.
evil
e. qi
yin e.
Eviprostat N
evodia
Evodia rutaecarpa
evoked potential
ewe daisy
EW Herbal Eyewash Formula
Ewing
E. sarcoma
E. tumor
Ex
extra point
exacerbated symptom
exaggeration
e. method
e. method joint mobilization
e. technique
e. treatment
examination
cytologic e.
energy e.
four e.'s: visual observation,
listening and smelling,
questioning, and physical
HNC e.
Naturopathic Physicians
Licensing E. (NPLEx)
osteopathic postural e.
osteopathic structural e.
plumb line e.
scanning e.
screening e.
static symmetric e.
structural e.
examiners
National Board of
Chiropractic E. (NBCE)
exarteritis
Ex-B
extra point on the back of the trunk
Ex-B 20 yaoqi

Ex-B 17 dingchuan
Ex-B 21 huatuojiaji
Ex-CA
   extra point on the chest and
   abdomen
excavatio
excavation
excavatum
   pectus e.
excentric amputation
excess
   e. condition
   e. disturbance
   shi e.
   state of e.
   stomach e.
   e. of vital energy
   yang e.
excessive
   e. energy
   e. energy buildup
   e. function
excess-type
   e.-t. condition
   e.-t. disturbance
   e.-t. symptom
exchange
   carbon dioxide e.
   respiratory gas e.
   yin and yang balance and e.
excision
excitation
excitatory
   e. feedback loop
   e. terminal
excited
   inhibited e.
excitomuscular
exclusion diet
excursion
Executive Stress Formula
exercise
   aerobic e.
   anaerobic e.
   angry cat e.
   bioenergetic e.
   biofeedback e.

e. bone
breathing e.
cat back e.
cervical isometric e.
dynamic e.
endurance e.
energy e.
exercise program e.
functional palpation e.
hamstring muscle e.
heel slide e.
hip adductor muscle e.
hip flexor stretching e.
Hoshino e.
isokinetic e.
isometric e.
isometric stabilizing e.
isotonic e.
Kegel e.
latissimus dorsi muscle e.
Lewit e.
Mackenzie extension
   program e.
mind-body e.
muscle-setting e.
Norwegian e.
pendulum e.
physical e.
piriformis muscle e.
e. program
psoas muscle e.
qigong e.
quadratus lumborum muscle e.
rectus femoris muscle e.
relaxing e.
retraining e.
reverse torso curl e.
self-mobilizing e.
SHQ breathing e.
sitting to kneeling e.
strengthening e.
therapeutic e.
e. therapy
toning e.
torso curl e.
torso extension e.
trunk control e.

E

NOTES

exercise *(continued)*
  trunk lift e.
  vital energy e.
  wall press e.
  warm-up e.
  William flexion e.
exercise-induced asthma
exertion
  dyspnea on e. (DOE)
exfoliative dermatitis
exhalation
  e. breath
  caught in e.
  e. phase
  e. restriction
  e. restriction, bucket-handle
    component
  e. restriction, pump-handle
    component
  e. rib
  voluntary e.
exhaustion
  e. condition
  e. of liver qi
  physical e.
  e. syndrome
Ex-HN
  extra point on the head and neck
  Ex-HN 8 anmian I
  Ex-HN 9 anmian II
  Ex-HN 5 jiachengjiang
  Ex-HN 4 qiuhou
  Ex-HN 6 sishencong
  Ex-HN 2 tai-yang
  Ex-HN 7 yiming
  Ex-HN 1 yintang
  Ex-HN 3 yuhao
exit foramen
Ex-LE
  extra point on the lower extremity
  Ex-LE 36 bafeng
  Ex-LE 31 heding
  Ex-LE 32 xiyan
exodic nerve
exogenous
  e. obesity
  e. toxicity
exoskeleton
exostosis, pl. **exostoses**
  hereditary multiple exostoses
  multiple exostoses

expansion
  extensor e.
  extensor digital e.
expectorant
expenditure
  energy e.
  musculoskeletal system
    energy e.
  nonresting energy e.
Experience oil
experiment
  control e.
experimental hypnosis
expiration abdominal stretch
expression
  emotional e.
exsanguinate
exsanguination
exsanguine
Exstress
extend
extended
  bilateral sacrum e.
  e. chi
  e. facet
  e., rotated, sidebent (ERS)
  e., rotated, sidebent dysfunction
  e., rotated, sidebent left
    (ERSL)
  e., rotated, sidebent right
    (ERSR)
  e., rotated and side bent
    vertebral
  e., rotated and side bent
    vertebral position
  sacrum e.
extensa
  manus e.
extensibility
  muscle e.
  e. of muscle
  e. testing
extension
  bilateral e.
  e. compression test
  craniosacral e.
  e. dysfunction of sacrum
  flexion, abduction, external
    rotation, e. (FABERE)
  full e.
  horizontal e.
  knee e.
  e. lesion of the sacrum

e. load
lumbar spine extension
   sacral e.
nail e.
neutral e.
regional e.
e. restriction
sacral e.
sagittal plane e.
e., sidebent right, rotated left
   (ESRRL)
skeletal e.
sphenobasilar e.
e. test for C2–7 motion
thoracic spine e.
torso e.
unilateral e.
wrist e.
extensor
e. aponeurosis
e. back muscle
e. carpi radialis brevis (ECRB)
e. carpi radialis brevis muscle
e. carpi radialis longus
   (ECRL)
e. carpi radialis longus muscle
e. carpi ulnaris
e. carpi ulnaris muscle
e. comminicus muscle
e. digital expansion
e. digiti minimi muscle
e. digiti quinti muscle
e. digitorum brevis (EDB)
e. digitorum brevis muscle
e. digitorum brevis muscle of
   hand
e. digitorum communis muscle
e. digitorum longus
e. digitorum longus muscle
e. digitorum muscle
e. expansion
extensor retinaculum e.
e. hallucis brevis muscle
e. hallucis longus
e. hallucis longus muscle
hip e.
e. indicis muscle

e. indicis proprius muscle
e. indicis proprius musculus
e. muscle of fingers
e. muscle of little finger
neck e.
e. neck muscle linear stretch
e. pollicis brevis muscle
e. pollicis longus muscle
extensorum
retinaculum musculorum e.
extensus
hallux e.
exterior
e. condition
externa
epicondylalgia e.
facies e.
hematorrhachis e.
membrana intercostalis e.
external
e. acoustic meatus
e. anal canal
e. auditory meatus
e. climatic influence
e. cold influence
e. collateral ligament of wrist
e. compression test
e. conjugate diameter
e. fixation
e. genitalia
e. heat
e. hydrotherapy
e. illness
e. intercostal membrane
e. intercostal muscle
e. jugular vein
e. layer of dura
e. lip of iliac crest
e. malleolus
e. oblique muscle
e. obturator muscle
e. occipital protuberance
e. pathogenic climatic factor
e. pathogenic factor
e. qigong
e. rib torsion
e. rotation

E

NOTES

external *(continued)*
    e. rotation with flexed hip
        muscle energy technique
    e. rotation with neutral hip
        muscle energy technique
    e. rotator muscle
    e. semilunar fibrocartilage
    e. surface
    e. surface of frontal bone
    e. surface of parietal bone
    e. torsion
    e. torsion dysfunction
    e. wind influence
externi
    musculus intercostalis e.
externus
    musculus obturator e.
    musculus thyroarytenoideus e.
    musculus vastus e.
extortor
extra
    e. point (Ex)
    e. point on the back of the
        trunk (Ex-B)
    e. point on the chest and
        abdomen (Ex-CA)
    e. point on the head and
        neck (Ex-HN)
    e. point on the lower
        extremity (Ex-LE)
    e. point on the upper
        extremity (Ex-UE)
extraarticular
extracaliceal
extracapsular
    e. ankylosis
    e. fracture
    e. ligament
extracarpal
extracellular fluid
extracorporeal
extract
    aged garlic e.
    apricot seed e.
    aqueous e.
    bilberry e.
    butcher's broom e. 4:1
    butterbur root e.
    catnip and fennel e.
    cat's claw inner bark e.
    celendine e.
    chondrus e.
    coneflower e.

    crataegus e.
    dandelion e.
    dong quai fluid e.
    ethanolic e.
    e. of *Ginkgo biloba* (EGb)
    ginkgo biloba e. (GBE)
    ginkgo biloba leaf e.
    goldenseal e. 4:1
    gotu kola gold e.
    grapeseed e.
    green tea e. (GTE)
    horse chestnut e.
    horse chestnut seed e.
    horsetail e.
    Irish moss e.
    kava kava e.
    lavender liquid e.
    licorice liquid e.
    licorice root e.
    liquid liver e. #521
    liver e.
    lobelia e.
    lyophilized aqueous root e.
    milk thistle e.
    milk thistle fluid e.
    mussel e.
    nettles liquid e.
    oat e.
    oyster e.
    plant e.
    plantago e.
    Pygeum africanum e. (PAE)
    sarsaparilla root e.
    saw palmetto liposterolic e.
    schisandra e.
    standardized e.
    tansy e.
    valerian e.
    valerian root e.
    white cohosh liquid e.
    yarrow grass e.
    yellowroot liquid e.
extraction
    supercritical fluid e. (SFE)
Extractum
    E. Filicis Aethereum
    E. Filicis Maris Tenue
    E. Rhei Liquidum
extradural
    e. anesthesia
    e. hematorrhachis
extrafusal fiber
extraligamentous

extramural
extraneous
extraordinary
  e. channel
  e. meridian (EM)
extrapoint neima
extratarsal
extratubal
extravasation
extravascular fluid
extravertebral joint
extra-virgin olive oil
extreme
  polar e.
extremital
extremitas
  e. acromialis claviculae
  e. anterior splenica
  e. inferior
  e. posterior splenica
  e. sternalis claviculae
extremity
  extra point on the lower e. (Ex-LE)
  extra point on the upper e. (Ex-UE)
  inferior e.
  lower e.
  lymphatic pump with lower e.
  lymphatic pump with upper e.
  short lower e.
  superior e.
  upper e.
extrinsic
  e. activating force
  e. chi
  e. corrective force
  e. muscle

extrinsic-applied thrusting force
extubate
extubation
exudate
  serosanguinous e.
exudation
exudative inflammation
exude
Ex-UE
  extra point on the upper extremity
  Ex-UE 28 baxie
eye
  e. balm
  clear e.
  crab's e.
  day's e.
  e. disorder
  doll's e.
  dominant e.
  knee e.
  e. movement
  pheasant's e.
  e. roll sign
  e. root
  Scotty dog's e.
  third e.
  Vital E.'s
  e. wash
eyebright
  e. compress
  meadow e.
  red e.
  e. tea
Eysenck Personality Inventory
EZ Lift table

E

NOTES

137

faba calabarica
fabella
FABERE
  flexion, abduction, external rotation, extension
    FABERE test
face
  cow f.
  dish f.
  f. needle
facehole
facespace
facet
  f. arthropathy
  articular f.
  f. asymmetry
  f. of atlas for dens
  cervical f.
  clavicular f.
  closed f.
  costal f.
  extended f.
  f. facing
  flexing f.
  f. joint
  Lenoir f.
  locked f.'s
  lumbar f.
  open f.
  opening f.
  f. orientation
  superior articular f.
  superior costal f.
  f. symmetry
  thoracic f.
  transverse costal f.
  f. tropism
  vertebral f.
facetectomy
facial
  f. bone
  f. injury
  f. nerve
  f. nerve paralysis
  f. paresis
  f. sauna
facialis
facies
  f. anterior
  f. articularis

f. bovina
f. dorsalis
f. externa
f. lateralis
f. medialis
f. posterior
facilitate
facilitated
  f. positional release (FPR)
  f. positional release treatment
  f. segment
  f. segmental release technique
facilitation
  heterosynaptic f.
  nervous system f.
  proprioceptor neuromuscular f.
facilitator
facing
  facet f.
faciodigitogenital dysplasia
facioscapulohumeral
  f. atrophy
  f. muscular dystrophy
factor
  accelerator f.
  angiogenesis f.
  Bifido F.
  bipolar f.
  causal f.
  Christmas f.
  clotting f.
  corticotropin-releasing f. (CRF)
  emotional f.
  endothelium-derived relaxing f. (EDRF)
  external pathogenic f.
  external pathogenic climatic f.
  glass f.
  homeopathic growth f.
  f. II
  Joint F.'s
  labile f.
  orthogonal risk f.
  osteoclast activating f.
  pathogenic f.
  platelet-activating f. (PAF)
  stable f.
  tumor necrosis f. (TNF)
facultative parasite

F

failed
   f. lower back syndrome
   f. test suggestion
failure
   acute renal f.
   congestive heart f. (CHF)
   heart f.
   kidney f.
   secondary f.
fainting
fairy cup
fairywand
faith
   f. healer
   f. healing
   F. and Health Consortium
   (FHC)
falcate
falces (*pl. of* falx)
falciform
   f. cartilage
   f. ligament
fall
   childhood f.
fallen
   f. arch
fallopian ligament
false
   f. aneurysm
   f. ankylosis
   f. cinnamon
   f. coltsfoot
   f. coxa vara
   f. hellebore
   f. indigo
   f. joint
   f. negative
   f. positive
   f. rib
   f. saffron
   f. suture
   f. unicorn root
   f. valerian
   f. vertebra
   f. white cedar
false-negative diagnosis
false-positive
   f.-p. diagnosis
falx, pl. **falces**
   f. aponeurotica
   f. cerebelli
   f. cerebri
   f. inguinalis

familial
   f. hypoparathyroidism
   f. spinal muscular atrophy
family
   mint f.
   omega-3 f.
   spurge f.
   sumac f.
fang
   f. feng
   f. ji
fangchi
   Aristolochia f.
fangji
   guang f.
fango
fantasy ability
Farabeuf triangle
faradomuscular
farasyon maiy
farfara
   Tussilago f.
farinosa
   Aletris f.
fascia, pl. **fasciae**
   antebrachial f.
   f. antebrachii
   f. axillaris
   bicipital f.
   brachial f.
   f. brachii
   broad f.
   f. cervicalis
   f. cervicalis profunda
   clavipectoral f.
   f. clavipectoralis
   Colles f.
   continuity of f.
   cribriform f.
   f. cribrosa
   crural f.
   f. cruris
   dartos f.
   deep f.
   deep cervical f.
   dense f.
   f. dorsalis manus
   f. dorsalis pedis
   Dupuytren f.
   f. of forearm
   Hesselbach f.
   iliac f.
   f. iliaca

iliopectineal f.
infraspinatus f.
integration of f.
intercolumnar fasciae
interosseous f.
investing f.
investing layer of cervical f.
f. lata
f. of leg
lumbodorsal f.
middle cervical f.
f. nuchae
nuchal f.
obturator f.
palmar f.
parietal pelvic f.
pectoral f.
f. pectoralis
pelvic f.
f. pelvis
f. pelvis parietalis
f. pelvis visceralis
pharyngobasilar f.
f. pharyngobasilaris
phrenicopleural f.
f. phrenicopleuralis
plantar f.
popliteal f.
Porter f.
pretracheal f.
prevertebral f.
prevertebral layer of cervical f.
f. profunda
semilunar f.
Sibson f.
subcutaneous f.
subsartorial f.
f. subserosa
subserous f.
superficial f.
f. superficialis
superficial layer of deep
  cervical f.
f. thoracolumbalis
thoracolumbar f.
vastoadductor f.
visceral pelvic f.

fascial
  f. barrier
  f. compartment
  f. creep
  f. dysfunction
  f. function
  f. injury
  f. layer
  f. pattern
  f. patterning of Zink
  f. plane
  f. release technique
  f. release treatment
  f. restriction
  f. semiconduction
  f. unwinding
fascicle
  muscle f.
fascicular degeneration
fasciculation
fasciculi
  transverse f.
fasciculus
  medial longitudinal f.
  semilunar f.
fasciitis
  plantar f.
fasciodesis
fasciorrhaphy
fasciotomy
fashion
  alternating f.
fast
  cleansing f.
  f. method of insertion
  f. twitch fiber
fasting
  controlled f.
  F. Plus
  f. therapy
fat
  monounsaturated f.
  polyunsaturated f.
  saturated f.
fatigability
fatigable

NOTES

F

fatigue
    f. fracture
    muscle f.
    f. strength
fat-pad
fatty
    f. acid
    f. acid metabolism
    f. replacement
faulty union
Fayette principles of rotation
FCER
    Foundation for Chiropractic
    Education and Research
FC with dong quai
FDA
    Food and Drug Administration
fear condition
feather
    goose f.
featherfoil
febrifuga
    Smilax f.
febrifuge plant
fecal incontinence
fechel
Federal Food, Drug, and Cosmetic Act
Federation of Chiropractic Licensing Boards
feedback
    auditory EMG f.
    autogenic f.
    biologic f.
    bioreceptor f.
    EEG f.
    EEG theta wave f.
    electromyograph f.
    finger pulse f.
    frontal electromyographic f.
    f. inhibition
    f. instrumentation
    kinesthetic f.
    f. look
    respiration f.
    sensory-motor-rhythm f.
    somatosensory f.
    temperature f.
    thermal f.
    visual f.
feel
    abnormal f.
    empty end f.

    end f.
    jerky f.
    jerky end f.
    loose f.
    normal f.
    rapidly ascending end f.
    soft f.
    spongy f.
    springy f.
    sticky f.
    tightening end f.
fei
    feng han su f.
    feng re fan f.
    f. qi xu
    tan shi zu f.
    f. yin xu
Feingold diet
feishu
    f. point
    ub 13 f.
Feiss line
feiyang
    ub 58 f.
Feldenkrais
    F. Awareness Through Movement
    F. bodywork
    F. method
    F. sequence
    F. technique
felon herb
felonwood
felonwort
feltwort
Fem
    F. Cal
    F. Mend
    F. Osteo HRT
    F. Prenatal
female regulator
Femcal Plus
femoral
    f. artery
    f. canal
    f. muscle
    f. nerve
    f. nerve entrapment
    f. opening
    f. region
    f. ring
    f. triangle
    f. trochanter

femorale
  calcar f.
  trigonum f.
femoralis
  canalis f.
  fovea f.
femoris
  biceps f.
  caput f.
  caput breve musculi bicipitis f.
  caput longum musculi
    bicipitis f.
  caput ossis f.
  collum f.
  collum ossis f.
  condylus lateralis f.
  condylus medialis f.
  corpus f.
  corpus ossis f.
  epicondylus lateralis ossis f.
  epicondylus medialis ossis f.
  fovea capitis f.
  inferior subtendinous bursa of
    biceps f.
  linea intercondylaris f.
  linea pectinea f.
  musculus biceps f.
  musculus quadratus f.
  musculus quadriceps f.
  musculus quadriceps
    extensor f.
  musculus rectus f.
  musculus tensor fasciae f.
  os f.
  quadriceps f.
  rectus f.
  regio f.
  short head of biceps f.
  trochlea f.
  tuberculum adductorium f.
femoroacetabular joint
femoropatellar joint
femorotibial joint
Fem-R
Femtrol
femur
  adductor tubercle of f.

  f. angle of inclination
  head of f.
  intercondylar line of f.
  lateral condyle of f.
  lateral epicondyle of f.
  longitudinal axis of f.
  medial condyle of f.
  medial epicondyle of f.
  neck of f.
  patellar surface of f.
  pectineal line of f.
  pit of head of f.
  popliteal plane of f.
  popliteal surface of f.
  round ligament of f.
  shaft of f.
femur-futu
  st 32 f.-f.
fencer's reflex
fenchelholz
fenestra
fenestrated
fenestration
feng
  fang f.
  f. han su fei
  f. re fan fei
  f. shui
  f. tsao
fengchi
  gb 20 f.
fengfu
  du 16 f.
fenglong
  st 40 f.
fengshi
  gb 31 f.
Fenn effect
fennel
  bitter f.
  common f.
  Florence f.
  garden f.
  large f.
  sweet f.
  f. tea

F

NOTES

fennel *(continued)*
   wild f.
   F./Wild Yam Supreme
fenouil
   aneth f.
fenouille
Fen-Phen
   Herbal F.-P.
fentanyl
fenugreek seed
Fenu-Thyme
fera
   Indigo f.
ferasyunu
   su f.
Ferguson
   angle of F.
   F. lumbosacral angle
fern
   male f.
   ostrich f.
   parsley f.
   scented f.
   shield f.
   sweet f.
ferox
   Datura f.
ferrous fumarate
ferrugineum
   Rhododendron f.
ferrum
   f. phos
   f. phosphoricum
Ferula assafoetida
festination
fetalis
   rachitis f.
fever
   big f.
   hay f.
   tidal f.
   f. tree
feverfew
   F. Glyc
   F. Nasal Mist
   F. Power
Feverfew/Dogwood Supreme
fevertree
feverwort
FHC
   Faith and Health Consortium
fiber
   A f.

C f.
   collagen f.
   efferent f.
   elastic f.
   extrafusal f.
   fast twitch f.
   flax f.
   Gerdy f.
   β-glucan soluble f.
   insoluble f.
   intercolumnar f.
   intrafusal f.
   motor f.
   muscle f.
   myelinated nerve f.
   nerve f.
   nuclear bag f.
   nuclear chain f.
   osteocollagenous f.
   osteogenetic f.
   pain f.
   perforating f.
   postganglionic motor f.
   preganglionic f.
   raphespinal f.
   reticular f.
   Sharpey f.
   skeletal muscle f.
   slow twitch f.
   soluble f.
   type Ia f.
   type II f.
   unmyelinated C f.
   Weitbrecht f.
fibra
fibrae intercrurales anuli inguinalis superficialis
fibrillary neuroma
fibrillation
   atrial f.
fibrinopurulent inflammation
fibrinous
   f. adhesion
   f. inflammation
fibroblast
fibrocartilage
   circumferential f.
   external semilunar f.
   interarticular f.
   semilunar f.
   stratiform f.
fibrocartilago
   f. basalis

f. interarticularis
f. intervertebralis
fibrocystic breast disease
fibrodysplasia ossificans progressiva
fibroelastic
fibroid
uterine f.
fibroma
nonossifying f.
nonosteogenic f.
fibromatosis
palmar f.
fibromuscular
fibromyalgia syndrome (FMS)
fibroneuroma
fibroplate
fibrosa
articulatio f.
capsula f.
junctura f.
localized osteitis f.
multifocal osteitis f.
tunica f.
fibrosis
annulus f.
cystic f.
interstitial f.
radiation f.
renal interstitial f.
fibrositis syndrome
fibrosus
lacertus f.
fibrous
f. adhesion
f. ankylosis
f. articular capsule
f. capsule
f. cartilage
f. cortical defect
f. digital sheaths of foot
f. digital sheaths of hand
f. dysplasia of bone
f. dysplasia of jaws
f. joint
f. layer
f. sheaths
f. tendon sheath

f. tissue
f. union
fibula
apex of head of f.
articular facet of head of f.
head of f.
interosseous border of f.
lateral surface of f.
malleolar articular surface of f.
medial crest of f.
medial surface of f.
neck of f.
posterior border of f.
posterior ligament of head
of f.
posterior surface of f.
shaft of f.
somatic dysfunction of f.
styloid process of f.
upper extremity of f.
fibulae
apex capitis f.
caput f.
collum f.
corpus f.
crista medialis f.
fossa malleoli f.
margo anterior f.
margo interosseus f.
margo posterior f.
fibular
f. artery
f. articular surface of tibia
f. collateral ligament
f. collateral ligament of ankle
f. head
f. head anterior
f. head dysfunction
f. head functional technique
f. head posterior
f. lymph node
f. malleolus
f. margin of foot
f. node
f. notch
f. somatic dysfunction

F

NOTES

fibularis
    incisura f.
fibularium
    retinaculum musculorum f.
fibulocalcaneal
ficaria
    Ranunculus f.
ficus
field
    bioenergetic f.
    bioenergy f.
    biomagnetic f.
    f. blam
    f. block
    f. block anesthesia
    electrical f.
    electromagnetic f. (EMF)
    electromagnetic energy f.
    energy f.
    human energy f.
    interference f.
    f. lady's mantle
    magnetic f.
    f. mallow
    osteopathy in the cranial f.
      (OCF)
    f. pansy
    perceptual f.
    f. poppy
    pulsed electromagnetic f.
    uneven energy f.
    weak energy f.
fieldlove
fifth
    f. chakra
    f. finger
    f. toe
fight-or-flight response
figure-of-eight bandage
figwort
    common f.
fila (*pl. of* filum)
filarial
    f. arthritis
    f. synovitis
filbert
filfil
filiform
    f. needle
    f. steel needle
Filipendula
filius ante patrem

filix-mas
    Dryopteris f.-m.
film
    backward-bending dynamic f.
    decubitus f.
    erect f.
    forward-bending dynamic f.
    lateral spot f.
    left oblique lumbar spine f.
    lumbosacral junction spot f.
    plain f.
    plain f.
    right oblique lumbar spine f.
    scout f.
    sidebending dynamic f.
    spot f.
filtrum
filum, pl. **fila**
    f. durae matris spinalis
    fila radicularia
    f. of spinal dura mater
    terminal f.
    f. terminale
fimbria
financial status
finasteride
finder
    point f.
finding
    palpable f.
finetune
finger
    abductor muscle of little f.
    baseball f.
    f. clubbing
    deep flexor muscle of f.
    drop f.
    extensor muscle of f.
    extensor muscle of little f.
    fifth f.
    first f.
    f. flexor muscle
    fourth f.
    hammer f.
    index f.
    jerk f.
    lateral surface of f.
    little f.
    lock f.
    mallet f.
    middle f.
    opposer muscle of little f.
    palmar surfaces of f.

pulp of f.
f. pulse feedback
ring f.
second f.
short flexor muscle of little f.
snap f.
spring f.
stuck f.
superficial flexor muscle of f.
f. temperature
third f.
trigger f.
vinculum breve of f.
vinculum longum of f.
web of f.'s
fingernail
fingerpad
finite skin contour
Finkelstein test
finocchio
fir
balsam f.
f. balsam
joint f.
f. pine
Scotch f.
silver f.
fire
f. element
gastric f.
heart f.
liver f.
ministerial f.
f. path
f. qi
f. rising
rising heart f.
rising liver f.
rising stomach f.
sovereign f.
stomach f.
fireweed
firing pattern
first
f. chakra
F. Color tea
f. cuneiform bone

f. dorsal interosseous muscle
of the hand
f. finger
f. metacarpal-carpal
f. rib
f. rib superior subluxation
first-aid plant
fish
deep-water ocean f.
f. killer
f. oil
f. oil supplement
f. poison tree
saltwater f.
fishberry
fishfuddle
fishskin disease
fish-wood
fissura
fissural
fissuration
fissure
anal f.
petrosquamous f.
fissured fracture
fistula
fit
epileptic f.
grand mal epileptic f.
Fitness Plus
five
f. center heat
F. Elements acupuncture
f. element theory
f. phase or five elements:
wood, fire, earth, metal, and
water
f. phases
f. shu point
five-fingers
fixation
external f.
internal f.
intraosseous f.
fixator muscle
fixed dressing

F

NOTES

fixus
radius f.
flag
blue f.
f. lily
poison f.
sweet f.
water f.
flail joint
flammable anesthetic
Flanders poppy
flank bone
flannel-leaf
flap
f. amputation
muscle f.
f. operation
flapless amputation
flare
innominate f.
flash
hot f.
flat
f. back posture
f. bone
f. chest
f. hand
f. spot
flatfoot
flattened
f. lower cervical spine
f. vertex
flattening
f. of lumbar lordosis
lumbar spine f.
thoracic spine f.
f. of thoracic spine
flatulence
Flatulex
flavescens
    Phoradendron f.
flavone
flavonoid glycoside
flax
f. fiber
f. lignan
mountain f.
Flax-O-Mega
flaxseed oil
fleaseed
flection
Fleet Castor Oil Emulsion
flesh and blood

Fletcher's Castoria
fleur-de-lis
fleur d'ulmaire
flex
flexa
manus f.
flexed
bilaterally f.
bilateral sacrum f.
f. knee muscle energy
technique
left sacrum f.
f., rotated, and side bend
vertebral
f., rotated, and side bend
vertebral position
f., rotated, sidebent (FRS)
f., rotated, sidebent dysfunction
f., rotated, sidebent left
(FRSL)
f., rotated, sidebent position
f., rotated, sidebent right
(FRSR)
sacrum f.
talus plantar f.
flexibilitas
cerea f.
f. cerea
flexible collodion
Flexi-Factors
fleximeter
flexing facet
flexion
f., abduction, external rotation,
extension (FABERE)
f. barrier
craniosacral f.
f. crease
f. dysfunction of sacrum
horizontal f.
knee f.
lateral f.
neutral f.
palmar f.
partial hip f.
f. phase
plantar f.
regional f.
restricted horizontal f.
f. restriction
sacral f.
sagittal plane f.

f., sidebent right, rotated left (FSRRL)
f. somatic dysfunction of the sacrum
sphenobasilar f.
f. test
unilateral sacral f.
flexion-distraction technique
flexion-extension
 f.-e. cervical injury
 f.-e. injury
 f.-e. movement
flexor
 f. carpi radialis
 f. carpi radialis muscle
 f. carpi ulnaris muscle
 deep neck f.
 f. digiti minimi brevis muscle of foot
 f. digiti minimi brevis muscle of hand
 f. digiti quinti muscle
 f. digitorum brevis muscle
 f. digitorum longus muscle
 f. digitorum profundus muscle
 f. digitorum superficialis muscle
 f. hallucis brevis muscle
 f. hallucis longus muscle
 hip f.
 f. muscle
 neck f.
 f. pollicis brevis muscle
 f. pollicis longus muscle
 f. reflex
 f. retinaculum
 f. retinaculum of forearm
 f. retinaculum of lower limb
 f. tendon
flexorum
 retinaculum musculorum f.
flexuosus
 Cymbopogon f.
flexura
flexural
flexure
 lumbar f.

flexus
 hallux f.
floating
 f. cartilage
 f. patella
 f. ribs [XI–XII]
Flood ligament
floor
flor
 f. de lis
 f. de prosepina
flora
 oral f.
Floradix Iron + Herbs
Florajen
floral water mist
Florence fennel
flores ulmariae
floribunda
 Dioscorea f.
floridum
 lignum f.
flour
 wheat f.
flow
 axoplasmic f.
 chi f.
 dural blood f.
 energetic f.
 gentle f.
 ionic f.
 f. of life force
 f. of qi
 peak f.
 peripheral blood f.
 qi f.
 f. rate
 self-regulation of blood f.
 thin f.
 venous f.
 vertebral artery f.
flower
 American cone f.
 arnica f.
 cardinal f.
 chamomile f.
 chocolate f.

F

NOTES

flower *(continued)*
    Christmas f.
    comb f.
    dagger f.
    dragon f.
    dried f.
    Easter f.
    elder f.
    f. essence
    helmet f.
    Indian f.
    jasmine f.
    jupiter f.
    lavender f.
    lime f.
    malva f.
    meadowsweet f.
    moccasin f.
    pasque f.
    passion f.
    pelican f.
    primrose f.
    f. remedy
    wild chrysanthemum f.
    wild passion f.
    yarrow f.
flowering top
flowing hyperostosis
flowmeter
flow-over vaporizer
flu
    Spanish f.
fluctuantes
    costae f. [XI–XII]
fluctuation
    cerebral spinal fluid f.
    cerebrospinal fluid f.
    f. of cerebrospinal fluid
    fluid f.
    fluid pattern f.
    lateral f.
fluid
    body f.
    cerebrospinal f. (CSF)
    extracellular f.
    extravascular f.
    f. fluctuation
    fluctuation of cerebrospinal f.
    f. fluctuation technique
    inflammatory f.
    interstitial f.
    intracellular f.
    intravascular f.

    lubricating f.
    movement of f.
    f. pattern fluctuation
    synovial f.
    yin f.
fluitantes
    costae f.
fluoridation
fluoride
fluoromethane
fluoroscope
fluoroscopic control
fluoroscopy
    video f.
fluoxetine
flush
    ascorbic acid f.
flushing
fly
    green blow f.
    f. larva
    Spanish f.
FMS
    fibromyalgia syndrome
foalswort
foam
    human fibrin f.
focal
    f. point
    f. point of concentration
focusing
    f. of breath
    f. of the conscious awareness
Foeniculum vulgare
foenum-graecum
    Trigonella f.-g.
foetida
    Cimicifuga f.
foetidum
    Dracontium f.
folate
    f. deficiency
    f. insufficiency
fold
    axillary f.
    gluteal f.
    inguinal aponeurotic f.
    interdigital f.
    opercular f.
    posterior axillary f.
    synovial f.
folding fracture
folia *(pl. of* folium)

folic acid
folinic acid
folium, pl. **folia**
folk
    f. healing
    f. medicine
    f. principle
    f. remedy
follicle
follicle-stimulating hormone (FSH)
follicular hyperkeratosis
followup organ
fomentation
fontanelle
    anterior f.
food
    f. additive
    f. allergy
    Body Language Essential
      Green F.'s
    carbohydrate-rich f.
    f. coloring
    F. and Drug Administration
      (FDA, USFDA)
    f. elimination diet
    functional f.
    Green Earth F.
    f. intolerance
    Now F.'s
    organically grown f.
    psyllium-enriched f.
    sulfur-containing f.'s
    unrefined f.
    whole f.'s
foodstuff
foot
    abductor digiti minimi muscle
      of f.
    accessory flexor muscle of f.
    f. arch
    arch of f.
    articulations of f.
    ass's f.
    ball of the f.
    bear's f.
    bird's f.
    cat's f.

dorsal fascia of f.
dorsal interossei interosseous
  muscles of f.
dorsal surface of digit of f.
dorsum of f.
dove's f.
drop f.
fibrous digital sheaths of f.
fibular margin of f.
flexor digiti minimi brevis
  muscle of f.
f. functional technique
fundiform ligament of f.
gallbladder meridian of f.
head of phalanx of hand or f.
interphalangeal joint of f.
intrinsic muscles of f.
joints of f.
kidney meridian of f.
lateral border of f.
lateral longitudinal arch of f.
lateral part of longitudinal
  arch of f.
liver meridian of f.
longitudinal arch of f.
lumbrical muscles of f.
medial arch of f.
medial border of f.
medial longitudinal arch of f.
medial part of longitudinal
  arch of f.
Morand f.
Morton f.
f. orthotic
f. orthotic device
f. placement
f. plate
f. process
pronated right f.
pronation of f.
f. pronation
f. reflexology
root of f.
short f.
sole of f.
spastic flat f.
spleen meridian of f.

F

NOTES

foot *(continued)*
    stomach meridian of f.
    f. strain
    f. supination
    supination of the f.
    synovial sheaths of digits
      of f.
    tibial border of f.
    transverse arch of f.
    tuberosity of distal phalanx of
      hand and f.
    urinary bladder meridian of f.
    weightbearing of f.
    white man's f.
    wolf's f.
football calf
footdrop
footplate
foramen, pl. **foramina**
    congenital sternal f.
    f. costotransversarium
    costotransverse f.
    exit f.
    greater sciatic f.
    internal auditory f.
    intervertebral f.
    f. intervertebrale
    lesser sciatic f.
    f. of Luschka
    f. of Magendie
    f. magnum
    mastoid f.
    f. nutricium
    nutrient f.
    obturator f.
    f. obturatum
    f. ovale
    parietal f.
    posterior condyloid f.
    f. processus transversi
    sacral foramina
    f. sacrale
    sciatic f.
    f. transversarium
    transverse f.
    f. of transverse process
    f. of vena cava
    vertebral f.
    f. vertebrale
    vertebroarterial f.
    f. vertebroarteriale
    Weitbrecht f.
foraminiferous

foraminulum
force
    activating f.
    animal f.
    compressive f.
    f. of consciousness
    coreolis f.
    corrective f.
    dark female f.
    elementary reproductive f.
    extrinsic activating f.
    extrinsic-applied thrusting f.
    extrinsic corrective f.
    flow of life f.
    guiding f.
    Immune F.
    impaction compressive f.
    inherent f.
    intrinsic activating f.
    intrinsic corrective f.
    life f.
    light male f.
    moment of f.
    pathogenic f.
    patient muscle f.
    protective f.
    pull f.
    pulsatile f.
    reserve f.
    respiratory f.
    shear f.
    springing f.
    structural f.
    thrust f.
    thrusting f.
    unifying f.
    f. vector
    vital f.
    yin f.
forcé
    redressement f.
force-counterforce
forceps
force-velocity curve
forearm
    deep fascia of f.
    dorsal f.
    fascia of f.
    flexor retinaculum of f.
    interosseous membrane of f.
    lateral border of f.
    medial border of f.

oblique cord of interosseous
  membrane of f.
posterior region of f.
posterior surface of f.
f. pronation
pronation of f.
radial border of f.
somatic dysfunction of f.
supination of the f.
f. supination
ulnar margin of f.
volar f.
forefinger
forehead
foreign body
forequarter amputation
forest mushroom
forking larkspur
form
  sustained-release f.
  tai chi f.
formaldehyde
  melamine f.
formononetin
formula
  Amara F.
  AntiAllergy f.
  ASTRA 8 f.
  Calms Forte Homeopathic F.
  Colloidal Energy F.
  cornsilk buchu f.
  DHEA Men's F.
  Dr. John R. Christopher F.
  electrical f.
  Entelev F. JS 114
  Essiac f.
  EW Herbal Eyewash F.
  Executive Stress F.
  GNC Menopause F.
  hawthorn f.
  Hayfever Homeopathic F.
  Heilig f.
  Herbal Eyebright F.
  Hoxsey f.
  KB F.
  kidney f.
  kidney tonic f.

liver f.
liver tonic f.
Macular Support F.
Men's Multiple F.
Mucolytic Drainage F.
Multigenics Intensive Care F.
Multigenics Maintenance F.
One-A-Day Energy F.
PEP F.
F. 600 Plus for Men
Quietude Homeopathic F.
Resistance Support F.
Rudolf Weiss F.
saw palmetto f.
Sheridan's F.
Traumeel Homeopathic F.
vertebral f.
Winter F.
fornicate
fornix, pl. **fornices**
forte
  AE Mulsion F.
  Bio-Cardiozyme F.
  Eugalan F.
  Gluco-Flex F.
  Infla-Zyme F.
  Intenzyme F.
  Megavital F.
  Oxy-5000 F.
  Tebonin f.
  Tentex F.
fortified cereal
fortify
forward
  f. bending
  f. bent
  f. head posture
  injury behind f.
  f. sacral torsion
  f. torsion
forward-bending
  f.-b. dynamic film
  f.-b. vertebral motion
forward-to-backward bending
FOS
  fructooligosaccharide

NOTES

153

fossa
acetabular f.
f. acetabuli
anconal f.
f. axillaris
axillary f.
Biesiadecki f.
f. condylaris
f. coronoidea humeri
f. cranii anterior
cubital f.
f. cubitalis
digital f.
glenoid f.
iliac f.
f. iliaca
iliacosubfascial f.
f. iliacosubfascialis
iliopectineal f.
infraclavicular f.
f. infraclavicularis
f. infraspinata
infraspinous f.
intercondylar f.
f. intercondylaris
intercondyloid f.
ischiorectal f.
Jobert de Lamballe f.
jugular f.
landmarks of ischiorectal f.
f. of lateral malleolus
lesser supraclavicular f.
f. malleoli fibulae
f. malleoli lateralis
mandible f.
mandibular f.
f. mandibularis
Mohrenheim f.
f. olecrani
olecranon f.
f. poplitea
popliteal f.
f. radialis humeri
f. scarpae major
subclavicular f.
subscapular f.
f. subscapularis
f. supraclavicularis minor
f. supraspinata
supraspinous f.
temporal f.
trochanteric f.
f. trochanterica

Fo-Ti
foulage
foul urine
foundation
F. for Chiropractic Education
and Research (FCER)
National Osteopathic F.
four
f. big symptoms
craniosacral vault f. (CV4)
f. diagnostic methods
f. examinations: visual
observation, listening and
smelling, questioning, and
physical
f. gates
F. Gentlemen Decoction
f. Rs
remove, replace, reinoculate,
repair
f. times a day (q.i.d.)
fourchée
main f.
four-point
f.-p. contact
f.-p. sacral motion test
fourth
f. chakra
f. finger
f. lumbar nerve [L4]
f. toe
f. ventricle of brain
f. ventricle of cerebrum
fourth-layer
f.-l. muscle
f.-l. spinal muscle
fovea, pl. **foveae**
f. articularis capitis radii
f. articularis inferior atlantis
f. articularis superior atlantis
f. capitis femoris
f. costalis inferior
f. costalis processus transversi
f. costalis superior
f. dentis atlantis
f. of the femoral head
f. femoralis
f. of radial head
foveated chest
foveola
f. coccygea
coccygeal f.
foveolar

Fowler position
foxberry
foxglove
fox's clote
FPR
  facilitated positional release
  FPR treatment
fraction
  Grifron-Pro Maitake D f.
  left ventricular ejection f.
fracture
  apophysial f.
  articular f.
  avulsion f.
  f. bed
  bending f.
  bimalleolar f.
  birth f.
  f. blister
  f. box
  boxer's f.
  capillary f.
  clay shoveler's f.
  closed f.
  closed reduction of f.
  comminuted f.
  complex f.
  compound f.
  dentate f.
  dislocation f.
  f. dislocation
  double f.
  epiphysial f.
  extracapsular f.
  fatigue f.
  fissured f.
  folding f.
  greenstick f.
  hairline f.
  hangman's f.
  impacted f.
  incomplete f.
  intertrochanteric f.
  intraarticular f.
  intracapsular f.
  linear f.
  longitudinal f.

  march f.
  multiple f.
  oblique f.
  occult f.
  f. of odontoid base
  open f.
  open reduction of f.
  parry f.
  pathologic f.
  pertrochanteric f.
  pilon f.
  segmental f.
  silver-fork f.
  simple f.
  spiral f.
  splintered f.
  spontaneous f.
  sprain f.
  stable f.
  stellate f.
  strain f.
  stress f.
  subcapital f.
  subperiosteal f.
  supracondylar f.
  torsion f.
  torus f.
  transcervical f.
  transcondylar f.
  trimalleolar f.
  tripod f.
  unstable f.
  ununited f.
fragment
  butterfly f.
fragrans
  Myristica f.
frame
framework
  body f.
  unitary person f.
francesa
  rosa f.
Frankenhäuser plexus
free
  f. border
  f. border of nail

F

NOTES

free *(continued)*
  Breeze F.
  F. & Easy Wanderer
  f. interval
  f. margin
  f. movement
  f. nerve ending
  Prost-Answer Alcohol F.
  f. radical
  f. radical damage
  Stone F.
  Stress F.
Freeda vitamin
freedom
  point of f.
  range of f.
free-form
  f.-f. amino acids
  f.-f. push hands
free-running circadian rhythm
freeze-dried
  echinacea fresh f.-d.
  f.-d. mussel
  f.-d. nettle
frena (*pl. of* frenum)
French
  F. honeysuckle
  F. lavender
  F. lilac
  F. marigold
  F. psyllium
  F. tarragon
frenulum, pl. frenula
  synovial frenula
frenulum of M'Dowel
frenum, pl. frena
  synovial frena
frequency
  high f.
  low f.
  pulse f.
frequency/intensity effect
frequency-pulling entrainment
fresh
  f. air
  f. blueberry
  f. carrot juice
  f. cell
  f. cell therapy
  f. water leech
  f. wheatgrass juice
fretting

friar's
  F. Balsam
  f. cap
friction
  dynamic f.
  f. massage
  starting f.
  static f.
Friedreich ataxia
frilosite
fringe
  synovial f.
  f. tree
  white f.
frog-leg lateral projection
frôlement
frondosa
  Grifola f.
frondosus
  Rubus f.
frons
frontad
frontal
  f. bone
  f. electromyographic feedback
  f. EMG biofeedback
  f. EMG signal
  f. margin
  f. plane
  f. posture variation
  f. section
  f. sinusitis
  f. and temporal theta wave
frontale
  os f.
frontalis
  margo f.
front-mu
  f.-m. point
frontozygomatic
frottage
frozen shoulder
FRS
  flexed, rotated, sidebent
    FRS dysfunction
    FRS position
    FRS vertebral
FRSL
  flexed, rotated, sidebent left
FRSR
  flexed, rotated, sidebent right
fructooligosaccharide (FOS)
fructose

fruit
ackee f.
ammi f.
anise f.
brier f.
chaste tree f.
colocynth f.
cranberry whole f.
dog rose f.
glaceed f.
morus f.
passion f.
f. paste
saw palmetto f.
St. Mary's thistle f.
sulfured f.
fruitarian
fruit-leather
fruit-shell
walnut f.-s.
frutescens
Capsicum f.
Perilla f.
fruticosus
Rubus f.
Fryette
F. law
F. principles I–III
FSH
follicle-stimulating hormone
FSRRL
flexion, sidebent right, rotated left
fu
gong f.
f. ling
f. mai tang
f. organ
f. peng zi
f. pen zi
xiang f.
f. xiao mai
yang ming f.
zang f.
f. zi
Fucus
F. serratus
F. vesiculosus

fuel
Ripped F.
fuge
devil's f.
fulcrum
pillow f.
Sutherland f.
fuliu
ki 7 f.
full
F. Bloom tea
f. body stretch
f. extension
F. Potency Licorice Root
Vegicaps
full-blown migraine
fuller's herb
fullness/emptiness pattern
fulminant hyperpyrexia
fulva
Ulmus f.
fumarate
dimethyl f.
ferrous f.
monoethyl f.
fumaric acid ester
fumitory
hedge f.
funcho
function
adrenal f.
circulatory f.
cognitive f.
excessive f.
fascial f.
harmonizing f.
immune f.
inadequate f.
integrated muscle f.
isomeric f.
Jebsen Test of Hand F.
mental f.
meridian f.
mitochondrial f.
muscle f.
neuroendocrine f.
neurological f.

F

NOTES

function *(continued)*
   normal f.
   proprioceptive f.
   reciprocal tension membrane f.
   renal f.
   segmental muscle f.
   synchronous f.
   trophic f.
   undisturbed f.
   visceral f.
   warming f.
   yang f.
functional
   f. anatomy
   f. brain scanning
   f. capacity
   f. contracture
   f. disorder
   f. disturbance
   f. food
   f. health problem
   f. hypertrophy
   f. indirect technique
   f. integration
   f. ligamentous balance
     technique
   f. nosology
   f. palpation exercise
   f. parameter
   f. pathology
   f. potential
   f. refractory period
   f. splint
   f. system
   f. technique
   f. treatment
   f. unit
functionality
functioning
   inadequate f.
fundi *(pl. of* fundus)
fundic
fundiform ligament of foot
fundus, pl. **fundi**

fungal infection
fungi *(pl. of* fungus)
fungicidal
fungicide
fungitoxic
fungitoxicity
fungoides
   mycosis f.
fungus, pl. **fungi**
   pasiania f.
   shelf fungi
funic
funicle
funicular
   f. myelitis
   f. myelosis
funiculus
   contralateral dorsolateral f.
   lateral f.
   posterior f.
funnel breast
furring of the tongue
furrow
   digital f.
furrowing of the tongue
furuncle
fusiform
   f. aneurysm
   f. muscle
   f. receptor
fusiformis
   musculus f.
fusimotor
fusion
   bone block f.
   spinal f.
   vertebral f.
fustigation
futu
   li 18 neck f.
Futurebiotics
fuyang

γ (*var. of* gamma)
G115
G/A
    Glandiet Powder G.
GABA
    gamma aminobutyric acid
gad
GAG
    glycosaminoglycan
      GAG synthesis
gagroot
gait
    g. analysis
    antalgic g.
    ataxic g.
    calcaneal g.
    cross-patterning of g.
    equine g.
    gluteus maximus g.
    gluteus medius g.
    helicopod g.
    hemiplegic g.
    high-steppage g.
    hysterical g.
    g. momentum
    osteoarthritis g.
    scissor g.
    shuffling g.
    stance phase of g.
    steppage g.
    swing phase of g.
    symmetrical g.
    g. training
    g. velocity
    waddling g.
galactogogue
galanga
    kaempferia g.
galangae
    rhizoma g.
galangal
galanthamine hydrobromide
Galbraith treatment
Galbreath mandibular drainage
galenical
galericulata
    Scutellaria g.
Galium
    G. *aparine*
    G. *odoratum*

gall
    elephant's g.
    oak g.
    g. weed
gallbladder
    g. channel (gb)
    damp heat in the liver and g.
    g. meridian
    g. meridian of foot
galli
    crista g.
Galloselect N
gallstone
    cholesterol g.
Galphimia glauca
GALT
    gut-associated lymphoid tissue
galvanic
    g. skin response
    g. skin response meter
galvanism
    high-volt g.
galvanometer
    d'Arsonval g.
galvanomuscular
galvanopalpation
galvanotonus
gamekeeper's thumb
gamma, γ
    g. aminobutyric acid (GABA)
    g. aminobutyric acid
      transaminase
    g. camera
    g. globulin
    g. hydroxybutyrate (GHB)
    g. linolenic acid (GLA)
    g. motor neuron
gammaglobulin
gan
    g. dan shi re
    g. di huang
    g. jiang
    g. qi yu jie
    g. shang yan
    g. xue xu
    g. yang shang kang
    g. yin xu
gang
    ba g.
ganga

G

ganglia (*pl. of* ganglion)
ganglial
gangliate
gangliform contracture
ganglioform
ganglion, pl. **ganglia, ganglions**
  aberrant g.
  autonomic g.
  basal g.
  Bock g.
  carotid g.
  celiac g.
  g. cervicale inferius
  g. cervicale medium
  g. cervicale superius
  cervicothoracic g.
  coccygeal g.
  collateral g.
  craniospinal sensory g.
  dorsal root g.
  g. geniculi
  hypogastric g.
  inferior cervical g.
  inferior mesenteric g.
  g. intermedia
  intervertebral g.
  lateral chain g.
  Laumonier g.
  g. lumbalia
  lumbar g.
  mesenteric g.
  middle cervical g.
  nerve g.
  parasympathetic g.
  paravertebral g.
  periosteal g.
  prevertebral g.
  sacral g.
  g. sacralia
  spinal g.
  g. spinale
  stellate g.
  g. stellatum
  superior cervical g.
  superior cervical g.
  superior mesenteric g.
  sympathetic g.
  sympathetic lateral chain g.
  thoracic g.
  g. thoracica
  thoracic lateral chain g.
  thoracolumbar g.

  vertebral g.
  g. vertebrale
ganglionic blockade
ganglionic-blocking effect
ganglions (*pl. of* ganglion)
ganglioplegic
ganglioside
Ganoderma lucidum
ganshu
  g. point
  ub 18 g.
Gantzer muscle
gap
  g. arthroplasty
  Bochdalek g.
gapping
  joint g.
garam masala
garance
Garcinia
  G. atriviridis
  G. cambogia
  G. indica
garden
  g. angelica
  g. basil
  g. celandine
  g. chervil
  g. cress
  g. endive
  g. fennel
  g. lavender
  g. lettuce
  g. marigold
  g. parsley
  g. patience
  g. rue
  g. sage
  g. sorrel
  g. spurge
  g. thyme
gargarizans
  Bufo bufo g.
garget
gargle
  pure tree tea oil and water g.
  witch hazel g.
garlic
  g. bulb
  g. capsule
  licorice and g.
  One-A-Day G.
  g. powder

processed g.
raw g.
g. sage
Garlic-Power
Garlique
gas
anesthetic g.
g. chromatographic-mass spectrometry (GCMS, GC-MS)
g. chromatography (GC)
laughing g.
ozone g.
Up Your G.
gaseous distention
Gasex
gastric
g. acid
g. acid secretion
g. fire
g. lavage
g. motility index
g. pacemaker
g. ulcer
g. upset
Gastricard N
gastritis
hyposecretory g.
gastrocnemii
caput laterale musculi g.
caput mediale musculi g.
gastrocnemius
g. muscle
musculus g.
gastrocsoleus muscle
Gastrodia elata
gastroenteritis
gastroenterological disorder
gastroesophageal reflux
gastrointestinal (GI)
g. bleeding
g. cancer
g. complaint
g. discomfort
g. lumen
gastroptosis
gastroscopic monitoring

gate
four g.'s
g. mechanism
spinal g.
g. theory of pain
gate-control
g.-c. hypothesis
g.-c. theory
g.-c. theory of pain
gathering qi
gatillier
gating
gato
una de g.
gaucha
nobleza g.
gaucho
gauge
gaultheria
g. oil
G. procumbens
gauntlet bandage
gauze dressing
gb
gallbladder channel
gb 26 daimai
gb 20 fengchi
gb 31 fengshi
gb 41 foot linqi
gb 37 guangming
gb 4 hanyan
gb 30 huantiao •
gb 21 jianjing
gb 25 jingmen
gb 40 qiuxu
gb 24 riyue
gb 8 shuaigu
gb 2 tinghui
gb 1 tongziliao
gb 12 wangu
gb 39 xuanzhong
gb 14 yangbai
gb 34 yanglingquan
GBE
ginkgo biloba extract
GBE 24
GB Tablets

NOTES

G

GC
  gas chromatography
GC-MS
  gas chromatographic-mass
  spectrometry
GCMS
  gas chromatographic-mass
  spectrometry
GE-132
ge
  g. gen tang
  g. shu point
  g. xian zhu yu tang
Geisteswissenschaften
gel
  All Natural Aloe Vera G.
  aloe vera g.
  Arniflora G.
  Oxy C-2 G.
  Rhuli G.
  Ssssting Stop Homeopathic G.
  Wonder G.
gelatin
  Chinese g.
  Japanese g.
  vegetable g.
gelsemium
Gelsemium sempervirens
gemellus
  g. inferior muscle
  g. muscle
  g. superior muscle
general
  g. adaptation response
  g. anatomy
  g. anesthesia
  g. anesthetic
  g. stimulant
  g. tonification point
generales
  termini g.
**generally recognized as safe
  (GRAS)**
generator
  aerosol g.
  pain g.
generic name
genetic disorder
geneticist
genetics
  advanced g.
  transplantation g.
genetotrophic disease

Gengivario
genicula (*pl. of* geniculum)
genicular
geniculate
geniculi
  ganglion g.
geniculum, pl. **genicula**
genievre
genista
genistein
genital herpes
genitalia
  external g.
  lymphatic drainage of
    external g.
genitofemoral nerve
gentian
  pale g.
  g. root
  stemless g.
  g. violet
  yellow g.
Gentiana
  G. lutea
  G. scabra
gentle
  g. flow
  g. manipulation
  g. soft tissue massage
genu
  g. recurvatum
  g. valgum
  g. varum
genual
genus
  articulatio g.
  musculus articularis g.
  rete articulare g.
George's Aloe Vera Juice
Geotran
geraniol
geranium
  G. maculatum
  G. robertianum
  rose g.
  scented g.
  wild g.
gerardiana
  Ephedra g.
Gerdy
  G. fibers
  G. ligament
  G. tubercle

geriatric massage
geriatrics
Geriforte
germ
    corn g.
    wheat g.
German
    G. chamomile
    G. lactucarium
    G. rue
    G. sarsaparilla
germander
    large-leaved g.
    wall g.
germanicum
    phu g.
germanium
germicidal
germicide
Gero Vita
Gerson diet
geshu
    ub 17 g.
geum
GH3 cream
GHB
    gamma hydroxybutyrate
ghee
ghost
    root of the Holy G.
GI
    gastrointestinal
        lower GI
        upper GI
giantism, gigantism
giant leech
gibbous
gibbus
gigantism (*var. of* giantism)
Gilead
    balm of G.
Gillenia trifoliata
Gillet test
Gincosan
Ginexin Remind
ginger
    cayenne g.

Chinese g.
Indian g.
g. peppermint combo
G. Power
g. rhizome
g. root
g. slice isolation
G. Trips
wild g.
Gingerall
gingivitis
    ulcerative g.
ginglymoarthrodial
ginglymoid joint
ginglymus
    helicoid g.
    lateral g.
Ginkai
ginkgo
    G. biloba
    g. biloba extract (GBE)
    g. biloba leaf extract
    G. Go
    g. leaf
    G. Phytosome
    G. Power
Ginkgo/Gotu Kola Supreme
Ginkgold
ginkgolide
    g. B
    g. C
    g. O
Ginkoba
ginkogink
ginkolide A
Ginkovit
Ginsana
    Neo G.
Ginsatonic
ginseng
    g. abuse syndrome
    American g.
    Asian g.
    Asiatic g.
    blue g.
    Brazilian g.
    Chinese g.

NOTES

G

ginseng *(continued)*
 g. complex
 Japanese g.
 Korean g.
 liquid g.
 Minadex Mix G.
 Oriental g.
 Panax g.
 radix g.
 g. root
 Rumanian g.
 Siberian g.
 Western g.
 women's g.
 yellow g.
ginsterkraut
girdle
 g. anesthesia
 anterior and inferior right
  shoulder g.
 joints of inferior limb g.
 joints of pectoral g.
 joints of pelvic g.
 joints of superior limb g.
 pectoral g.
 sea g.
 shoulder g.
 thoracic g.
 g. vessel
GLA
 gamma linolenic acid
glabella
glabra
 Chelone g.
 Glycyrrhiza g.
glaceed fruit
gladiate
gladiolus
gland
 accessory g.
 adrenal g.
 arteriococcygeal g.
 body of sweat g.
 brachial g.
 cervical g.
 coccygeal g.
 Gley g.
 glomiform g.
 levator muscle of thyroid g.
 meibomian g.
 parathyroid g.
 pectoral g.
 pineal g.

 sebaceous g.
 sheath of thyroid g.
 sudiferous g.
 sweat g.
 thymus g.
 thyroid g.
 Wölfler g.
Glandiet
 G. Powder G/A
 G. Powder P/T
Glandiet Supplement A
Glandiet Supplement G
Glandiet Supplement P
Glandiet Supplement T
glandula
 g. parathyroidea
 g. thyroidea
 g. thyroidea accessoria
glandulae
 g. cervicales uteri
 g. tarsales
glandular
 NZ g.
 raw pituitary g.
 raw spleen g.
 g. therapy
glandule
glass
 g. factor
 soluble g.
 water g.
glauca
 Galphimia g.
 Yucca g.
glaucoma
Glechoma hederacea
glenohumeral
 g. articulation
 g. joint
 g. joint functional technique
 g. joint glenoid labrum
  technique
 g. ligament
 g. seven step Spencer
  technique
glenoid
 g. fossa
 g. labrum of scapula
 g. labrum technique
 g. ligament
 g. surface
glenoidal lip
Gley gland

glial limiting membrane
glide
  anterior g.
  anteroposterior g.
  condylar g.
  dorsal to plantar g.
  supine condylar g.
gliding joint
glioma of the spinal cord
Globase
globeberry
globular receptor
globulin
  accelerator g.
  gamma g.
  serum g.
  serum accelerator g.
globulus
  Eucalyptus g.
globus
glomal
glome
glomera (*pl. of* glomus)
glomerular filtration rate
glomerule
glomerulonephritis
glomerulose
glomerulus
  malpighian g.
glomiform gland
glomus, pl. **glomera**
  g. body
glory
  morning g.
glossopharyngeal nerve
glossopharyngeus
  musculus g.
glucan
  beta g.
  1,3 beta g.
Gluco-Flex Forte
glucomannan
gluconeogenesis
Glucoprime
GlucosaMend
glucosamine (GS)
  g. complex

  G. Mega
  g. sulfate
glucose
  blood g.
  hypertonic g.
  g. metabolism
  g. tolerance
glucose-6-phosphate dehydrogenase
  (G6PD, G-6-PD)
Glucosim
glue
  bee g.
glutamic acid
glutamine synthetase enzyme
glutathione
  g. peroxidase
  g. peroxidase level
gluteae
  lineae g.
gluteal
  g. fold
  g. lines
  g. lymph node
  g. muscle
  g. region
  g. surface of ilium
gluten
gluten-free vegan diet
gluteofemoral bursa
gluteoinguinal
gluteus
  g. maximus
  g. maximus gait
  g. maximus muscle
  g. maximus muscle retraining
  g. medius bursae
  g. medius gait
  g. medius muscle
  g. medius muscle retraining
  g. minimus
  g. minimus bursa
  g. minimus muscle
  g. muscle
glutinosa
  Rehmannia g.
glutinosum
  Eriodictyon g.

G

NOTES

Glyc
  Feverfew G.
glycation
  protein g.
glycerine
Glycerite
  Echinacea G.
glycerol
glycine
  g. max
  zinc gluconate g. (ZGG)
glycogenolytic
glycolytic metabolic pathway
glycosaminoglycan (GAG)
glycoside
  anthroquinone g.
  cardiac g.
  digitalis g.
  flavonoid g.
Glycyrrhiza
  G. glabra
  G. palidiflora
  G. uralensis
glycyrrhizae radix
glycyrrhizin
glycyrrhizinic acid
Gnaphalium
  G. polycephalum
  G. uliginosum
GNC
  GNC Liquid Shark Cartilage
  GNC Menopause Formula
gnome's calf
go
  Ginkgo G.
  Whey to G.
goatnut
goat's
  g. milk
  g. rue
  g. thorn
goatweed
gobo
  wild g.
god
  grace of G.
  nectar of the g.'s
goddess circle
God's
  G. tree
  G. wonder plant
goiter
  iodine-deficient g.

gokshura
gold
  China G.
  g. needle
golden
  g. apple
  g. bough
  g. button
  g. grondsel
  g. ragwort
  g. rocket
  G. Salve
  g. senecio
goldenrod
  g.-horsetail compound
  sweet g.
goldenseal
  g. compress
  g. extract 4:1
  g. power
  g. root
  g. tea
goldsiegel
goldy star
golfer's elbow
Golgi
  G. tendon apparatus
  G. tendon organ
  G. tendon reflex
goma alatira
gomishi
gommelaque
gompholic joint
gomphosis
gonadal plexus
gonalgia
gonarthritis
gonarthrosis
gonarthrotomy
gonatagra
gonatocele
gong
  chi g.
  g. fu
  qi g., chi kung
gongsun
  sp 4 g.
goniometer
gonococcal arthritis
Gonolobus
  G. condurango
  G. condurango (Triana)
  nichols

gonorrhea
gonorrheal arthritis
Gonstead technique
gonycampsis
good posture
goose
    g. feather
    g. grass
    wild g.
gooseberry
    Indian g.
goosewort
Gossypium
gossypium
    Cochlospermum g.
gossypol
gotu
    g. kola
    g. kola gold extract
    g. kola herb
gouge
gout
    articular g.
    tophaceous g.
gouty arthritis
Govallo immunoembryotherapy
governing
    g. meridian
    g. point
    g. vessel (gv)
governor vessel
G6PD, G-6-PD
    glucose-6-phosphate dehydrogenase
    G6PD deficiency
    G6PD deficient
grab
    needle g.
grace
    g. of God
    herb of the g.
gracile nucleus
gracilis
    g. muscle
    g. muscle
    musculus g.
    musculus tibialis g.
    g. syndrome

gradient
    morphogen g.
    phase g.
graft
    bone g.
    dowel g.
    muscle pedicle bone g.
    tendon g.
grain
    unrefined g.
gram-negative
    g.-n. bacilli
    g.-n. bacteria
gram-positive bacteria
granadilla
granatum
grand
    g. mal epilepsy
    g. mal epileptic fit
Grande
    Aloe G.
    Chamomile G.
grandfather peyote
grandiflora
    Hydrangea g.
grandiflorum
    Epimedium g.
    Jasminum g.
    Platycodon g.
    Trillium g.
grandiflorus
    Cereus g.
    Selenicereus g.
granulation
    arachnoid g.
    tissue g.
    g. tissue
granule
    Black Draught G.'s
    Senokot G.
granulestin
grape
    bear's g.
    mountain g.
    Oregon g.
    sea g.

G

NOTES

grapeseed
    g. extract
    g. oil
grapple plant
GRAS
    generally recognized as safe
grasp
grass
    ague g.
    barley g.
    g. carp
    couch g.
    dog g.
    East Indian lemon g.
    goose g.
    moon g.
    pigeon g.
    pudding g.
    quack g.
    ripple g.
    scurvy g.
    shave g.
    spring g.
    star g.
    sweet vernal g.
    tongue g.
    wheat g.
Gratiola
gratus
    Strophanthus g.
gravel
    kidney g.
    g. root
graveolens
    Anethum g.
    Apium g.
    Pelargonium g.
    Ruta g.
gravis
    myasthenia g.
gravitational
    g. line
    g. stress
gravity
    line of g.
    g. lumbar traction
    G. Lumbar Traction system
    g. stressor
gray
    g. aura
    g. degeneration
    g. matter
    periaqueductal g. (PAG)

graybeard
greasewood
great
    g. adductor muscle
    g. bur
    g. burdock
    g. lobelia
    g. mullein
    g. scarlet poppy
    g. sciatic nerve
    g. sundew
    g. toe
    g. wild valerian
    g. wing
    g. wing of sphenoid
greater
    g. ammi
    g. celandine
    g. circulation
    g. multangular bone
    g. nettle
    g. pectoral muscle
    g. peritoneal cavity
    g. plantain
    g. prickly lettuce
    g. psoas muscle
    g. rhomboid muscle
    g. sciatic foramen
    g. sciatic notch
    g. trochanter
    g. tubercle of humerus
    g. tuberosity of humerus
    g. yang
    g. yin
Greek hayseed
green
    g. arrow
    g. blow fly
    dandelion g.'s
    g. dragon
    g. drink
    G. Earth Food
    g. endive
    G. glenoid labrum technique
    g. hellebore
    g. leafy vegetable
    g. mint
    g. oats
    poke g.'s
    g. sorrel
    g. tea
    g. tea extract (GTE)
    g. tongue

greensauce
greenstick fracture
griffe
   main en g.
Grifola frondosa
Grifron-Pro Maitake D fraction
grindelia
   hardy g.
grinding
   tooth g.
grip
   single finger g.
   g. strength
gristle
groats
groin
gromwell
grondsel
   golden g.
groove
   bicipital g.
   carpal g.
   costal g.
   interosseous g.
   intertubercular g.
   lateral bicipital g.
   Lucas g.
   medial g.
   medial bicipital g.
   musculospiral g.
   obturator g.
   popliteal g.
   Sibson g.
   spiral g.
   subclavian g.
   subcostal g.
   supraacetabular g.
   vertebral g.
gross motion testing
ground
   g. cinchona bark
   g. hemlock
   g. holly
   g. ivy
   g. juniper
   g. lily

   g. raspberry
   g. substance
grounding pad electrode
group
   blood g.
   control g.
   g. curve assessment
   g. dysfunction
   hamstring muscle g.
   quadriceps g.
   g. of ribs
growth
   appositional g.
   g. arrest lines
   g. hormone
   g. hormone secretion
   g. hormone therapy
grub
Gruber cul-de-sac
Grynfeltt triangle
GS
   glucosamine
GSR meter
gt
   drop
GTE
   green tea extract
gtt
   drops
gu
   hua g.
   g. jing tsao
   long g.
   g. sui bu
guaiac
guaiacum
   g. complex
   G. officinale
gua luo xie bai bai jiu tang
guan
guanchong
guang fangji
guangming
   gb 37 g.
guanmutong
guanyuan
   ren 4 g.

G

NOTES

guanyuanshu
 ub 26 g.
guarana
 g. gum
 g. paste
 G. Plus
 g. rush
 g. seed
guard
 Cell G.
guardian qi
guarding
 muscle g.
guar gum
Guatemala lemongrass
guayusa
 Ilex g.
guayusa leaf
guduchi
Guggal-Lip
guggulipid, gugulipid
gui
 dang g.
 g. pi tang
 g. yang tang
 g. zhi
 g. zhi tang
guide
 g. ingredient
 spirit g.
guided imagery
guideline
 therapeutic g.'s
guiding force
guilai
 st 29 g.
guild
 American Herbalists G.
 g. certification
 g. certified
Guillain-Barré syndrome
guillotine amputation
gum
 Acacia g.
 g. arabic
 g. benjamin

bleeding g.'s
Brain G.
g. dragon
guar g.
guarana g.
hog g.
karaya g.
g. myrrh
myrrh g.
g. opium
g. plant
sterculia g.
Tasmanian blue g.
g. thus
g. tragacanth
g. tree
g. turpentine
gumball
 Peace of Mind g.'s
gummatous abscess
gummifer
 Astragalus g.
 Atractylis g.
gummi tragacanthae
gum-resin
 myrrh g.-r.
gunstock deformity
Günz ligament
gut-associated lymphoid tissue
 (GALT)
gutter
 paravertebral g.
 vertebral g.
Guyon
 canal of G.
 tunnel of G.
gv
 governing vessel
gynecological
 g. disorder
 g. tumor
gynocardia oil
Gyoxylide
gypsum pillow
gypsyweed
gyrate

H7 acupuncture point
HAB 1
habena, pl. habenae
habenal
habenula, pl. habenulae
habit scoliosis
habituation to monotonous stimuli
habitus
    body h.
Hackett sacroiliac cinch belt
hacking
hackmatack
Haementeria
Hagenia abyssinica
hai
    qi h.
    h. zao
hai-erh-ch'a
Hain Pumpkin Seed Oil Caps
hair
    h. analysis
    Ultra H.
hairline fracture
Hakomi bodywork
Haldane effect
half-life
    plasma h.-l.
halisteresis
halisteretic
Haller
    H. arch
    H. insula
hallex
hallfoot
hallices (*pl. of* hallux)
hallucal
hallucination
    hypnotic h.
    stump h.
hallucinogen
    botanical h.
hallucis
    caput obliquum musculi
      adductoris h.
    caput transversum musculi
      adductoris h.
    musculus abductor h.
    musculus adductor h.
    musculus flexor brevis h.
    musculus flexor longus h.

hallus
hallux, pl. hallices
    h. dolorosus
    h. extensus
    h. flexus
    h. malleus
    h. rigidus
    h. valgus
    h. varus
halo
    h. cast
    h. traction
halosteresis
halothane-induced hepatitis
ham
hamamelis
    H. virginiana
    h. water
hamate
    h. bone
    hook of h.
hamatum
    os h.
Hamilton Rating Scale for
  Depression
hammer
    h. finger
    h. toe
hammerhead shark
Hamon No. 14
hamstring
    h. length
    h. muscle
    h. muscle exercise
    h. muscle group
    h. muscle stretch
    h. tendon
hamular
hamulus
han
    h. disturbance
    h. shi kun pi
    h. zhi gan mai
hand
    abductor digiti minimi muscle
      of h.
    accoucheur h.
    ape h.
    articulations of h.
    cleft h.

H

hand *(continued)*
    common flexor sheath of h.
    h. diagnosis
    dorsal fascia of h.
    dorsal interossei interosseous muscles of h.
    dorsal surface of digit of h.
    dorsum of h.
    extensor digitorum brevis muscle of h.
    fibrous digital sheaths of h.
    first dorsal interosseous muscle of the h.
    flat h.
    flexor digiti minimi brevis muscle of h.
    free-form push h.'s
    h. functional technique
    heart meridian of h.
    interphalangeal joint of h.
    joints of h.
    large intestine meridian of h.
    laying on of h.'s
    listening h.
    lumbrical muscles of h.
    lung meridian of h.
    monkey h.
    h. myofascial release technique
    Naeser laser home treatment program for the h.
    navicular bone of h.
    obstetric h.
    opera-glass h.
    pericardium meridian of h.
    prehensile motion of h.
    h. ratio
    h. region myofascial release technique
    sanjiao meridian of h.
    skeleton h.
    small intestine meridian of h.
    h. somatic dysfunction
    spade h.
    split h.
    synovial sheaths of digits of h.
    trident h.
    writing h.
handbag muscle
hand-eye coordination
handle
    wire webbing h.
hands-off test

hands-on
    h.-o. application
    h.-o. approach
hangman's fracture
Hanout
    Ras El H.
hanyan
    gb 4 h.
hao
    qing h.
haplocalyx
    Mentha h.
happy
    h. major
    H. Motion
hardening of the arteries
hardock
hardy grindelia
harmala alkaloid
harmonex
harmonious
    h. energy state
    h. sexuality
harmonize
harmonizing
    h. effect
    h. function
    h. influence
    h. point
harmony
    psychic h.
Harmonyl
harness
    Pavlik h.
haronga
    h. bark
    h. leaf
harp
    Jew's h.
Harpagophytum procumbens
Harris lines
hartsthorn
Harungana madagascariensis
Harvard
    H. Group Scale of Hypnotic Susceptibility (HGSHS)
    H. Group Scale of Hypnotic Susceptibility, Form A (HGSHS:A)
harvest
Harvest oil
hashish
Hatha yoga

Haus
    Salus H.
haver
haver-corn
haversian space
haw
    black h.
    sweet h.
hawkweed
    mouse-ear h.
hawthorn, hawthorne
    h. berry
    h. formula
    h. heart
    h. leaf
Hawthorne
    H. Phytosome
    H. Power
hay fever
Hayfever Homeopathic Formula
haymaids
hayseed
    Greek h.
hazel
    snapping h.
    witch h.
HCB
    hexachlorobenzene
HCl
    hydrochloride
        L-cysteine HCl
        L-lysine HCl
        L-ornithine HCl
        Yohimbine HCl
HDL
    high-density lipoprotein
he
    heart channel
        he che da zao wan
        he point
        he sea point
        he 9 shaochong
        he 8 shaofu
        he 3 shaohai
        he 7 shenmen
        he shou wu

        he 5 tongli
        he 6 yinxi
head
    anterior fibular h.
    biceps femoris muscle long h.
    biceps femoris muscle short h.
    h. carriage
    crown of h.
    h. of femur
    h. of fibula
    fibular h.
    fovea of the femoral h.
    fovea of radial h.
    h. halter cervical traction
    humeral h.
    h. of humerus
    Indian h.
    intraarticular ligament of
      costal h.
    lateral h.
    H. law
    long h.
    h. of malleus
    h. of mandible
    medial h.
    h. of metacarpal
    h. of metatarsal
    metatarsal h.
    h. mobility
    motion of radial h.
    oblique h.
    h. of phalanx of hand or foot
    phlegm affecting the h.
    posterior fibular h.
    radial h.
    h. of radius
    h. of rib
    semispinal muscle of h.
    short h.
    splenius muscle of h.
    h. of stapes
    h. of talus
    h. of thigh bone
    transverse h.
    h. of ulna
    ulnar h.

NOTES

H

173

headache
    chronic h.
    h. diary
    hemicephalgic h.
    hypotension h.
    migraine h.
    muscle-contraction h.
    shao-yang type h.
    sinusitis h.
    spinal h.
    tai-yang type h.
    tension h.
    tonic h.
    traction h.
    vascular h.
    yang-ming type h.
Headaid
heal
    h. all
    hind h.
healer
    faith h.
healing
    absent h.
    h. art
    bioenergy h.
    breath-directed inner h.
    color h.
    communal h.
    conditioned h.
    crystal h.
    deficient wound h.
    directed h.
    distant h.
    h. energy
    esoteric h.
    faith h.
    folk h.
    h. imagery
    indigenous h.
    magnetic h.
    manual h.
    h. meditation
    mental h.
    paranormal h.
    h. quality
    remote h.
    shamanic h.
    spiritual h.
    h. touch
    h. visualization
    wound h.

health
    h. enhancement counseling
    H. From the Sun
    One-A-Day Cholesterol H.
    One-A-Day Menopause H.
    One-A-Day Prostate H.
    Touch for H.
    whole life h.
heart
    h. attack
    bleeding h.
    bursting h.
    h. chakra
    h. channel (he)
    h. energy
    h. energy center
    h. failure
    h. fire
    hawthorn h.
    h. meridian
    h. meridian of hand
    mother's h.
    h. point
    h. qi
    H. Science
    sternocostal surface of h.
    h. yang xu
heart-brain synchronization
Heartcare
Heartcin
heartsease
heat
    ba gang diagnostic criteria: yin and yang, interior and exterior, deficiency and excess, cold and h.
    h. bi
    damp h.
    h. disturbance
    dry h.
    external h.
    five center h.
    inner h.
    internal h.
    kidney yin xu with empty h.
    moist h.
    h. pad
    h. stress detoxification
    h. therapy
    xue-stage h.
    yang ming h.
heat-based hydrotherapy
heather

heating
　　tissue h.
heat-type disturbance
heaven
　　key of h.
Hebe (*var. of Veronica*)
Heberden node
hectogram
hectoliter
hederacea
　　Glechoma h.
Hedera senticosa
hedge
　　h. fumitory
　　h. woundwort
hedgehog
hedgemaids
heding
　　Ex-LE 31 h.
heel
　　h. bone
　　h. jar
　　h. lift
　　h. pad
　　h. pain
　　painful h.
　　prominent h.
　　h. slide exercise
　　h. spur
　　h. strike
　　h. tendon
heerabol
hegu
　　li 4 h.
height
Heilig
　　H. formula
　　H. formula for lift therapy
heiligenwurzel
helecho macho
helenium
　　Inula h.
Helianthus annuus
heliao
　　li 19 nose h.
helical axis

helicis
　　h. major muscle
　　h. minor muscle
Helicobacter pylori
helicoid ginglymus
helicopod gait
helicopodia
heliotherapy
heliotrope
Heliotropium
helium neon laser
helix
　　large muscle of h.
hellebore
　　black h.
　　European white h.
　　false h.
　　green h.
　　swamp h.
　　white h.
Hellerwork
helmetflower, helmet flower
helotomy
helper T cell
helvetica
　　Ephedra h.
hemal
　　h. arch
　　h. spine
hemanalysis
hemangiectatic hypertrophy
hemangiomas
　　dyschondroplasia with h.
hemarthrosis
hematic
hematocrit
hematogenic oxidation therapy
hematogenous osteitis
hematologist
hematology
hematoma
　　subdural h.
hematomyelia
hematomyelopore
hematopathology
hematorrhachis
　　h. externa

NOTES

H

175

hematorrhachis *(continued)*
  extradural h.
  h. interna
  subdural h.
hematostatic
hematosteon
hematuria
hemiacrosomia
hemiarthroplasty
hemicellulose
hemicentrum
hemicephalgic headache
Hemidesmus indicus
hemilateral
hemimelia
  dysplasia epiphysialis h.
hemiparesis
  posttraumatic h.
hemiplegia
hemiplegic
  h. amyotrophy
  h. apoplexia
  h. gait
hemiseptum
hemisphere
hemispherium
hemithoracic duct
hemithoracicus
  ductus h.
hemithorax
hemivertebra
hemlock
  ground h.
  poison h.
  sweet h.
  water h.
hemochromatosis
Hemo Cleen
Hemodren Simple
hemodynamic
hemoglobin
hemology
Hemoluol
hemolytic anemia
hemopathology
hemoperfusion
  charcoal h.
hemophilic
  h. arthritis
  h. joint
hemorrhage
  cerebral h.
  trauma with h.

hemorrhagic
  h. anemia
  h. diathesis
  h. rickets
hemorrhoid
  H. Tea
hemostasis
  local h.
hemostatic collodion
hemostyptic
hemothorax
hemp
  Indian h.
  h. tree
henbane
heparin
hepatic lesion
Hepatico Tonic Pills
hepatitis
  h. A
  acute viral h.
  h. B
  h. B surface antigen
  h. C
  chronic h.
  h. C virus
  h. D
  drug-induced h.
  h. E
  halothane-induced h.
  shark cartilage-induced h.
  viral h.
hepatobiliary
hepatocellular dysfunction
hepatoencephalopathy
hepatoprotectant
hepatoprotection
Hepato-Pure
hepatotoxic
hepatotoxicity
  carbon tetrachloride-induced h.
heptaphylla
  Tabebuia h.
heracleifolia
  Cimicifuga h.
herb
  Benedict's h.
  h. bennet
  bitter h.
  blessed thistle h.
  carpenter's h.
  catnip h.
  Detox Blend Bulk H.'s

dried h.
Egyptian's h.
Eight Precious H.'s
enchanter's h.
felon h.
Floradix Iron + H.'s
fuller's h.
gotu kola h.
h. of the grace
holy h.
horehound h.
kidney tonic h.'s
king h.
loose h.
lubricative h.'s
marsh h.
meadowsweet h.
medicinal h.
moxa h.
Nu Veg goldenseal h.
parsley h.
h. Peter
h. Robert
sarothamni h.
scullcap h.
UniTea H.'s
witches' h.
woman's sexuality h.
herba
h. benedicta
h. de la pastora
h. ephedrae
h. veneris
Herbaderm
herbal
h. agent
h. bath
h. bath therapy
h. cigarette
h. decoction
H. Diuretic Complex
H. Eyebright Formula
H. Fen-Phen
h. flea-repellent pet collar
Insure H.
K'an H.'s
h. medicine

Nytol H.
h. pillow
RidgeCrest H.'s
H. Slim
h. soup
h. therapy
h. tonic
h. treatment
H. Trim
H. Uprising
h. water mist
Herbalene
herbalism
herbalist
Chinese h.
clinical h.
master h.
medical h.
herbe
christe h.
h. sacree
herb-of-grace
herbology
Herb Trade Association (HTA)
herbygrass
Hercule's club
hereditary
h. deforming chondrodystrophy
h. multiple exostoses
h. progressive
arthroophthalmopathy
h. qi
h. spinal ataxia
Hering-Breuer inflation reflex
hermeneutic circle
hermeneutics
hernia
hiatal h.
meningeal h.
muscle h.
synovial h.
hernial aneurysm
herniated
h. disk
h. intervertebral disk
h. nucleus pulposus (HNP)

NOTES

H

herniation
   central disk h.
   contained disk h.
   disk h.
   noncontained disk h.
heroin
herpanacine
herpes
   genital h.
   h. infection
   h. simplex
   h. simplex labialis
   h. simplex type I virus (HSV-I)
   h. simplex type II virus (HSV-II)
   h. simplex virus (HSV)
   h. zoster
   h. zoster infection
herpetic labialis
herrabol
hertz (Hz)
hesitancy
   urinary h.
hesperidin
Hesselbach fascia
hetastarch
heterocheiral
heterolateral
heterosynaptic facilitation
heterotopic bone
heterotropoides
   Asarum h.
Hevert-Carmin
hexachlorobenzene (HCB)
hexadactyly
hexandrum
   podophyllum h.
Hey ligament
HGSHS
   Harvard Group Scale of Hypnotic Susceptibility
HGSHS:A
   Harvard Group Scale of Hypnotic Susceptibility, Form A
hiatal hernia
hiatus
   adductor h.
   h. adductorius
   aortic h.
   esophageal h.
   inferior vena cava h.
   sacral h.

   h. sacralis
   h. saphenus
   scalene h.
   h. tendineus
   tendinous h.
   h. totalis sacralis
Hibiscus sabdariffa
hieracifolia
   Erechtites h.
Hierochloe odorata
high
   h. cholesterol
   h. colonic
   h. cranberry
   h. frequency
   h. hypnotic ability
   h. intensity
   h. lordosis
   h. mallow
   h. molecular weight polysaccharide
   h. spinal anesthesia
   h. stimulus intensity
   h. velocity low amplitude thrust technique
   h. velocity thrust technique
   h. veronica
high-density lipoprotein (HDL)
high-dose
   h.-d. nutrient therapy
   h.-d. vitamin therapy
high-frequency
   h.-f. jet ventilation
   h.-f. low-intensity analgesia
   h.-f. low-intensity electrical stimulation
   h.-f. low-intensity needling
   h.-f. low-intensity stimulation
   h.-f. stimulation
high-intensity progressive resistance training
high-performance liquid chromatography (HPLC)
high-risk model of threat perception (HRMTP)
high-steppage gait
high-velocity
   h.-v. low-amplitude (HVLA)
   h.-v. low-amplitude joint mobilization
   h.-v. low-amplitude technique
   h.-v. short-amplitude thrust
   h.-v. thrust

high-voltage pulsed current
high-volt galvanism
Higtaper
hila (*pl. of* hilum)
hilar
hillock
    seminal h.
HiLo
    H. BodyTable
    H. MultiPro table
    H. PowerTilt
    H. table
hilum, pl. **hila**
Himalayan rhubarb
Himbin
    Dayto H.
hindberry
hind heal
hindquarter amputation
hinge joint
hini
hinojo
hintsam
HIP
    Hypnotic Induction Profile
hip
    h. adductor muscle
    h. adductor muscle exercise
    h. bone
    h. capsular pattern
    h. dislocation
    drop test of h.
    h. drop test
    h. dysfunction
    h. extensor
    h. flexor
    h. flexor stretching exercise
    h. functional technique
    internal rotation with flexed
      hip muscle energy
      technique h.
    h. joint
    h. joint abduction
    h. joint adduction
    h. joint capsular pattern
    h. joint disorder
    h. joint dysfunction

    h. joint firing pattern
    h. joint play
    h. myofascial technique
    h. reduction
    retinaculum of articular capsule
      of h.
    rose h.'s
    rotator muscle of h.
    h. shift
    snapping h.
    h. somatic dysfunction
    h. synovitis
    h. tender point
    transient synovitis of h.
    triceps muscle of h.
    vitamin C with rose h.'s
hipberries
hippocastanum
    Aesculus h.
Hipposelinum
hippotherapy
hircus, pl. **hirci**
hirta
    Euphorbia h.
hirtha
    Carex h.
hirudin
    recombinant h.
    subcutaneous h.
hirudinization
Hirudo medicinalis
Hiss plantar whip
histamine
histidine
histiocyte
histocompatibility
    h. testing
Histo-Fluine P
histoincompatibility
histology
history
    psychosocial h.
hit
    direct h.
hitchhiker's thumb
hitching
    joint h.

NOTES

H

HIV
  human immunodeficiency virus
hive dross
hives
HM
  home management
HNC
  holistic nurse certification
  holistic nurse certified
    HNC examination
HNP
  herniated nucleus pulposus
hoarhound (*var. of* horehound)
hoarseness
hockle elderberry
Hodgkin disease
hog
  h. apple
  h. gum
hogberry
hogweed
hoja
  la h.
hoku-gomishi
hold
  vault h.
Holden line
holism
holistic
  h. assessment
  h. communication
  h. concept
  h. ethics
  h. massage
  h. nurse certification (HNC)
  h. nurse certified (HNC)
  h. nursing
  h. nursing diagnosis
  h. pattern
  h. yoga
hollow
  h. back
  h. bone
  bump and h.
  h. organ
holly
  box h.
  ground h.
  knee h.
  sea h.
holly-leaved barberry
holme
  sea h.

holocord
holorachischisis
holotelencephaly
holotropic breathwork
holt thistle
holy
  h. basil
  h. herb
  h. thistle
  h. weed
homalocephalous
home
  h. management (HM)
  h. training
homeopath
homeopathic
  Cinchona H.
  h. clearing
  h. growth factor
  h. immunotherapy
  h. potency
  h. remedy
  Spongia Tosta H.
  h. tincture
  h. vaccination
homeopathy
  classical h.
  isopathic h.
homeostasis
  systemic h.
homeostatic
  h. balance
  h. change
  h. effect
  h. mechanism
  h. meridian
  h. point
homeovitic medicine
HomeoViticS
homework
homing value
homocysteine
  h. pathway
  plasma h.
  plasma total h.
homolateral
homomorphic
homonomous
homonomy
homonymous
homotopic
homotoxicology
homotype

homotypic
homozygous achondroplasia
homuncular acupuncture
Honduran sarsaparilla
honey
   Oats and H.
honeysuckle
   French h.
   Jamaican h.
hong hua
hood
   dorsal h.
hoodwort
hoof
   horse h.
hook
   h. and back up
   h. of hamate
   nine h.'s
hooked
   h. bone
   h. needle
Hooke law
hoop
   sacred h.
Hoover test
Hopkins Symptom Checklist
   (HSCL)
ho point
hops
Hordeum vulgare
horehound, hoarhound
   common h.
   h. herb
   h. tea
   water h.
   white h.
horizontal
   h. axis
   h. cun
   h. extension
   h. external rotation
   h. flexion
   h. internal rotation
   h. plane
   h. plane postural
     decompensation

horizontalis
hormion
hormonal
hormone
   adrenal h.
   adrenocorticotrophic h. (ACTH)
   adrenocorticotropic h. (ACTH)
   cortical adrenal h.
   corticotropin-releasing h.
   follicle-stimulating h. (FSH)
   growth h.
   hydrophilic h.
   luteinizing h. (LH)
   melanocyte-stimulating h.
   parathyroid h.
   h. replacement therapy
   steroid h.
   stress h.
   thyroid h.
   thyroid-stimulating h. (TSH)
   thyrotropin-releasing h.
Hormozon
horn
   dorsal h.
   sacral h.
   h.'s of saphenous opening
   ventral h.
Horner syndrome
horridus
   Oplopanax h.
horse
   h. balm
   charley h.
   h. chestnut
   h. chestnut extract
   h. chestnut seed
   h. chestnut seed extract
   h. fly weed
   h. hoof
   h. savin
   yellow h.
horseheal
horsepower
horseradish root
horsetail extract
horseweed
Horsley bone wax

NOTES

H

hortensis
  Satureja h.
Hoshino exercise
host-defense agent
host resistance
hot
  h. abscess
  h. air sterilizer
  h. castor oil pack
  h. energy
  h. flash
  h. ginger tea
  h. moist pack
  h. pack
  h. pepper
  h. phlegm
  h. tub
hot/cold pattern
hot-cold tissue texture abnormality
hourglass vertebra
hourly point
housemaid's knee
houxi
  si 3 h.
Hoxsey formula
Hoyer canal
HP
  No Pain HP
HPA
  hypothalamic-pituitary-adrenal
  HPA axis
HPLC
  high-performance liquid
  chromatography
HPT
  hypothalamic-pituitary-thyroid
HR
  HR 129 Serene
  HR 133 Stress
HRMTP
  high-risk model of threat perception
HRT
  Fem Osteo HRT
HSCL
  Hopkins Symptom Checklist
H-shape vertebra
hsia ku ts' ao
hsiang
  h. dan
  h. rua
hsien mao
HSV
  herpes simplex virus

HSV-I
  herpes simplex type I virus
HSV-II
  herpes simplex type II virus
HTA
  Herb Trade Association
HTN
  hypertension
hu
  h. jian wan
  h. tao ren
hua
  h. gu
  hong h.
  jin chien h.
  kuandong h.
  h. toe jia jie point
  h. wang
hualtata
huan
  jin bu h.
huang
  h. bai
  cao ma h.
  h. di nei jing
  gan di h.
  jian h.
  h. lian
  h. lian jie tu tang
  H. Lian Su Tablets
  ma h.
  muzei mu h.
  h. qi gui zhi tang
  h. qin
  sheng di h.
  h. t'eng ken
  h. tsao
  zhi bai di h.
  zhi bei di h.
huantiao
  gb 30 h.
huatuojiaji
  Ex-B 21 h.
  h. point
huatuo point
hu-chiao
huckleberry
Hueter-Volkman principle
hui xue point
huiyin cavity
huizong
hulver
  sea h.

human
    h. cytomegalovirus
    h. ecology
    h. energy field
    h. fibrin foam
    h. immunodeficiency virus
      (HIV)
    h. response pattern
    h. thrombin
humanistic therapy
humanology
humeral
    h. artery
    h. articulation
    h. head
humerale
    caput h.
humeri (*pl. of* humerus)
humeroradial
    h. articulation
    h. joint
humeroradialis
    articulatio h.
humeroscapular
humeroscapularis
    periarthritis h.
humeroulnar
    h. articulation
    h. joint
humeroulnaris
    articulatio h.
humerus, pl. humeri
    anatomical neck of h.
    articulatio humeri
    capitulum of h.
    capitulum humeri
    caput humeri
    collum humeri
    collum anatomicum humeri
    collum chirurgicum humeri
    condyle of h.
    condylus humeri
    coronoid fossa of h.
    corpus humeri
    deltoid tuberosity of h.
    epicondylus lateralis humeri
    epicondylus medialis humeri

    fossa coronoidea humeri
    fossa radialis humeri
    greater tubercle of h.
    greater tuberosity of h.
    head of h.
    lateral border of h.
    lateral epicondyle of h.
    lesser tubercle of h.
    lesser tuberosity of h.
    little head of h.
    margo lateralis humeri
    margo medialis humeri
    medial border of h.
    medial epicondyle of h.
    neck of h.
    posterior surface of shaft
      of h.
    pulley of h.
    radial fossa of h.
    shaft of h.
    supracondylar process of h.
    surgical neck of h.
    trochlea humeri
    trochlea of h.
    tuberculum majus humeri
    tuberculum minus humeri
    tuberositas deltoidea humeri
humidity
    absolute h.
    relative h.
hummaidh
humoral
    h. immunity
    h. therapy
humor therapy
humpback
Humphry ligament
Humulus lupulus
hunchback
Huneke phenomenon
Hungarian chamomile
hunger
    narcotic h.
Hunter canal
Huntington chorea
huo
    chiang h.

NOTES

huo *(continued)*
h. lou xiao ling dan
h. ma ren
ming men h.
qiang h.
yin yang h.
husk
psyllium h.
HVLA
high-velocity low-amplitude
HVLA technique
HVLA thrusting technique
hyaline cartilage
hyaluronic acid
hyaluronidase
hybrid acupuncture
hydnocarpus oil
hydrangea
H. arborescens
H. grandiflora
mountain h.
hydrarthrodial
hydrarthrosis
intermittent h.
hydrastine
Hydrastis canadensis
hydrazine sulfate
Hydro Bonnet
hydrobromide
galanthamine h.
hydrocephalus
hydrochloride (HCl)
betaine h.
lidocaine h.
urea h.
Yohimbine h.
Hydrocil
hydrocollator pack
hydrocotyle
hydrogen peroxide
hydrokinetic
H. Vichy shower
hydromassage
hydrophilia
Aeromonas h.
hydrophilic hormone
hydrophobia
hydrosyringomyelia
hydrotherapy
cold-based h.
colon h.
external h.
heat-based h.

internal h.
h. tub
hydroxide
calcium h.
hydroxocobalamin
hydroxybutyrate
gamma h. (GHB)
5-hydroxytryptophan
hydroxyzine
hygiene
dental h.
hygienist
colonic h.
Hygl
Hylands
hymenology
hymenosepalus
Rumex h.
hyoid
hyoideum
os h.
hyopharyngeus
hyoscine poisoning
Hyoscyamus niger
hypalbuminemia
hyparterial
hypaxial
hyperabduction test
hyperacidity
hyperactive
hyperactivity
hyperacute rejection
hyperalgesia
hyperargininemia
hyperbaric
h. anesthesia
h. oxygen
h. oxygenation
h. oxygen therapy
h. spinal anesthesia
hyperbrachycephaly
hypercalcemia
hypercalciuria
Hypercalm
hypercapnia
hypercarbia
hypercholesterolemia
hyperextension
hypertrophy h.
lumbopelvic h.
hyperextension-hyperflexion injury
hyperflexion
hyperglycemia

hyperhomocystinemia
  vascular toxic h.
hypericin
hypericum
  H. 0.3
  h. extract capsule
  H. perforatum
hyperkalemia
  systemic h.
hyperkeratosis
  follicular h.
hyperkinesis
hyperlipidemia
hyperlipidemic
hyperlipoproteinemia
hyper liver yang ascending
hyperlordosis
hypermenorrhea
hypermetabolism
hypermobile joint
hypermobility
  compensatory h.
  physiologic h.
  secondary h.
  h. of segment
hypermorph
hyperosteoidosis
hyperostosis
  ankylosing h.
  h. corticalis deformans
  diffuse idiopathic skeletal h.
  flowing h.
  streak h.
hyperostotic spondylosis
hyperoxaluria
hyperoxygenation
Hyper-Oxy portable hyperbaric
  chamber
hyperphosphatasia
hyperpigmentation
hyperplasia
  benign prostatic h. (BPH)
hyperplastic osteoarthritis
hyperpyrexia
  fulminant h.
hyperresponsiveness
  bronchial h.

hypersensitivity response
hypersthenia
hypersthenic
hypersympathetic syndrome
hypertension (HTN)
  accelerated h.
  benign intracranial h.
  diastolic h.
  drug-induced h.
  essential h.
  isolated systolic h.
  labile h.
  pulmonary h.
  resistant h.
hypertensive encephalopathy
hyperthermia
  induced h.
  malignant h.
hyperthyroidism
hypertonia
hypertonic
  h. glucose
  h. muscle
hypertonicity
  muscle h.
  spine muscle h.
  trapezius muscle h.
  unilateral erector spinal
    muscle h.
  unilateral upper trapezius
    muscle h.
hypertonus
hypertrophic
  h. arthritis
  h. pulmonary osteoarthropathy
hypertrophy
  benign prostatic h. (BPH)
  h. dysfunction screening
  endemic h.
  functional h.
  hemangiectatic h.
  h. hyperextension
  left ventricular h.
  physiologic h.
  vicarious h.
hypertyrosinemia
hyperuricemia

NOTES

H

hyperuricemic syndrome
hyperventilation
hypervitaminosis
  h. A
  h. D
hyphema
hypnoanalgesia
  surgical h.
hypnosis
  American Board of Dental H.
  American Board of
    Medical H.
  American Board of
    Psychological H. (ABPH)
  American Boards of H.
  American Society of
    Clinical H.
  American Society of
    Clinical H.
  clinical h.
  dental h.
  experimental h.
  International Society of H.
  medical h.
  Society for Clinical and
    Experimental H.
hypnotherapeutic
hypnotherapist
hypnotherapy
  adjunctive h.
  clinical h.
  nonspecific h.
  specific h.
hypnotic
  h. ability
  h. analgesia
  h. behavior
  h. capacity
  h. depth measurement
  h. hallucination
  h. induction
  H. Induction Profile (HIP)
  h. induction ritual
  h. instruction
  h. mode of information
    processing
  h. performance
  h. procedure
  h. responsiveness
  h. suggestion
  h. trance
hypnotist

hypnotizability
hypoactivity
hypoallergenic
hypobaric spinal anesthesia
hypocalcemia
hypocalcification
hypocapnia
hypocarbia
hypochondriac
  h. area
  h. pain
  h. region
hypochondriaca
  regio h.
hypochondrium
hypochondroplasia
hypoderm
hypodermis
hypodynamia
hypoesthesia
hypofunction
hypogastric
  h. ganglion
  h. plexus
hypoglossal nerve
hypoglycemia
hypoglycemic
hypokalemia
hypokalemic paralysis
hypokinesis
hypokinetic disease
hypomelia
hypomobile joint
hypomobility
hypomorph
hypomotility
hypomyotonia
hyponatremia
hyponychial
hyponychium
hypoparathyroidism
  familial h.
hypophalangism
hypophosphatasia
  adult h.
hypoplastic fetal chondrodystrophy
hyposecretory gastritis
hypostatic abscess
hypostosis
hypotension
  h. headache
  induced h.

hypotensive anesthesia
hypothalamic-pituitary-adrenal
(HPA)
   h.-p.-a. axis
hypothalamic-pituitary-thyroid (HPT)
   h.-p.-t. axis
hypothalamus
hypothalamus-pituitary
hypothenar
   h. eminence
   h. muscle
   h. prominence
hypothenaris
   eminentia h.
hypothermia
   accidental h.
   moderate h.
   profound h.
   regional h.
   total body h.
hypothermic anesthesia
hypothesis
   gate-control h.
   neurological h.
   sliding filament h.

hypothyroidism
   congenital h.
hypotonia
hypotonicity
hypotonic muscle tone
hypoventilation
hypovolemia
hypoxia
   hypoxic h.
   ischemic h.
hypoxic hypoxia
hypsiloid
   h. cartilage
   h. ligament
hyssop
   wild h.
Hyssopus officinalis
hysteresis
hysterical
   h. gait
   h. joint
hysteromyoma
Hz
   hertz

NOTES

H

I
    indirect treatment
    resultant current
IAT
    immunoaugmentative therapy
iatrogenic
    i. affect
    i. drug interaction
    i. illness
IBD
    inflammatory bowel disease
IBS
    irritable bowel syndrome
ibuprofen
IC
    integrated care
ICA
    International Chiropractic
    Association
ice
    i. massage
    i. pack
    i. tongs motion
Iceland
    I. lichen
    I. moss
ichnogram
ichthyosis
ICS
    intercostal space
Ida
    bramble of Mount I.
idaeus
    Rubus i.
IDDM
    insulin-dependent diabetes mellitus
idea
    traditional i.
identifiable cause
identification
    diagnostic i.
identity
idiomuscular contraction
idiopathic
    i. bone cavity
    i. hypertrophic osteoarthropathy
    i. low back pain
    i. nocturnal urticaria
IDS 89

Ig
    immunoglobulin
IgA
    immunoglobulin A
    IgA nephropathy
    secretory IgA
IgM
    immunoglobulin M
ignatia
Ignatia amara
ILA
    inferior lateral angle
ileus
    adynamic i.
    postfracture i.
    postoperative i.
    i. tender point
Ilex
    I. aquifolium
    I. cassine
    I. guayusa
    I. paraguariensis
    I. vomitoria
ilia (*pl. of* ilium)
iliac
    i. artery
    i. bone
    i. bursa
    i. colon
    i. crest
    i. crest levelness test
    i. fascia
    i. fossa
    i. muscle
    i. muscle energy technique
    i. nervous plexus
    i. region
    i. spine
    i. tubercle
    i. tuberosity
iliaca
    crista i.
    fascia i.
    fossa i.
    tuberositas i.
iliacae
    labium externum cristae i.
    labium internum cristae i.
    linea intermedia cristae i.
iliacosubfascial fossa

iliacosubfascialis
   fossa i.
iliacum
   os i.
   tuberculum i.
iliacus
   i. minor muscle
   i. muscle
   musculus i.
ilial motion
ilii
   ala ossis i.
   corpus ossis i.
   osteitis condensans i.
iliocapsularis
   musculus i.
iliococcygeal muscle
iliococcygeus muscle
iliocostalis
   i. cervicis muscle
   i. lumborum muscle
   i. muscle
   musculus i.
   i. thoracis muscle
iliocostal muscle
iliofemoral
   i. ligament
   i. triangle
iliofemoroplasty
iliohypogastric
   i. nerve
   i. nerve entrapment
iliolumbar ligament
iliometer
iliopagus
iliopectineal
   i. arch
   i. bursa
   i. eminence
   i. fascia
   i. fossa
   i. ligament
   i. line
iliopectineus
   arcus i.
iliopsoas
   i. muscle
   musculus i.
iliopubica
   eminentia i.
iliopubic eminence
iliosacral
   i. caudad shear

   i. cephalic shear
   i. dysfunction
   i. functional technique
   i. inferior shear
   i. inflare
   i. joint
   i. joint dysfunction
   i. joint mobilization
   i. joint movement
   i. motion
   i. outflare
   i. rotated laterally
   i. rotated medially
   i. rotational dysfunction
   i. somatic dysfunction
   i. superior shear
iliosciatic notch
iliospinal
iliothoracopagus
iliotibial
   i. band
   i. band friction syndrome
   i. band syndrome
   i. tract
iliotibialis
   tractus i.
iliotrochanteric ligament
ilioxiphopagus
ilium, pl. ilia
   anterior i.
   gluteal surface of i.
   inferior i.
   inflare of i.
   left posterior i.
   os i.
   outflare of i.
   posterior i.
   right anterior i.
   sacropelvic surface of i.
   somatic dysfunction of i.
   weightbearing of i.
   wing of i.
illness
   biao i.
   external i.
   iatrogenic i.
   internal i.
   li i.
   malignant i.
   systemic i.
imagery
   anodyne i.
   guided i.

healing i.
interactive guided i.
mental i.
transpersonal i.
imaging
    magnetic resonance i. (MRI)
    i. procedure
Im-Aid
imbalance
    chi i.
    dosha i.
    emotional i.
    energetic i.
    energy i.
    metabolic i.
    muscle i.
    pitta i.
    postural i.
    posture i.
    spiritual i.
    i. test
imedeen
immediate amputation
immersion
    i. bath
    whole-body i.
immobilization
    i. technique
immortality
    plant of i.
immovable
    i. bandage
    i. joint
ImmuBoost
Immunaid
immune
    i. dysregulation
    i. dysregulation disorder
    i. enhancement
    I. Force
    i. function
    i. protein
    i. rejection reaction
    i. response
    i. stimulant
    i. system
    Target I.

immune-complex vasculitis
immune-enhancing
    i.-e. effect
    i.-e. point
    i.-e. property
immune-regulatory
immunity
    cell-mediated i.
    humoral i.
immunoaugmentative therapy (IAT)
immunocompetence
immunocompromise
immunocyte
immunodiffusion
immunodysfunction
immunoembryotherapy
    Govallo i.
immunoglobulin (Ig)
    i. A (IgA)
    i. E antiserum
    i. M (IgM)
immunological change
immunomodulation
immunomodulatory
Immuno-Nourish
immunoreactivity
    type I immediate i.
    type IV delayed i.
immunoresponsive
immunostimulant
immunostimulation
immunosuppressant
immunosuppression
immunotherapy
    homeopathic i.
    venom i.
immunotonic mushroom
impact
    I. of Events Scale
impacted fracture
impaction compressive force
impairment rating
imperfecta
    osteogenesis i.
impersistence
    motor i.

NOTES

Pain Disability I. (PDI)
pelvic i.
ponderal i.
Röhrer i.
i. of suspicion
therapeutic i.
tibiofemoral i.
India
  mora de la I.
Indian
  I. apple
  I. arrowwood
  I. balm
  I. balsam
  I. berry
  I. chakra system
  I. dye
  I. elm
  I. flower
  I. ginger
  I. gooseberry
  I. head
  I. hemp
  I. indigo
  I. medicine
  I. mulberry
  I. mustard
  I. paint
  I. pennywort
  I. pink
  I. plantago
  I. plantago seed
  I. poke
  I. saffron
  I. sage
  I. shamrock
  I. snakeroot
  I. squill
  I. tobacco
  I. tragacanth
  I. turmeric
  I. valerian
  I. water navelwort
indica
  Azadirachta i.
  Cannabis i.
  Garcinia i.

Tamarindus i.
Urginea i.
indication
  acupuncture i.
indicator muscle
indices (*pl. of* index)
indicis (*gen. of* index)
indicum
  Nerium i.
indicus
  Cocculus i.
  Hemidesmus i.
indigenous healing
indigestion
  aluminum free i.
  I. Mixture
Indigo
  I. fera
  I. tinctoria
indigo
  common i.
  false i.
  Indian i.
  i. weed
  wild i.
  yellow i.
indirect
  i. action technique
  i. balance procedure
  i. barrier
  i. energy
  i. infrared radiation
  i. intersegmental motion testing
  i. ligamentous balance
    technique
  i. method
  i. method joint mobilization
  i. motion technique
  i. moxibustion
  i. moxibustion with ginger
    slice isolation
  i. moxibustion with moxa
    cigar
  i. OMT
  i. technique
  i. treatment (I, IND)

NOTES

individuality
    biochemical i.
individual vertebral motion testing
indomethacin
induced
    i. apnea
    i. hyperthermia
    i. hypotension
    i. motion
induction (IND)
    hypnotic i.
    i. process
    qigong i.
    waking hypnotic i.
industrial accident
infantile idiopathic scoliosis
infarct
    bone i.
infarction
    cardiac i.
    cerebral i.
    circadian pattern of onset of
       myocardial i.
    myocardial i. (MI)
infection
    candida i.
    Epstein-Barr viral i.
    fungal i.
    herpes i.
    herpes zoster i.
    pyogenic i.
    stomatologic i.
    upper respiratory i. (URI)
    upper respiratory tract i.
    urinary i.
    urinary tract i. (UTI)
    viral i.
infectious arthritis
inferior
    apertura thoracis i.
    arcus palpebralis i.
    i. border
    i. border of mandible
    i. branch
    i. cervical ganglion
    i. extensor retinaculum
    extremitas i.
    i. extremity
    i. facet joint
    fovea costalis i.
    i. gemellus muscle
    i. hypogastric plexus
    i. ilium

    i. lateral angle (ILA)
    i. lateral angle of sacrum
    i. lateral angle test
    i. limb
    linea glutea i.
    i. margin
    margo i.
    i. mesenteric ganglion
    musculus gemellus i.
    musculus obliquus capitis i.
    musculus serratus posterior i.
    musculus tarsalis i.
    i. nuchal line
    pars i.
    i. part
    i. petrosal sinus
    i. pole
    i. posterior serratus muscle
    i. pubic dysfunction
    i. pubis
    i. radioulnar joint
    i. retinaculum of extensor
       muscles
    right symphysis i.
    i. sagittal sinus
    spina iliaca anterior i.
    spina iliaca posterior i.
    i. subtendinous bursa of biceps
       femoris
    i. tarsal muscle
    i. temporal line
    i. thyroid tubercle
    i. tibiofibular joint
    i. transverse axis
    i. transverse scapular ligament
    i. trunk of brachial plexus
    i. ulnar collateral artery
    i. vena cava hiatus
    i. zygapophysial joint
inferioris
    articulationes cinguli membri i.
    cingulum membri i.
    ossa membri i.
    regiones membri i.
    retinaculum musculorum
       flexorum membri i.
inferius
    ganglion cervicale i.
    membrum i.
    retinaculum musculorum
       extensorum i.
    segmentum renale anterius i.
    trigonum lumbale i.

inferno
infertility
infiltration
 i. anesthesia
 trigger point i.
inflammable
inflammation
 chronic i.
 exudative i.
 fibrinopurulent i.
 fibrinous i.
 ocular i.
 purulent i.
 serofibrinous i.
 serous i.
 suppurative i.
 urinary tract i.
inflammatory
 i. alteration
 i. arthritis
 i. bowel disease (IBD)
 i. fluid
 i. joint disease
 i. process
 i. vascularization
inflare
 iliosacral i.
 i. of ilium
 right innominate i.
inflata
 Lobelia i.
inflatable splint
inflatum
 Rapuntium i.
Infla-Zyme Forte
influence
 external climatic i.
 external cold i.
 external wind i.
 harmonizing i.
 pathogenic i.
 pathogenic wind i.
influential
 i. point
 i. point of blood
 i. point of the bone
 i. point of the marrow

 i. point of tendon
 i. point of the vessel
influenza
 Spanish i.
 i. virus
information
 afferent i.
 inhibitory i.
 i. processing
 i. transfer
Informed Nutrition Shark Cartilage
infraaxillary
infraclavicular
 i. fossa
 i. triangle
infraclavicularis
 fossa i.
 regio i.
infracortical
infracostal
infracostalis
 musculus i.
infraction
infracture
infraglenoid
 i. tubercle of scapula
infrahyoid node technique
inframarginal
infraorbital
infrapatellar bursitis
infrapatellare
 corpus adiposum i.
infrapatellaris
 plica synovialis i.
infrared
 i. heat lamp
 i. laser
 i. microscope
 i. moxibustion
 i. radiation
infrared-beam diode laser
infrascapularis
 regio i.
infrascapular region
infraspinata
 fossa i.

NOTES

infraspinatus
  i. fascia
  i. muscle
  musculus i.
infraspinous fossa
infrasternal angle
infrasternalis
  angulus i.
infratonic QGM
infundibula
infundibular
infundibuliform
infundibulum
infusion
  lyophilized i.
infusion-aspiration drainage
ingredient
  adjutant i.
  assistant i.
  associate i.
  deputy i.
  envoy i.
  guide i.
ingrowing toenail
ingrown nail
inguinal
  i. aponeurotic fold
  i. ligament
  i. ligament tender point
inguinalis
  falx i.
inhalation
  i. analgesia
  i. anesthesia
  i. anesthetic
  caught in i.
  i. phase
  i. restriction
  i. rib
  steam i.
  i. therapy
  voluntary i.
inhaler
inherent
  i. body rhythm
  i. bone motility
  i. force
  i. mobility
  i. mobility of brain and spinal cord
  i. motion
  i. movement
  i. tissue motion

inhibited
  i. excited
  i. gluteus muscle
  i. muscle symptoms
  i. rectus abdominis muscle
  i. tibialis anterior muscle
inhibition
  competitive i.
  feedback i.
  postsynaptic i.
  presynaptic i.
  reciprocal i.
  recurrent i.
  reflex i.
  serotonin reuptake i.
  soft muscle i.
  soft tissue i.
inhibitor
  dopa decarboxylase i.
  MAO i.
  monoamine oxidase i.
inhibitory
  i. feedback loop
  i. information
  i. myofascial technique
  i. terminal
inion
initiate muscle action
injectable medication
injection
  diagnostic i.
  intracavitary i.
  intrathecal i.
  liver extract i.
  sacroiliac i.
  sclerosant i.
  i. technique
  i. therapy for trigger points
  trigger point i.
injury
  i. above downward
  i. before backward
  i. behind forward
  i. below upward
  closed-head i.
  degloving i.
  facial i.
  fascial i.
  flexion-extension i.
  flexion-extension cervical i.
  hyperextension-hyperflexion i.
  i. left to right
  pneumatic tire i.

reperfusion i.
repetitive strain i. (RSI)
repetitive stress i. (RSI)
i. right to left
sacroiliac joint i.
soft tissue i.
sports i.
traumatic brain i. (TBI)
whiplash i.
inkberry
inlay
inlet
    thoracic i.
innate intelligence
inner
    i. bark
    i. core
    i. heat
    i. malleolus
    i. strength
    I. Voice tea
Innerfresh Pro
innermost intercostal muscle
innervate
innervation
    autonomic i.
    bladder i.
    cutaneous i.
    diaphragm i.
    dural i.
    i. of female pelvis
    nasal sinus i.
    reciprocal i.
    segmental i.
    sympathetic i.
    temporomandibular ligament i.
    i. of thorax
innominatal
innominate
    i. anatomy
    anteriorly rotated i.
    anteriorly rotated right i.
    i. axis
    i. bone
    i. flare
    left posterior i.
    i. motion testing

posteriorly rotated left i.
right anterior i.
rotated i.
shear of i.
i. shear
i. shear dysfunction
i. shear technique
upslipped i.
i. vein
innominatum
    os i.
Inokiton
inorganic germanium dioxide
inosine prabonex
Inosiplex
inositol nicotinate
inotropic
inquiline parasite
INR
    international normalized ratio
inscription
    tendinous i.
inscriptio tendinea
insertion
    aponeurosis of i.
    depth of needle i.
    fast method of i.
    oblique i.
    perpendicular i.
    separation of muscle origin
      and i.
    slow i.
    slow method of i.
    tangential i.
    tendon i.
Insight tea
insole
    magnetic i.'s
insoluble fiber
insomnia
    Self-Rating of I.
    sleep onset i.
inspiration
    i. rib isometrics
    i. rib stretch
instability
    vasomotor i.

NOTES

instantaneous axis of rotation
instep
instillation of anesthetic
institute
    National Heart, Lung, and
      Blood I. (NHLBI)
instruction
    hypnotic i.
    task motivational i.
instrument
    Profile of Mood State i.
instrumentation
    American Association for
      Medical I. (AAMI)
    biofeedback i.
    feedback i.
insufficiency
    cardiac i.
    cerebral i.
    folate i.
    muscle i.
insufflate
insufflation anesthesia
insufflator
insula
    Haller i.
insular
insulin
    i. deficiency
    i. sensitivity
    i. shock
insulin-dependent diabetes mellitus
  (IDDM)
insult
    cerebral i.
Insure Herbal
intake
    caloric i.
integral
    i. traditional Chinese medicine
      (ITCM)
    I. yoga
integrate
integrated
    i. care (IC)
    i. muscle function
    i. neuromusculoskeletal release
    i. unit
integrating chakra
integration
    energy i.
    i. of fascia

functional i.
I. of Natural Systems Theory
neuromuscular i.
postural i.
Rolfing movement i.
soma neuromuscular i.
structural i.
Trager psychophysical i.
integrative
    i. breathwork
    i. health care
    i. massage
    i. medicine
    i. physician
integrifolium
    Parthenium i.
integrity
    structural i.
integument
integumentary
integumentum commune
intelligence
    innate i.
intensify
intensity
    contraction i.
    current i.
    current/voltage i.
    EA i.
    high i.
    high stimulus i.
    i. knob
    low i.
    milliwatt i.
    mW i.
    voltage i.
intensive
    i. cooperation
    i. manipulation
intention
intentional touch
Intenzyme Forte
interaction
    drug i.
    drug-herb i.
    iatrogenic drug i.
    mind-body i.
interactive guided imagery
interannular
interarticular
    i. fibrocartilage
    i. joint

I

interarticularis
fibrocartilago i.
pars i.
interbody
intercalated
intercanalicular
intercarpal
i. joint
i. ligament
intercarpales
articulationes i.
intercartilaginous
intercavernous
intercellular communication
intercentral
intercessor
intercessory prayer
interchondral
i. articulation
i. joint
interchondrales
articulationes i.
interclavicular
i. ligament
i. notch
intercoccygeal
intercolumnar
i. fasciae
i. fiber
intercondylar
i. eminence
i. fossa
i. line of femur
i. tubercle
intercondylaris
eminentia i.
fossa i.
intercondyloid
i. fossa
i. notch
intercondyloidea
eminentia i.
interconnectedness
interconnection
intercornual ligament
intercostal
i. anesthesia

i. arteries
i. ligament
i. membrane
i. muscle
i. nerve entrapment
i. neuralgia
i. space (ICS)
intercostale
spatium i.
intercostales
membranae i.
intercostohumeral
intercostohumeralis
intercristal
intercrural fibers of superficial ring
intercuneiform
i. joint
i. ligament
interdigit
interdigital
i. fold
interdigitalis
plica i.
interface
electrode-to-skin i.
structure-function i.
interfemoral
interference field
interferential
i. current
i. electrotherapy
interior
i. cold
interior/exterior pattern
interischiadic
interlamellar
interleukin
interleukin-1
interlobar
interlobular
intermalleolar
intermaxillary suture
intermedia
crista sacralis i.
ganglion i.
pars i.
intermediary

NOTES

199

intermediate
  i. amputation
  i. cuneiform bone
  i. great muscle
  i. lacunar node
  i. line of iliac crest
  i. part
  i. sacral crest
  i. vastus muscle
intermediolateral cell column
intermedium
  os i.
  os cuneiforme i.
intermedius
  i. muscle
  musculus vastus i.
  vastus i.
intermembranous
intermetacarpales
  articulationes i.
intermetacarpal joint
intermetameric
intermetatarsal
  i. articulation
  i. joint
intermetatarsales
  articulationes i.
intermetatarseum
  os i.
intermittens
  dyskinesia i.
intermittent
  i. arthralgia
  i. claudication
  i. hydrarthrosis
intermuscular
  i. gluteal bursa
  i. septum
intermusculare
  septum i.
interna
  hematorrhachis i.
  membrana intercostalis i.
internal
  i. agitation
  i. auditory foramen
  i. carotid artery
  i. carotid nerve
  i. chi
  i. collateral ligament of the wrist
  i. disturbance
  i. fixation

  i. heat
  i. hydrotherapy
  i. illness
  i. intercostal membrane
  i. intercostal muscle
  i. jugular vein
  i. lip of iliac crest
  i. malleolus
  i. medicine
  i. milieu
  i. oblique muscle
  i. obturator muscle
  i. qigong
  i. rotation with flexed hip muscle energy technique hip
  i. rotation with neutral hip muscle energy technique
  i. rotator muscle
  i. semilunar fibrocartilage of knee joint
  i. viscera
internally
  liver wind moving i.
internasal suture
international
  I. Chiropractic Association (ICA)
  i. normalized ratio (INR)
  I. Prostate Symptom Score (IPSS)
  I. Society of Hypnosis
  i. unit (IU)
interneuron
internum
  perimysium i.
internus
  musculus intercostalis i.
  musculus obturator i.
  musculus thyroarytenoideus i.
  musculus vastus i.
interobserver error
interosseal
interossei
  musculi i.
interosseous
  i. border
  i. border of fibula
  i. border of radius
  i. border of tibia
  i. border of ulna
  i. bursa of elbow
  i. cartilage
  i. crest

i. cuneocuboid ligament
i. cuneometatarsal ligament
i. fascia
i. groove
i. groove of calcaneus
i. groove of talus
i. margin
i. membrane of forearm
i. membrane of leg
i. metacarpal ligament
i. metacarpal space
i. metatarsal ligament
i. metatarsal space
i. muscle
i. sacroiliac ligament
i. talocalcaneal ligament
i. tibiofibular ligament
interosseus, pl. **interossei**
    margo i.
interpectoral lymph node
interpediculate
interpeduncular
interphalangeal
    i. articulation
    i. joint
    i. joint of foot
    i. joint of hand
interposition arthroplasty
interpromotion
interproximal
interpubic disk
interpubicus
    discus i.
interradial
interradicular septa of maxilla and
   mandible
interrelationship
    structure-function i.
interscalene triangle
interscapular
interscapulothoracic amputation
interscapulum
intersciatic
intersectio, pl. **intersectiones**
    i. tendinea
intersection
    tendinous i.

intersegmental
    i. motion
    i. motion testing
interseptal
interseptum
interspace
interspinal
    i. line
    i. muscle
    i. plane
interspinale
    planum i.
interspinales
    i. lumborum muscle
    musculi i.
interspinalis
    linea i.
interspinous
    i. ligament
    i. space
interstice
interstitial
    i. cystitis
    i. fibrosis
    i. fluid
    i. fluid colloid osmotic
      pressure
    i. fluid pressure
    i. lamella
interstitium
intertarsal
    i. articulation
    i. joint
intertarseae
    articulationes i.
intertendineus
    conexus i.
intertendinous connections of
   extensor digitorum
intertragic notch
intertransversalis
intertransversarii
    i. laterales musculi
    i. mediales lumborum musculi
    i. muscle
    musculi i.

NOTES

intertransverse
  i. ligament
  i. muscle
intertrochanteric
  i. crest
  i. fracture
  i. line
intertrochanterica
  crista i.
  linea i.
intertubercular
  i. groove
  i. line
  i. plane
  i. sulcus
  i. tendon sheath
intertuberculare
  planum i.
intertubercularis
  linea i.
  sulcus i.
intertubular
interval
  free i.
intervening muscle
intervenous tubercle of right
  atrium
intervention
intervertebral
  i. canal
  i. cartilage
  i. derangement
  i. disk
  i. foramen
  i. ganglion
  i. motion
  i. notch
  i. symphysis
intervertebrale
  foramen i.
intervertebralis
  anulus fibrosus disci i.
  calcinosis i.
  discus i.
  fibrocartilago i.
  symphysis i.
intervillous
interzonal mesenchyme
Intestaprime
intestinal
  i. absorption
  i. biosis

  i. motion
  i. mucosa
intestine motility
intimal tear
intimus
  musculus intercostalis i.
intoe
intolerance
  carbohydrate i.
  food i.
intortor
intoxication
  mushroom i.
intraarticular
  i. cartilage
  i. fracture
  i. ligament of costal head
  i. orgotein
  i. sternocostal ligament
intrabuccal wound
intracanalicular
intracapsular
  i. ankylosis
  i. fracture
  i. ligament
intracarpal
intracartilaginous
intracavitary injection
intracelial
intracellulare
  Mycobacterium i.
intracellular fluid
intracerebroventricular
intracorporeal
intracostal
intracranial
  i. bleed
  i. congestion
  i. membrane
  i. mobility
  i. part of vertebral artery
  i. pressure
intractable pain
intracutaneous
intrad
intradermal
intraduct
intrafascicular
intrafusal fiber
intraglandular
intraligamentous
intralobar
intralobular

...

I

intralocular
intraluminal
intramedullary
  i. anesthesia
  i. reamer
intrameningeal
intramural bleeding
intramuscular
  i. B$_{12}$
  i. trigger point
intranasal anesthesia
intraobserver error
intraocular pressure
intraoral
  i. anesthesia
  i. muscle
intraosseous
  i. anesthesia
  i. fixation
intraosteal
intraparietal
intrapsychic stressor
intrarrhachidian
intraspinal
  i. anesthesia
  i. membrane mobility
intraspinous muscle
intrastromal
intrasynovial
intratarsal
intratendinous bursa of elbow
intrathecal injection
intrathoracic
intrathyroid cartilage
intratracheal
  i. anesthesia
  i. intubation
  i. tube
intratubal
intratubular
intrauterina
  rachitis i.
intravaginal electrical stimulation
intravascular fluid
intravenous (IV)
  i. anesthesia
  i. anesthetic

i. bolus
i. drip
i. nutrient therapy
i. overdose
i. regional anesthesia
i. vitamin C
intravitreous
intrinsic
  i. activating force
  i. chi
  i. chi method
  i. corrective force
  i. muscle
  i. muscle
  i. muscles of foot
introducer
introflection
introitus
intubate
intubation
  blind nasotracheal i.
  endotracheal i.
  intratracheal i.
  nasotracheal i.
  orotracheal i.
  tracheal i.
intubator
intuition
  transcendent i.
intumescence
intumescent
intumescentia lumbosacralis
intybus
  Chicorium i.
  Cichorium i.
Inula helenium
invasion
  wind-cold i.
  wind-heat i.
invasive procedure
Inventory
  Beck Anxiety I.
  Beck Depression I. (BDI)
  California Personality I. (CPI)
  Daily Stress I.
  Eysenck Personality I.
  Meyers Briggs I.

NOTES

Inventory *(continued)*
    Minnesota Multiphasic
      Personality I. (MMPI)
    NEO Personality I.
    Neuroticism, Extroversion, and
      Openness Personality I.
    State-Trait Anxiety I.
    Wickram Experience I.
inverse
    i. correlation
    i. stretch reflex
inversion-eversion
inverted talus
invertor
investigational new drug (IND)
investing
    i. cartilage
    i. fascia
    i. layer of cervical fascia
investment
    aponeurosis of i.
invisible infrared laser
involucrum, involucre, pl. **involucra**
involuntary
    i. component
    i. mechanism
    i. motion
    i. movement
    i. nutation-counternutation
      movement
iodine
    Kelp Natural I.
    molecular i.
iodine-deficient goiter
iodophor
iodum
ion
    ammonium i.
ionic
    i. flow
    i. migration
ionized magnesium
IPA
    independent practice association
ipecac syrup
ipecacuanha
    Cephaelis i.
ipe roxo
Ipomoea purpurea
ipsilateral flexor reflex
IPSS
    International Prostate Symptom
      Score

Iridin
iridology
iris
    wild i.
Irish
    I. broom top
    I. moss
    I. moss extract
Irisin
Iris versicolor
iron cookware
iron-deficiency anemia
irradiate
irradiation
    laser i.
irregular
    i. bone
    i. channel
irregulare
    os i.
irresuscitable
irreversible
    i. condition
    i. reaction
irrigation
    bladder i.
    colonic i.
    drip-suck i.
irritability
    electric i.
    myotatic i.
irritable
    i. bladder
    i. bowel
    i. bowel syndrome (IBS)
irritation
    sciatic nerve i.
Iscador
ischemia
    muscle i.
    postural i.
    vertebrobasilar i.
ischemic
    i. heart disease
    i. hypoxia
    i. lumbago
    i. muscular atrophy
    i. myocardium
    i. pain
ischia (*pl. of* ischium)
ischiadic
    i. plexus
    i. spine

ischiadica
spina i.
ischiadicum
tuber i.
ischiadicus
ischial
i. bone
i. bursa
i. bursitis
i. ramus
i. spine
i. tuberosity
i. tuberosity level test
ischialgia
ischiatic notch
ischii
corpus ossis i.
os i.
ischioanal
ischiobulbar
ischiocapsular ligament
ischiocavernosus
ischiocavernous
ischiococcygeal
ischiococcygeus muscle
ischiocondylar part
ischiodynia
ischiofemoral ligament
ischiofibular
ischiogluteal bursitis
ischionitis
ischiopagus
ischioperineal
ischiopubic ramus
ischiorectal fossa
ischiosacral
ischiotibial
ischiovaginal
ischiovertebral
ischium, pl. **ischia**
body of i.
tuber of i.
isinglass
Japanese i.
island
bone i.

islandica
Cetraria i.
islet
isobaric spinal anesthesia
isodactylism
isode
isoflavone
isokarpalo
isokinetic
i. exercise
i. muscle strength
i. resistance
isolated systolic hypertension
isolation
ginger slice i.
indirect moxibustion with
ginger slice i.
moxibustion with ginger
slice i.
isoleucine
isolytic
i. contraction
i. muscle contraction
i. procedure
isomeric function
isometric
i. contraction
i. exercise
i. muscle contraction
i. muscle strength
i. relaxation
i. resistance
i. stabilizing exercise
i. strengthening position sitting
i. therapy
i. traction
isometrics
inspiration rib i.
isomorphism
isoPAG
phenylacetylisoglutamine
isopathic homeopathy
isopathy
isoprinosine
IsoProtein Plus
isoproterenol
isorhamnetin

NOTES

isothiocyanate
    phenethyl i. (PEITC)
isotonic
    i. contraction
    i. exercise
    i. muscle contraction
    i. traction
isotretinoin
ispaghula
    i. seed
    i. seed-shell
ISP Nutrition
isthmic spondylolisthesis
isthmus
itch-weed
ITCM
    integral traditional Chinese medicine
iter

iteral
ITO
    ITO laser pen
Ito needle
IU
    international unit
IV
    intravenous
        IV phentolamine test
        IV regional block
ivory vertebra
ivy
    ground i.
    poison i.
ixine
    Kramena i.
Iyengar-style yoga

jaborandi
    pernambuco J.
    Pilocarpus j.
    J. tree
Jacob's
    J. ladder
    J. staff
Jacobson relaxation technique
Jacuzzi
Jade Screen Immune Tonic
jaguar
jalap
    cancer j.
    j. resin
    true j.
Jamaica
    J. pepper
    J. quassia
Jamaican
    J. dogwood
    J. honeysuckle
    J. sarsaparilla
jamba
jambolana
    Eugenia j.
jambolanum
    Syzygium j.
jambolao
jambool
jambu
jambul
jambula
jambulon plum
Jamestown weed
jamguarandi
Janda
    J. lower crossed syndrome
    scientific-clinical theory of J.
    J. upper crossed syndrome
Japanese
    J. gelatin
    J. ginseng
    J. isinglass
    J. meridian acupuncture
    J. method
Japa yoga
japon
    colle du j.
japonica
    Chaenomeles j.

Cydonia j.
Eriobotrya j.
Lonicera j.
japonicus
    Ophiopogon j.
jar
    heel j.
jasmine flower
Jasminum
    J. grandiflorum
    J. sambac
Jason Winter's Tea Tree oil
jathar agni
jaundice
    j. berry
    j. root
java plum
jaw
    fibrous dysplasia of j.'s
Jazzercise
JCAHO
    Joint Commission on Accreditation
    of Healthcare Organizations
Jebsen Test of Hand Function
Jeco-peptol
jejuni
    Campylobacter j.
jejunum
jelly
    aloe vera j.
    petroleum j.
    queen bee j.
    royal j.
jen chung
jenn
    j. mai
    j. mo
jequirity seed
jerk finger
jerky
    j. end feel
    j. feel
Jerusalem
    J. Balsam
    J. cowslip
    J. sage
jessamine
    j. rhizome
    j. yellow

J

Jesuit's
    J. bark
    J. tea
jet
    j. lag
    j. nebulizer
jewelry
    magnetic j.
jewelweed
Jew's
    J. harp
    J. myrtle
ji
    bai j.
    fang j., fangji
    j. ming san
    j. xue teng
jiache
    st 6 j.
jiachengjiang
    Ex-HN 5 j.
jiang
    gan j.
    j. huang turmeric
    shan sheng j.
    yi guan j.
jian huang
jianjing
    gb 21 j.
jianliao
    sj 14 j.
jianshe
    pe 5 j.
jianyu
    li 15 j.
jianzhen
    si 9 j.
jiao
    e j.
    ling yang j.
    lower j.
    middle j.
    san j.
    shui niu j.
    xi j.
    yu niu j.
jiaoxin
    ki 8 j.
jie
    gan qi yu j.
jiexi
    st 41 j.
jiggling hands syndrome

jihva
Jim's Juice
jimson weed
jin
    j. bu huan
    J. Bu Huan Anodyne tablet
    j. chien hua
    j. gui shen qi tang
    J. Shin Acutouch
    j. shin do
    J. Shin Do Bodymind
        Acupressure
    j. shin jyutsu
    j. ye
jing
    j. deficiency
    deficiency of kidney j.
    huang di nei j.
    kidney j.
    j. point
    j. qi
    j. wei tang
    j. well point
    yang ming j.
    j. yin zi
jingbamai
    qi j.
jinggu
jing-luo
    j.-l. system
jingmen
    gb 25 j.
jingming
    ub 1 j.
jiu
    zhen j.
    j. zi
jiuwei
    ren 15 j.
jizhong
    du 6 j.
Jnana yoga
Jobert de Lamballe fossa
jobi
    Coix lachryma j.
Joe-pye weed
Joe Weider
Johnny-jump-up
joint
    acromioclavicular j.
    ankle j.
    arthrodial j.

articular disk of
  acromioclavicular j.
articular disk of distal
  radioulnar j.
articular disk of
  sternoclavicular j.
asymmetrical j.
atlantoaxial j.
atlantooccipital j.
ball and socket j.
biaxial j.
bicondylar j.
bilocular j.
j. block
j. blockage
j. branch
calcaneocuboid j.
capitular j.
capsular portion of sacroiliac j.
j. capsule
j. capsule barrier
carpal j.
carpometacarpal j.
cartilaginous j.
Chopart j.
j. click
Clutton j.
coccygeal j.
J. Commission on
  Accreditation of Healthcare
  Organizations (JCAHO)
composite j.
compound j.
condylar j.
costochondral j.
costosternal j.
costotransverse j.
costovertebral j.
cotyloid j.
Cruveilhier j.
cubital j.
cuboideonavicular j.
cuneocuboid j.
cuneometatarsal j.
cuneonavicular j.
diarthrodial j.
digital j.

distal interphalangeal j.
distal radioulnar j.
distal tibiofibular j.
j. distraction
j. dysfunction
elbow j.
ellipsoidal j.
enarthrodial j.
extravertebral j.
facet j.
J. Factors
false j.
femoroacetabular j.
femoropatellar j.
femorotibial j.
fibrous j.
j. fir
flail j.
j.'s of foot
j.'s of free inferior limb
j.'s of free superior limb
j. gapping
ginglymoid j.
glenohumeral j.
gliding j.
gompholic j.
j.'s of hand
j.'s of head of rib
hemophilic j.
hinge j.
hip j.
j. hitching
humeroradial j.
humeroulnar j.
hypermobile j.
hypomobile j.
hysterical j.
iliosacral j.
immovable j.
incudomalleolar j.
inferior facet j.
j.'s of inferior limb girdle
inferior radioulnar j.
inferior tibiofibular j.
inferior zygapophysial j.
interarticular j.
intercarpal j.

NOTES

joint (*continued*)
interchondral j.
intercuneiform j.
intermetacarpal j.
intermetatarsal j.
internal semilunar fibrocartilage
of knee j.
interphalangeal j.
intertarsal j.
knee j.
lateral atlantoaxial j.
lateral atlantoepistrophic j.
lateral ligament of
temporomandibular j.
Lisfranc j.
j. lock
lumbosacral j.
Luschka j.
j. of Luschka
mandibular j.
manubriosternal j.
medial ligament of talocrural j.
median atlantoaxial j.
metacarpal j.
metacarpal-carpal j.
metacarpophalangeal j.
metatarsophalangeal j.
midcarpal j.
middle atlantoepistrophic j.
middle carpal j.
middle radioulnar j.
midtarsal j.
j. mobility
j. mobilization
j. mobilization procedure
mortise j.
j. motion
movable j.
multiaxial j.
J. and Muscle Relief Cream
neurocentral j.
neuropathic j.
oblique ligament of elbow j.
occipitoatlantal j.
j. oil
j.'s of pectoral girdle
peg-and-socket j.
j.'s of pelvic girdle
phalangeal j.
pisotriquetral j.
pivot j.
plane j.
plane of j.

j. play
j. play loss
polyaxial j.
j. pop
posterior intraoccipital j.
proximal interphalangeal j.
proximal radioulnar j.
proximal tibiofibular j.
radial collateral ligament of
elbow j.
radial collateral ligament of
wrist j.
radiocarpal j.
radiohumeral j.
radioulnar j.
rotary j.
round ligament of elbow j.
sacciform recess of distal
radioulnar j.
sacrococcygeal j.
sacroiliac j.
saddle j.
scapulothoracic j.
schindyletic j.
shoulder j.
simple j.
j. slack
socket j.
somatic dysfunction of
carpometacarpal j.
spheroidal j.
spiral j.
j. stacking
sternal j.
sternoclavicular j.
sternocostal j.
sternomanubrial j.
subtalar j.
j.'s of superior limb girdle
superior radioulnar j.
superior tibiofibular j.
superior zygapophysial j.
J. Support
suprahumeral j.
j. surface barrier
suture j.
synarthrodial j.
synchondrodial j.
syndesmodial j.
synovial j.
synovial extremity j.
talocalcaneal j.
talocalcaneonavicular j.

J

talocrural j.
talonavicular j.
talotibial j.
tarsal j.
tarsometatarsal j.
tarsometatarsal j.
tectorial membrane of median
atlantoaxial j.
temporomandibular j. (TMJ)
thigh j.
tibiofibular j.
j. tracking
transverse tarsal j.
trochoid j.
true arthrodial j.
ulnar collateral ligament of
elbow j.
ulnar collateral ligament of
wrist j.
ulnohumeral j.
ulnomeniscotriquetral j.
unciform j.
uncinate Luschka j.
uncovertebral j.
uniaxial j.
unstable hypermobile j.
wedge-and-groove j.
wrist j.
xiphisternal j.
zygapophysial j.
JointAssure
jojoba
Jones
J. tender point
J. tenderpoint
J. test
jong point
Josephing technique
Joshua tree
joule
joy
simpler's j.
juarandi
jue-yin, jueyin
j.-y. axis
j.-y. channel axis

jueyinshu
ub 14 j.
juga alveolaria
jugal
jugale
Juglans
J. nigra
J. regia
jugular
j. fossa
j. vein
juguloomohyoid node
jugum sphenoidale
juice
aloe vera j.
bean j.
cranberry j.
fresh carrot j.
fresh wheatgrass j.
George's Aloe Vera J.
Jim's J.
live j.
Mega J.
orange j.
prune j.
raw potato j.
Tahitian noni j.
j. therapy
wheatgrass j.
whole leaf aloe vera j.
juicing
jujube
Chinese j.
Ziziphus j.
juliao
st 3 j.
juncea
Brassica j.
junceum
Spartium j.
junction
costochondral j.
craniocervical j.
cranio-occipital j.
lumbosacral j.
manubriosternal j.
musculotendinous j.

NOTES

junction *(continued)*
  myotendinous j.
  sacrococcygeal j.
  scapulocostal j.
  sphenobasilar j.
  sternal-xiphoid j.
  sternomanubrial j.
junctional region
junctura
  j. cartilaginea
  j. fibrosa
  j. lumbosacralis
  j. sacrococcygea
  j. synovialis
juncturae
  j. membri inferioris liberi
  j. membri superioris
  j. membri superioris liberi
  j. ossium
  j. tendinum
  j. zygapophysiales
juncture
jung
  du j.
Jungian theory
Jüngling disease
Jungmann pelvic index

juniper
  baccal j.
  j. berry
  common j.
  ground j.
  j. mistletoe
Juniperus
juniros
  boca j.
jupiter flower
juque
  ren 14 j.
juvenile
  j. arthritis
  j. kyphosis
  j. muscular atrophy
  j. osteoporosis
  j. scoliosis
juvenilis
  osteochondritis deformans j.
juxtacortical
  j. chondroma
  j. osteogenic sarcoma
jyotisha
jyutsu
  jin shin j.

K_2
vitamin K_2
K3 acupuncture point
kadaram
kadaya
kadira
kaempferia galanga
kaempferol
Kaffree Tea
kaht
kai
K. Kit Pill
k. kit wan
K. Yeung Pill
Kalash-4
Maharishi Amrit K. (MAK-4)
Kalash-5
Maharishi Amrit K. (MAK-5)
kale
kali carb
kamphor balm
kang
gan yang shang k.
K'an Herbals
kan-li
kanpo
Kansas snakeroot
kapha
k. dosha
k. vata
Kaposi sarcoma
karaya
k. gum
k. self-adhesive conductive
material
k. tree
kardobenediktenkraut
karela
Karma yoga
Kasabach-Merritt syndrome
Kashin-Bek disease
kat
katechu
k. akazie
pegu k.
katesu
Katha
katila
katzenwurzel

kava
k. dermopathy
kava k.
k. kava extract
k. kava rhizome
k. root
kavapyrone
Kavasedon
Kavasporal
Kavatino
kawa
kawaratake mushroom
kayacikitsa
KB Formula
K cal, Kcal, kcal
kilocalorie
keeled chest
Kegel exercise
kelecin
kelp
K. Combination Tabs
K./Lecithin/B6
K. Natural Iodine
Norwegian K.
Pacific k.
kelpware
ken
huang t'eng k.
keratan sulfate
keratogenous membrane
Kerckring center
Kernosan Elixir
ketira
shagal el k.
ketorolac
keuschbaum
kew
key
k. of heaven
Our Lady's k.'s
k. rib
Key-E suppository
keyflower
khair
khat leaf
khella
khellin
ki
kidney channel
ki 4 dazhong

K

ki *(continued)*
  ki 7 fuliu
  ki 8 jiaoxin
  ki 5 shuiquan
  ki 3 taixi
  ki 10 yingu
  ki 1 yongquan
  ki 6 zhaohai
kidney
  k. bean
  k. and bladder tendinomuscular meridian
  k. channel (ki)
  k. energy
  k. essence
  k. failure
  k. formula
  k. gravel
  k. jing
  k. meridian
  k. meridian of foot
  k. stone
  k. stone pain
  k. tonic formula
  k. tonic herbs
  k. water
  k. yang
  k. yang deficiency
  k. yang xu
  k. yin
  k. yin xu with empty heat
kidney-heart
  k.-h. channel
  k.-h. meridian
Kidney-Liver Complex #406
kif
killer
  fish k.
  natural k. (NK)
  pain k.
kilocalorie (K cal, Kcal, kcal)
kilogram-meter
Kilose
kimono robe
kinematics
kinemometer
kineplastic amputation
kineplastics
kinesalgia
kinesialgia
kinesiatrics
kinesimeter

kinesiologist
  applied k.
kinesiology
  applied k.
  dental k.
kinesiometer
kinesipathist
kinesis
kinesitherapy
kinesthesia
kinesthesiometer
kinesthetic
  k. balance
  k. biofeedback
  k. feedback
  k. sense
kinetic
  k. energy
  k. system
kinetics
kinetogenic
kinetoscope
king
  k. herb
  k. of mushrooms
  k. point
  k. of spices
  tao te k.
King's-cure-all
kininogen
kinnikinnick, kinnikinnik
kino
  American k.
kinomometer
Kira
Kirksville Krunch
Kirlian photography
ki-shiatsu bodywork therapy
kita-gomishi
kiva
kivircik labada
klamath weed
klapping
kleeblattschädel
Klosterfrau Magentonikum
knapperty
  shepherd's k.
knead
kneading
knee
  articular muscle of k.
  collateral ligament of k.
  coronary ligament of k.

k. counterstrain
cruciate ligaments of k.
k. disarticulation amputation
drawer test of k.
k. extension
k. eye
k. flexion
k. functional technique
k. holly
housemaid's k.
k. joint
k. joint dysfunction
k. joint motion
lateral ligament of k.
locked k.
medial ligament of k.
posterior drawer test of k.
posterior ligament of k.
retraining position hands
and k.'s
rotary instability testing of k.
runner's k.
k. somatic dysfunction
k. tender point
k. torque unwinding
transverse ligament of k.
valgus stress testing of k.
varus stress testing of k.
k. wedge
knee-ankle-foot orthosis
kneecap
kneeling
self-stretch position k.
knife
cartilage k.
knight
Balsam of the Holy
Victorious K.
knit
loosely k.
knitbone
knitting
knob
intensity k.
k. root
k. weed
knoblaunch

knock-knee
knot
muscle k.
k. root
shepherd's k.
knotted marjoram
knotty brake
knotweed
knuckle pads
Koflet
Kofutu touch
koilosternia
kojic acid
kola
gotu k.
k. nut
kombu
kombucha
k. mushroom
k. tea
Kondremul with Cascara
kongzui
lu 6 k.
konjac mannan
Konsyl
Koong Yick Hung Fa oil
Korean
K. ginseng
K. hand acupuncture
Koryo
kosho
kousso
k. tree
Kramena ixine
krameria root
krapp
Krause bone
Kraus-Weber test
krestin
Kripalu yoga
krishnadi
kriyas
Kriya yoga
Krunch
Kirksville K.
kuandong hua
kubjelle

K

NOTES

kudzu treatment
kuei
   tian k.
Kühne plate
kullo
kummel
kummelol
kun bu
Kundalini
   K. trauma
   K. yoga
kung
   chi k.
kunlun
   ub 60 k.

kutzu
Kwai
Kyo-Dophilus
Kyo-Green
Kyolic
kypholordotic posture
kyphos
kyphoscoliosis
kyphoscoliotic pelvis
kyphosis
   juvenile k.
   posterior k.
kyphotic pelvis
kyphotone
kyushin

L3
 weightbearing line of L.
la
 l. hoja
 l. mulata
 l. pacho
 l. tranquera
labada
 kivircik l.
Laban movement analysis
Labbé triangle
labia (*pl. of* labium)
labial
labialis
 herpes simplex l.
 herpetic l.
labially
labiatic acid
labile
 l. factor
 l. hypertension
labium, pl. labia
 l. externum cristae iliacae
 l. internum cristae iliacae
 l. laterale lineae asperae
 l. mediale lineae asperae
laboratory testing
labra (*pl. of* labrum)
Labrada
Labrador Tea
labrum, pl. labra
 acetabular l.
 l. acetabulare
 articular l.
 l. articulare
 l. glenoidale scapulae
labyrinth
labyrinthine
labyrinthitis
labyrinthus
lac
lacca
lace
 Queen Anne's l.
lacertus
 l. cordis
 l. fibrosus
 l. medius
L-acetylcarnitine
Lachman test

laciniate ligament
lacrimal bone
lacrimale
 os l.
lacrimation
LactAid
lactic acid
lactiflora
 Paeonia l.
Lactinex
Lactobacillus
 L. acidophilus
 L. bifidus
 L. bulgaricus
lactone
 sesquiterpene l.
 terpene l.
lactoovovegetarian
lactose
lactovegetarian
Lactuca
 L. capitata
 L. sagittata
 L. sativa
 L. serriola
 L. virosa
lactucarium
 German l.
Lactucerin
lacuna
 muscular l.
 l. musculorum
lacunar
lacunule
lacus
lada
ladder
 Jacob's l.
 l. splint
ladder-to-heaven
ladies'-delight
lad's love
lady's
 l. mantle
 l. slipper
 l. thistle
 l. washbowl
laetrile
laevigata
 Crataegus l.

L

lag
    jet l.
lagena
lagenaria
    Cydonia l.
Laitan
lake
Lallouette pyramid
Lamaze
lambda
lambdoidal suture
lambdoid suture
lamb mint
lamb's quarters
lamella
    articular l.
    l. of bone
    circumferential l.
    concentric l.
    interstitial l.
lamellar bone
lamellate
lamina
    deep l.
    l. perpendicularis
    l. profunda
    l. propria
    superficial l.
    l. superficialis
    l. superficialis fasciae cervicalis
    l. superficialis fasciae
    temporalis
    l. of vertebral arch
    l. visceralis
laminar
Laminaria
laminated
lamination
laminotomy
lamp
    infrared heat l.
lanceolata
    Plantago l.
landmark
    anatomical l.
    l.'s of ischiorectal fossa
    rib l.
Landry-Guillain-Barré syndrome
Langenbeck triangle
Langer
    L. arch
    L. lines
    L. muscle

Langhans cells
Langhans-type giant cells
langwort
lanolin
lanten
lanulosa
    Achillea l.
Lanz line
laogong
    pe 8 l.
lapacho
    l. colorado
    l. morado
    purple l.
    red l.
lapachol
lappa
    Arctium l.
    Aucklandia l.
large
    l. fennel
    l. granular lymphocyte
    l. intestine channel (li)
    l. intestine meridian
    l. intestine meridian of hand
    l. intestine point
    l. muscle of helix
    l. pudendal lip
    l. yin axis
large-fiber stimulation
large-flowered cactus
large-leaved germander
L-arginine
larkspur
    forking l.
Larrea
    L. divaricata
    L. mexicana
    L. tridentata
larva
    fly l.
larvicidal
laryngeal mask
laryngitis
laryngopharynx
laryngospasm
Lasadoron
Lasègue sign
laser
    l. acupuncture
    Dynatronics Model 1620 l.
    helium neon l.
    infrared l.

infrared-beam diode l.
invisible infrared l.
l. irradiation
l. light
l. microscope
red-beam l.
soft l.
l. treatment
L-asparagine
L-aspartic acid
la-suan
lata
fascia l.
tensor of fascia l.
tensor muscle of fascia l.
latae
musculus tensor fasciae l.
tensor fasciae l.
latent energy
laterad
lateral
l. abdominal region
l. angle of scapula
l. arcuate ligament
l. atlantoaxial joint
l. atlantoepistrophic joint
l. bicipital groove
l. border
l. border of foot
l. border of forearm
l. border of humerus
l. border of nail
l. border of scapula
l. bucket-handle range
l. cartilaginous plate
l. central palmar space
l. chain ganglion
l. collateral ligament of ankle
l. column
l. condyle
l. condyle of femur
l. condyle of tibia
l. cord of brachial plexus
l. corticospinal tract
l. costotransverse ligament
l. crus
l. cun

l. cuneiform bone
l. curvature
l. cutaneous branch
l. cutaneous femoral nerve
l. direction
l. epicondylar crest
l. epicondylar ridge
l. epicondyle
l. epicondyle of femur
l. epicondyle of humerus
l. femoral condyle
l. femoral tuberosity
l. flexed rib
l. flexion
l. fluctuation
l. funiculus
l. ginglymus
l. great muscle
l. head
l. humeral epicondylitis
l. lacunar lymph node
l. lacunar node
l. ligament of elbow
l. ligament of knee
l. ligament of malleus
l. ligament of temporomandibular joint
l. ligament of wrist
l. limb
l. lip of linea aspera
l. longitudinal arch of foot
l. and longitudinal stretch
l. lumbar intertransversarii muscle
l. lumbar intertransverse muscle
l. lumbar spine
l. lumbocostal arch
l. malleolar ligament
l. malleolar network
l. malleolar surface of talus
l. malleolus
l. margin
l. mass
l. mass of atlas
l. meniscal tracking
l. meniscus

L

NOTES

lateral *(continued)*
  l. meniscus technique
  l. midpalmar space
  l. part of longitudinal arch of foot
  l. part of sacrum
  l. patellar retinaculum
  l. pelvic tilt functional curve
  l. process of calcaneal tuberosity
  l. process of talus
  l. pterygoid muscle
  l. pyramidal tract
  l. recess stenosis
  l. recumbent
  l. recumbent position
  l. recumbent thrust technique
  l. region of neck
  l. rib compression
  l. sacrococcygeal ligament
  l. segment
  l. spinal stenosis
  l. spinothalamic tract
  l. spot film
  l. strain
  l. stretch
  l. supracondylar crest
  l. supracondylar ridge
  l. surface
  l. surface of arm
  l. surface of fibula
  l. surface of finger
  l. surface of leg
  l. surface of lower limb
  l. surface of tibia
  l. surface of toe
  l. talocalcaneal ligament
  l. temporomandibular ligament
  l. translation test
  l. tubercle of posterior process of talus
  l. vastus muscle
  l. weightbearing arch
  l. xiyan point
laterale
  caput l.
  crus l.
  os cuneiforme l.
  rete malleolare l.
  retinaculum patellae l.
  tuberculum intercondylare mediale et l.

lateralis
  arcus lumbocostalis l.
  arcus pedis longitudinalis pars l.
  articulatio atlantoaxialis l.
  condylus l.
  crista sacralis l.
  crista supracondylaris l.
  facies l.
  fossa malleoli l.
  malleolus l.
  margo l.
  meniscus l.
  musculus vastus l.
  regio cervicalis l.
  sulcus bicipitalis l.
  vastus l.
laterally
  l. flexed superior rib
  iliosacral rotated l.
  translation l.
laterifolia
  Scutellaria l.
lateroduction
latherwort
latifolia
  Arnica l.
  Lavandula l.
latissimus
  l. dorsi
  l. dorsi muscle
  l. dorsi muscle exercise
  l. dorsi tender point
latus
  metatarsus l.
laughing gas
laughter therapy
Laumonier ganglion
laurel
  bay l.
  l. camphor
  rosa l.
Laurelis nobilis
laurier rose
Laurus nobilis
Lauth ligament
lavage
  gastric l.
lavanda
lavandin
Lavandula
  L. angustifolia
  L. latifolia

L. officinalis
L. stoechas
lavandulifolia
   Salvia l.
lavendel
   echter l.
lavender
   English l.
   l. essential oil
   l. flower
   French l.
   garden l.
   l. liquid extract
   l. oil
   l. petal
   Spanish l.
   spike l.
   true l.
law
   l. of approximation
   l. of detorsion
   Fryette l.
   Head l.
   Hooke l.
   mother-son l.
   l.'s of motion
   l.'s of myokinematics
   Ohm l.
   L. of Proving
   Rosenbach l.
   Sherrington l.
   L. of Similars
   Stokes l.
   Wolff l.
Laxacil Bulk
laxative
   bulk l.
   magnesium-containing l.
laxity
   pain-free l.
laxum
   Viscum l.
Laya yoga
layer
   arachnoid l.
   deep l.
   dura l.

dural l.
fascial l.
fibrous l.
meningeal l.
osteogenetic l.
l. palpation
parietal l.
pia l.
subserous l.
superficial l.
l. syndrome
visceral l.
layered muscles
laying on of hands
layor carang
L-carnitine
   acetyl L.-c.
LC Tone
L-cysteine HCl
LDL
   low-density lipoprotein
   LDL apoprotein B
   LDL cholesterol
LDL/HDL ratio
lead poisoning
leaf
   bay l.
   bearberry l.
   betel pepper l.
   Bible l.
   birch l.
   black nightshade l.
   boldo l.
   borage l.
   buchu l.
   ch'an su l.
   coca l.
   damiana l.
   elder l.
   ginkgo l.
   guayusa l.
   haronga l.
   hawthorn l.
   khat l.
   love l.
   Mexican flame l.
   moxa l.

L

NOTES

leaf *(continued)*
    mullein l.
    nettle l.
    parsley l.
    patchouli l.
    red raspberry l.
    sage l.
    senna l.
    seven l.
    strawberry l.
    tobacco l.
    wintergreen l.
    yaupon l.
leakage
    energy l.
lean muscle mass
learning
    cognitive l.
learning-based treatment
Leci-PC Liquid
lecithin
    egg l.
    soy l.
    soybean l.
lecithol
Ledebouriella divaricata
ledge
    Easter l.
ledgeriana
    Cinchona l.
Ledum palustre
leech
    fresh water l.
    giant l.
    medicinal l.
leferoot
left
    l. arm left sacral torsion
    l. branch
    l. cervical scoliosis
    easy normal l. (ENL)
    extended, rotated, sidebent l.
      (ERSL)
    extension, sidebent right,
      rotated l. (ESRRL)
    flexed, rotated, sidebent l.
      (FRSL)
    flexion, sidebent right,
      rotated l. (FSRRL)
    injury right to l.
    l. innominate externally rotated
    l. innominate outflare
    l. lumbar scoliosis

    neutral, sidebent right,
      rotated l. (NSRRL)
    l. oblique lumbar spine film
    l. on left forward sacral
      torsion
    l. on right torsion functional
      technique
    l. posterior ilium
    l. posterior innominate
    rotation l.
    rotation vertebral motion l.
    sacroiliac torsioned anteriorly
      left on l.
    sacroiliac torsioned posteriorly
      right on l.
    l. sacrum flexed
    l. sacrum flexed functional
      technique
    sidebending l.
    sidebending vertebral motion l.
    l. superior innominate shear
      dysfunction
    l. superior pubes
    l. superior symphysis
    l. unilateral anterior nutated
      sacrum
    l. ventricular ejection fraction
    l. ventricular hypertrophy
left-handed
left-on-left sacral torsion
left-on-right sacral torsion
left-sidedness
leg
    cruciate ligament of l.
    deep fascia of l.
    fascia of l.
    l. functional technique
    interosseous membrane of l.
    lateral surface of l.
    l. length at medial malleolus
      test
    l. length discrepancy
    l. length test
    posterior region of l.
    posterior surface of l.
    rider's l.
    tennis l.
    transverse ligament of l.
Legg-Calvé-Perthes disease
leggings
    pressurized l.
legume
lei gong teng

leiomyoma
uterine l.
lemon
l. balm
l. essential oil
l. verbena
Vita L.
water l.
wild l.
lemongrass
British Indian l.
cochin l.
Guatemala l.
Madagascar l.
l. tea
length
hamstring l.
psoralen plus ultraviolet light
of A wave l. (PUVA)
resting l.
l. of stride
l. test
Lenoir facet
lenticular
l. apophysis
l. process of incus
lenticularis
dystonia l.
lentiform bone
lentiginosis
centrofacial l.
lentil
lentinan
Lentinus edodes
Lent lily
leontopodium
Leonurus cardiaca
leopard's bane
leprosy
leptandra
Leptandra virginica
leptomeningeal carcinomatosis
leptopodia
Lequesne index score
LeShan
L. Method
L. therapy

lesion
anterior fat pad l.
atherosclerotic l.
brain l.
cord l.
erythematous l.
hepatic l.
manipulable l.
muscular l.
nodular l.
osteopathic l.
rib l.
skin l.
lesioned component
lesioning
lesser
l. burnet
l. celandine
l. centaury
l. multangular bone
l. peritoneal cavity
l. rhomboid muscle
l. sciatic foramen
l. sciatic notch
l. supraclavicular fossa
l. trochanter
l. trochanter pubic bone
l. tubercle of humerus
l. tuberosity of humerus
l. yang
l. yin
Lesshaft triangle
lethal dose
lettuce
acrid l.
bitter l.
garden l.
greater prickly l.
l. opium
romaine l.
strong-scented l.
wild l.
lettuce-leaf cigarette
Lettucine
leucadendron
Melaleuca l.

L

NOTES

leucarpum
 Phoradendron l.
leucine
leucodelphinidin
leucopelargonidin
leukemia
 acute lymphoblastic l. (ALL)
 acute promyelocytic l. (APL)
leukocyte
 polymorphonuclear l.
leukocytoblast
leukocytogenesis
leukocytosis
 neutrophil l.
leukocytotoxic testing
leukoderma
leukoencephalitis
 perivenous l.
leukomyelopathy
leukopenia
leukoplakia
 oral l.
leukorrhea
Leukorrhea Pills
leukosis
leukotriene synthesis
levamisole
levant
 l. berry
 l. wormseed
levator
 l. ani
 l. costales muscle
 l. muscle of thyroid gland
 l. scapulae
 l. scapulae muscle
 l. swelling
levatores
 l. costarum
 l. costarum muscle
level
 channel-structural l.
 cord l.
 dermatomal l.
 l. of ear
 energy-functional l.
 erythrocyte copper l.
 erythrocyte magnesium l.
 glutathione peroxidase l.
 lipoprotein l.
 l. of manifestation
 meridian l.
 organ l.

 l. of pelvis
 plasma l.
 relaxin l.
 serum cholesterol l.
 serum fatty acid l.
 serum magnesium l.
 serum melatonin l.
 shoulder l.
 thyroid hormone l.
 tissue l.
 voltage current l.
lever
 long l.
 Newton laws of l.
 short l.
leverage technique
Levisticum officinale
Levitor orthotic
levodopa
Lewit exercise
Lexat
L-glutamic acid
L-glutamine
 L-g. pantothenic acid
LH
 luteinizing hormone
Lhermitte sign
L-histidine
li
 large intestine channel
 li disturbance
 li 4 hegu
 li illness
 li 15 jianyu
 my li
 li 18 neck futu
 li 19 nose heliao
 li 11 quchi
 li 20 wingxiang
 li zhong tang
lian
 huang l.
 l. xin
liangmen
 st 21 l.
liangqiu
lianquan
 ren 23 l.
lib
 ad l.
libanotica
 Puschkina scilloides l.

Libbe lower bowel evacuation device
liber
    margo l.
liberi
    articulationes membri inferioris l.
    articulationes membri superioris l.
    juncturae membri inferioris l.
    juncturae membri superioris l.
libido
Libocedrus descurrens
lichen
    Iceland l.
lichwort
licorice
    l. ATC concentrate
    Chinese l.
    deglycyrrhizinated l. (DGL)
    l. and garlic
    l. liquid extract
    Persian l.
    l. root
    l. root extract
    l. root tea
    Russian l.
    Spanish l.
lidocaine hydrochloride
lieque
    lu 7 l.
li-fa-fang-yao
life
    breath of l.
    L. Change
    l. essence
    l. everlasting
    L. Experiences Survey
    l. force
    primary machinery of l.
    l. process
    L. Pulse
    River of L.
    l. root
    science of l.
    seed of l.
    Skin Gel Aloe L.

    Turlington's Balsam of L.
    water of l.
life-force line
life-giving vine of Peru
Lifepak
Lifestart
lifestyle counseling
lift
    heel l.
    mesenteric l.
    l. technique
    temporal l.
    l. therapy
    l. therapy sequence
ligament
    accessory l.
    accessory plantar l.
    accessory volar l.
    acromioclavicular l.
    alar l.
    anococcygeal l.
    anular l.
    arcuate l.
    arcuate popliteal l.
    arcuate pubic l.
    Bardinet l.
    Barkow l.
    l. barrier
    Bellini l.
    Bertin l.
    Bichat l.
    bifurcate l.
    Bigelow l.
    Bourgery l.
    Brodie l.
    Burns l.
    calcaneocuboid l.
    calcaneofibular l.
    calcaneonavicular l.
    calcaneotibial l.
    Caldani l.
    Campbell l.
    capsular l.
    caroticoclinoid l.
    caudal l.
    chondroxiphoid l.
    collateral l.

L

NOTES

ligament *(continued)*
    conoid l.
    Cooper l.
    coracoacromial l.
    coracoclavicular l.
    coracohumeral l.
    costoclavicular l.
    costotransverse l.
    costovertebral l.
    costoxiphoid l.
    cotyloid l.
    cruciate l.
    Cruveilhier l.
    cuboideonavicular l.
    cuneocuboid l.
    cuneonavicular l.
    deep posterior
      sacrococcygeal l.
    deep transverse metacarpal l.
    deep transverse metatarsal l.
    deltoid l.
    Denucé l.
    dorsal calcaneocuboid l.
    dorsal carpal l.
    dorsal carpometacarpal l.
    dorsal cuboideonavicular l.
    dorsal cuneocuboid l.
    dorsal cuneonavicular l.
    dorsal metacarpal l.
    dorsal metatarsal l.
    dorsal radiocarpal l.
    dorsal sacroiliac l.
    extracapsular l.
    falciform l.
    fallopian l.
    fibular collateral l.
    Flood l.
    Gerdy l.
    glenohumeral l.
    glenoid l.
    Günz l.
    Hey l.
    Humphry l.
    hypsiloid l.
    iliofemoral l.
    iliolumbar l.
    iliopectineal l.
    iliotrochanteric l.
    impression for
      costoclavicular l.
    inferior transverse scapular l.
    inguinal l.
    intercarpal l.

interclavicular l.
intercornual l.
intercostal l.
intercuneiform l.
interosseous cuneocuboid l.
interosseous cuneometatarsal l.
interosseous metacarpal l.
interosseous metatarsal l.
interosseous sacroiliac l.
interosseous talocalcaneal l.
interosseous tibiofibular l.
interspinous l.
intertransverse l.
intraarticular sternocostal l.
intracapsular l.
ischiocapsular l.
ischiofemoral l.
laciniate l.
lateral arcuate l.
lateral costotransverse l.
lateral malleolar l.
lateral sacrococcygeal l.
lateral talocalcaneal l.
lateral temporomandibular l.
Lauth l.
Lisfranc l.
longitudinal l.
long plantar l.
lumbocostal l.
medial arcuate l.
medial talocalcaneal l.
meniscofemoral l.
middle costotransverse l.
nuchal l.
oblique popliteal l.
orbicular l.
palmar l.
palmar carpal l.
palmar carpometacarpal l.
palmar metacarpal l.
palmar radiocarpal l.
palmar ulnocarpal l.
l. palpation
patellar l.
pectineal l.
pelvic l.
pisohamate l.
pisometacarpal l.
pisounciform l.
pisouncinate l.
plantar l.
plantar l.
plantar calcaneocuboid l.

plantar calcaneonavicular l.
plantar cuboideonavicular l.
plantar cuneocuboid l.
plantar cuneonavicular l.
plantar metatarsal l.
posterior costotransverse l.
posterior cruciate l.
posterior longitudinal l.
posterior meniscofemoral l.
posterior occipitoaxial l.
posterior sacroiliac l.
posterior sacrosciatic l.
posterior sternoclavicular l.
posterior talofibular l.
posterior talotibial l.
posterior tibiofibular l.
posterior tibiotalar l.
posterior tibiotalar part of
  deltoid l.
pterygospinal l.
pubocapsular l.
pubofemoral l.
quadrate l.
radial collateral l.
radiate l.
radiate sternocostal l.
Retzius l.
rhomboid l.
ring l.
sacrodural l.
sacroiliac l.
sacrospinous l.
sacrotuberous l.
serous l.
sheath l.
spinoglenoid l.
spring l.
stabilizing l.
Stanley cervical l.
stellate l.
sternoclavicular l.
sternopericardial l.
superficial dorsal
  sacrococcygeal l.
superficial posterior
  sacrococcygeal l.

superficial transverse
  metacarpal l.
superficial transverse
  metatarsal l.
superior costotransverse l.
superior transverse scapular l.
suprascapular l.
supraspinous l.
synovial l.
talocalcaneal l.
talofibular l.
talonavicular l.
tarsal l.
tarsometatarsal l.
temporomandibular l.
tibial collateral l.
tibial lateral l.
tibiocalcaneal l.
tibiocalcaneal part of deltoid l.
tibiofibular l.
tibionavicular l.
tibionavicular part of deltoid l.
transcarpal l.
transverse atlantal l.
transverse atlas l.
transverse carpal l.
transverse crural l.
transverse genicular l.
transverse humeral l.
transverse metacarpal l.
transverse metatarsal l.
transverse tibiofibular l.
trapezoid l.
triangular deltoid l.
ulnar collateral l.
ventral sacrococcygeal l.
ventral sacroiliac l.
vertebropelvic l.
volar carpal l.
Weitbrecht l.
Winslow l.
Wrisberg l.
yellow l.
Y-shaped l.
Zaglas l.
ligamenta

L

NOTES

ligamentous
l. articular strain
l. articular strain technique
l. attachment
l. damage
l. lock
l. stability
l. strain
l. tear
ligamentum
ligature
light
l. box
laser l.
low-intensity laser l.
l. male force
primary line of l.
l. therapy
l. touch
ultraviolet l.
lightheadedness
lighting
artificial l.
lightning bonesetter
lignan
flax l.
lignin
lignum
l. floridum
l. sassafras
l. vitae
ligou
Ligusticum chuanxiong
Ligustrum lucidum
like
like cures l.
lilac
French l.
lilliflora
Magnolia l.
lily
constancy l.
l. of the desert
flag l.
ground l.
Lent l.
liver l.
male l.
May l.
snake l.
l. of the valley
limb
bone of inferior l.

bone of lower l.
bone of superior l.
bone of upper l.
flexor retinaculum of lower l.
inferior l.
joints of free inferior l.
joints of free superior l.
lateral l.
lateral surface of lower l.
lincolnesque l.'s
lower l.
medial l.
pelvic l.
phantom l.
posterior surface of lower l.
regions of inferior l.
regions of lower l.
regions of superior l.
regions of upper l.
skeleton of free inferior l.
skeleton of free superior l.
superior l.
synovial joints of free
  lower l.
synovial joints of free
  upper l.
thoracic l.
upper l.
limb-girdle muscular dystrophy
limbic system
lime
bird l.
l. blossom
l. flower
l. paste
l. tree
l. water
limen
liminal
liminometer
limit of movement
limonine
limp
lin
san l.
lincolnesque limbs
lincomycin
linden
l. capsule
European l.
l. flower tea
l. lotion
l. tea

line

axillary l.
cement l.
cleavage l.
costoclavicular l.
Crampton l.
Daubenton l.
epiphysial l.
Feiss l.
gluteal l.'s
gravitational l.
l. of gravity
growth arrest l.'s
Harris l.'s
Holden l.
iliopectineal l.
inferior nuchal l.
inferior temporal l.
interspinal l.
intertrochanteric l.
intertubercular l.
Langer l.'s
Lanz l.
life-force l.
Looser l.'s
McKee l.
median l.
midaxillary l.
midclavicular l.
middle axillary l.
midheel l.
midmalleolar l.
Monro l.
Monro-Richter l.
Nélaton l.
oblique l.
parasternal l.
paravertebral l.
plumb l.
popliteal l.
postaxillary l.
posterior axillary l.
posterior median l.
Poupart l.
preaxillary l.
Richter-Monro l.
Roser-Nélaton l.

rough l.
sagittal l.
scapular l.
soleal l.
l. for soleus muscle
spiral l.
sternal l.
subcostal l.
superior temporal l.
supracrestal l.
supreme nuchal l.
temporal l.
terminal l.
trapezoid l.
Ullmann l.

linea, gen. and pl. **lineae**
l. aspera
l. axillaris anterior
l. axillaris media
l. axillaris posterior
l. epiphysialis
l. glutea anterior
lineae gluteae
l. glutea inferior
l. glutea posterior
l. intercondylaris femoris
l. intermedia cristae iliacae
l. interspinalis
l. intertrochanterica
l. intertubercularis
l. mediana anterior
l. mediana posterior
l. medio-axillaris
l. medioclavicularis
l. musculi solei
l. obliqua
l. obliqua cartilaginis
thyroideae
l. obliqua mandibulae
l. parasternalis
l. paravertebralis
l. pectinea femoris
l. poplitea
l. postaxillaris
l. preaxillaris
l. scapularis
l. sternalis

L

NOTES

linea *(continued)*
 l. subcostalis
 l. supracristalis
 l. terminalis of pelvis
 lineae transversae ossis sacri
 l. trapezoidea
linear
 l. amputation
 l. fracture
 l. streak
 l. stretch
 l. traction
linearis
 Aspalathus l.
ling
 fu l.
 l. jiao gou teng tang
 l. yang ge gen tang
 l. yang jiao
lingism
link
 endorphinergic l.
 mechanical l.
linoleic acid
linolenic acid (LNA)
linqi
 gb 41 foot l.
linseed
lint bells
linum
lion's-ear
lion's-foot
lion's-tail
lion's-tart
lion's tooth
lip
 acetabular l.
 articular l.
 glenoidal l.
 large pudendal l.
 small pudendal l.
lipid
 blood l.
 brain l.
 l. lowering agent
 l. peroxidation
 plasma l.
 l. pneumonia
 serum l.
lipidosterolic extract of *Serosa*
 repens **(LSESR)**
lipoic acid

lipoid
 l. pneumonia
 l. proteinosis
lipolysis
lipolytic
lipoma arborescens
lipomatosa
 macrodystrophia l.
lipopenia
lipoprotein
 high-density l. (HDL)
 l. level
 low-density l. (LDL)
5-lipoxygenase
Lippia citriodora
lipping
Liquescence
 Allergy L.
liquid
 aloe vera l.
 echinacea care l.
 l. ecstasy
 l. ginseng
 l. glucosamine sulfate
 Leci-PC L.
 l. liver extract #521
 l. solution
 l. stool incontinence
 therapeutic l.
 Traumeel oral l.
 witch hazel l.
Liquidambar
 L. orientalis
 L. styraciflua
Liquidum
 Extractum Rhei L.
liquor cotunnii
Liriosma ovata
lis
 flor de l.
Lisfranc
 L. joint
 L. ligament
 scalene tubercle of L.
 L. tubercle
L-isoleucine
lissive
list
 Munich Quality of Life
 Dimensions L.
listening hand
Lister tubercle
listlessness

lithium
Lithospermum officinale
little
 l. finger
 l. head of humerus
Little Leaguer's elbow
Liujingao
 Dahuang L.
liu wei di huang wan
liv
 liver channel
 liv 52
 liv 1 dadun
 liv 14 qimen
 liv 8 ququan
 liv 3 taichong
 liv 2 xingjian
 liv 13 zhangmen
 liv 6 zhongdu
live
 l. cell therapy
 l. enzyme analysis
 l. juice
liver
 l. channel (liv)
 desiccated l.
 l. detoxification
 l. disturbance
 l. extract
 l. extract injection
 l. fire
 l. fire rising
 l. formula
 gan feng nei dong
 l. lily
 l. meridian
 l. meridian of foot
 l. point
 l. qi
 l. qi congestion
 l. stagnation
 l. tonic formula
 l. tonic tea
 l. wind
 l. wind moving internally
 l. yang
 l. yang rising

 l. yin
 l. yin deficiency
Liverite
Liverprime
liverwort
living
 activities of daily l. (ADL)
 L. Air XL-15 unit
 l. antiseptic
Livingston treatment
Livingston-Wheeler
 L.-W. regimen
 L.-W. therapy
Livit-1
Livit-2
L-leucine
Lloyd flexion distraction table
L1–L5 vertebrae
L-lysine
 L.-l. cream
 L.-l. dihydrochloride
 L.-l. HCl
 L.-l. monohydrochloride
 L.-l. monoorotate
 L.-l. succinate
L-methionine
LNA
 linolenic acid
load
 extension l.
 l. reflex
 toxin l.
load-and-shift maneuver
loading
 tissue l.
lobar
Lobaria pulmonaria
lobata
 Pueraria l.
lobe
lobelia
 l. capsule
 l. extract
 great l.
 L. inflata
 l. tincture
Lobeline Lozenges

NOTES

lobi (*pl.* *of* lobus)
Lobidram Computabs
lobo
   menta de l.
lobster-claw deformity
lobster flower plant
lobular
lobulate
lobule
lobulet
lobulus
lobus, pl. lobi
local
   l. acupuncture point
   l. anemia
   l. anesthesia
   l. anesthetic
   l. anesthetic reaction
   l. effect
   l. hemostasis
   l. point
   l. segmental needling
   l. stimulant
localization
localized
   l. nodular tenosynovitis
   l. osteitis fibrosa
location of pain
lock
   bony l.
   l. finger
   joint l.
   ligamentous l.
locked
   l. facets
   l. knee
locking maneuver
locomotion
locomotor disorder
loco seed
locoweed
locular
locus
   l. dolendi
   l. dolendi point
lodestone
lodge
   purification l.
   sweat l.
Logan basic technique
logic
   nonlinear l.
   trance l.

logical incongruities
loin pain/hematuria syndrome
loins
   quadrate muscle of l.
Lomatol
lomilomi massage
long
   l. abductor muscle of thumb
   l. adductor muscle
   l. axis
   l. axis of body
   l. axis longitudinal stretch
   l. bone
   l. dan xie gan tang
   l. dong xie gan tang
   l. extensor muscle of great toe
   l. extensor muscle of thumb
   l. extensor muscle of toe
   l. fibular muscle
   l. flexor muscle of great toe
   l. flexor muscle of thumb
   l. flexor muscle of toe
   l. gu
   l. head
   l. levatores costarum muscle
   l. lever
   l. muscle barrier
   l. muscle of neck
   l. palmar muscle
   l. peroneal muscle
   l. plantar ligament
   l. radial extensor muscle of wrist
   l. restrictive barrier
   l. retention of the needle
   l. thoracic nerve palsy
longa
   Curcuma l.
longana
   Euphorbia l.
longevity
   Smart L.
longi
   musculi levatores costarum l.
   sulcus tendinis musculi fibularis l.
   sulcus tendinis musculi flexoris hallucis l.
   sulcus tendinis musculi peronei l.
   vagina tendinis musculi extensoris hallucis l.

vagina tendinis musculi
  extensoris pollicis l.
vagina tendinis musculi flexoris
  hallucis l.
vagina tendinis musculi flexoris
  pollicis l.
vagina tendinum musculi
  extensoris digitorum pedis l.
vagina tendinum musculi
  flexoris digitorum pedis l.
longissimus
  l. capitis muscle
  l. capitis musculus
  l. cervicis muscle
  l. cervicis musculus
  l. muscle
  musculus l.
  l. thoracis muscle
longitudinal
  l. arch of foot
  l. axis
  l. axis of femur
  l. bands of cruciform ligament
    of atlas
  l. fracture
  l. ligament
  l. section
  l. stretch
longitudinales
  sinus vertebrales l.
longitudinalis
  arcus pedis l.
  pars lateralis arcus pedis l.
  pars medialis arcus pedis l.
long-lasting success
long-leg arthropathy
long-lever
  l.-l. manipulation
  l.-l. technique
long-standing paresis
long-term
  l.-t. case
  l.-t. treatment
longum
  caput l.
  os l.
  Piper l.

longus
  l. capitis muscle
  l. capitis musculus
  l. cervicis muscle
  l. colli muscle
  extensor carpi radialis l.
    (ECRL)
  extensor digitorum l.
  extensor hallucis l.
  musculus abductor pollicis l.
  musculus adductor l.
  musculus extensor carpi
    radialis l.
  musculus extensor digitorum l.
  musculus extensor hallucis l.
  musculus extensor pollicis l.
  musculus fibularis l.
  musculus flexor digitorum l.
  musculus flexor hallucis l.
  musculus flexor pollicis l.
  musculus palmaris l.
  musculus peroneus l.
  palmaris l.
longwort
Lonicera japonica
lonjazo
look
  feedback l.
loop
  cervical l.
  excitatory feedback l.
  inhibitory feedback l.
  negative feedback l.
  l.'s of spinal nerves
  subclavian l.
  Vieussens l.
loose
  l. areolar tissue
  l. body
  l. cartilage
  l. connective tissue
  l. feel
  l. herb
  l. pack
  l. stool
loosely knit

L

NOTES

looseness
    deep-level l.
    soft tissue l.
Looser
    L. lines
    L. zones
loosestrife
LoowenWork therapy
Lopium
lo point
lordoscoliosis
lordosis, pl. lordoses
    cervical and lumbar lordoses
    flattening of lumbar l.
    high l.
    lumbar l.
    lumbar spine l.
    upper cervical l.
lordotic
    l. albuminuria
    l. curve
    l. pelvis
Lorenzo's oil
lorgnette
    main en l.
L-ornithine HCl
loss
    joint play l.
    l. of joint play
    major motion l.
    minimal motion l.
    motion l.
    sensory l.
lotion
    Aveeno L.
    calamine l.
    linden l.
    pau d'arco l.
    tea tree oil l.
    tei fu massage l.
lotus plumule
Louie
    lump of L.
louisa
Louis angle
louseberry
lovage
love
    l. bean
    boy's l.
    lad's l.
    l. leaf

low
    l. amplitude
    l. back dysfunction
    l. back pain
    l. frequency
    l. hypnotic ability
    l. immune resistance
    l. intensity
    l. spinal anesthesia
low-amplitude
    high-velocity l.-a. (HVLA)
low-density lipoprotein (LDL)
low-energy laser system
lower
    l. burner
    l. chakra
    l. crossed syndrome
    l. extremity
    l. extremity dermatome
    l. extremity dysfunction
    l. extremity screen
    l. GI
    l. jiao
    l. limb
    l. neck linear traction
    l. part
    l. thoracic scoliosis convex to right
    L. tubercle
    l. urinary tract symptom (LUTS)
lowest
    l. lumbar arteries
    l. thyroid artery
low-frequency
    l.-f., high-intensity analgesia
    l.-f., high-intensity electrical stimulation
    l.-f., high-intensity needling
    l.-f., high-intensity stimulation
    l.-f. pulsed current
    l.-f. stimulation
low-intensity
    l.-i. direct current
    l.-i. laser light
low-level electricity
lozenge
    Echinacea Herbal Comfort L.'s
    Lobeline L.'s
    tree tea oil l.'s
    Ultimate Zinc-C L.'s
    zinc l.
    zinc gluconate l.

L-phenylalanine
L-proline
L-propionylcarnitine
L-serine
LSESR
    lipidosterolic extract of *Serosa*
    repens
LT
    L-tryptophan
L-tetrahydropalmatine
L-tryptophan (LT)
L-tyrosine
lu
    lung channel
      lu 5 chize
      lu 6 kongzui
      lu 7 lieque
      lu 11 shaoshang
      lu 9 taiyuan
      lu 2 yunmen
      lu 1 zhongfu
lubricating fluid
lubricative herbs
Lucas groove
lucidum
    Ganoderma l.
    Ligustrum l.
Ludloff sign
Ludoxin
Ludwig angle
lu-hui
lumbago
    ischemic l.
lumbale
    tetragon l.
lumbales
    vertebrae l. [L1–L5]
lumbalia
    ganglion l.
lumbalis
    regio l.
lumbar
    l. articulatory technique
    l. cistern
    l. corset
    l. dermatome
    l. disk

l. diskogenic pain syndrome
l. erector spinae muscle
l. facet
l. flexure
l. ganglion
l. iliocostal muscle
l. interspinal muscle
l. lordosis
l. lymphatic trunk
l. lymph node
l. motion
l. myelogram
l. nerves [L1–L5]
l. nervous plexus
l. part of spinal cord
l. pillow
l. plexus
l. puncture
l. quadrate muscle
l. radiculopathy
l. region
l. rib
l. roll
l. rotator muscle
l. rotoscoliosis
l. scoliosis
l. spine
l. spine extension sacral
    extension
l. spine flattening
l. spine flexed, rotated,
    sidebent dysfunction
l. spine FRS dysfunction
l. spine functional technique
l. spine layer syndrome
l. spine lordosis
l. spine motion
l. spine motion testing
l. spine muscle energy
    technique
l. spine osteology
l. spine somatic dysfunction
l. spring test
l. tender point
l. tissue texture changes
l. triangle
l. vertebrae [L1–L5]

L

NOTES

lumbarization
lumbar-pelvic rhythm
lumbi (*pl. of* lumbus)
lumboabdominal
lumbocostal
    l. ligament
    l. trigone
lumbocostoabdominal triangle
lumbodorsal fascia
lumboiliac
lumboinguinal
lumboovarian
lumbopelvic hyperextension
lumborum
    musculi intertransversarii
      laterales l.
    musculi intertransversarii
      mediales l.
    musculi rotatores l.
    musculus iliocostalis l.
    musculus interspinalis l.
    musculus quadratus l.
    quadratus l.
lumbosacral
    l. angle
    l. enlargement
    l. enlargement of spinal cord
    l. joint
    l. junction
    l. junction motion
    l. junction spot film
    l. lordotic angle
    l. nerve trunk
    l. nervous plexus
    l. plexus
    l. spine
    l. spine myofascial release
      technique
lumbosacralis
    articulatio l.
    intumescentia l.
    junctura l.
lumbrical
    l. muscle
    l. muscles of foot
    l. muscles of hand
lumbricalis muscle
lumbricals
lumbricoides
    Ascaris l.
lumbus, pl. **lumbi**
lumen
    gastrointestinal l.

luminal size
lump of Louie
lunaception
lunate
    l. bone
    l. surface of acetabulum
lunatomalacia
lunatum
    os l.
lung
    l. channel (lu)
    L. Complex #407
    deficiency l.
    l. meridian
    l. meridian of hand
    l. moss
    oak l.
    phlegm obstructs the l.
    l. qi
    l. qi stagnation
    L. Tan Xie Gan Pill
    wind-cold affects the l.
    wind-heat affects the l.
    yin deficiency of the l.
lungs of oak
lungwort
    l. compound
    l. moss
lunula
luo
    l. connecting point
    l. connecting vessel
    l. connection
    l. point
    l. vessel
lupulus
    Humulus l.
lupus erythematosus
lu rong
Luschka
    foramen of L.
    joint of L.
    L. joint
    uncovertebral joint of L.
lutea
    Gentiana l.
luteinizing hormone (LH)
luteum
    Chamaelirium l.
LUTS
    lower urinary tract symptom
luxans
    coxa vara l.

luxatio
   l. erecta
   l. perinealis
luxation
Lycium chinensis
lycopene
lycopodium
Lycopodium clavatum
Lycopus europaeus
lymph
   l. circulation
   l. drainage therapy
   l. node
   l. nodes of elbow
   l. pump
lymphadenosis
lymphatic
   l. channel
   l. drainage
   l. drainage of external
      genitalia
   l. element
   l. massage
   l. obstruction
   l. pump
   l. pumping
   l. pump procedure
   l. pump treatment

   l. pump with lower extremity
   l. pump with upper extremity
   l. system
lymphatics
   nerve, artery, vein, empty
      space, l. (NAVEL)
   regional l.
lymphocyte
   B l.
   large granular l.
   l. stimulation response
   T l.
lymphoduct
lymphoglandula
lympholeukocyte
lymphoma
   malignant l.
lymphopenia
lyophilized
   l. aqueous root extract
   l. infusion
lysinate
   calcium l.
lysine
   l. acetylsalicylate
   l. prophylaxis
lysortine
Lytta (Cantharis) vesicatoria

NOTES

L

mA
    milliamp
ma
    m. huang
    m. huang xi xin fu zi tang
    xian m.
    m. xing shi gan tang
maag
MacDougall diet
mace
machine
    Rife m.
    TENS m.
    Voll m.
    white sound m.
macho
    helecho m.
machona
macis
Mackenzie extension program exercise
mackerel
macrobiotic
    m. diet
    m. shiatsu
macrobiotics
macrobrachia
macrocarpon
    Vaccinium m.
macrocephala
    Atractylodes m.
macrocheiria
macrocnemia
macrocosmic energy system
Macrocystis pyrifera
macrodactylia
macrodystrophia lipomatosa
macromelia
macronutrient
macrophage
    alveolar m.
macrophyllum
    Phoradendron m.
macrorrhizos
    Alocasia m.
macroscelia
macroscopic
macular
    m. degeneration
    M. Support Formula

maculata
    Cicuta m.
maculatum
    Conium m.
    Geranium m.
Macuna Plus
Madagascar
    M. lemongrass
    M. periwinkle
madagascariensis
    Commiphora m.
    Harungana m.
mad apple
madder
    dyer's m.
    m. root
mad-dog weed
madrugada
Maen
    Sanvita M.
Maffioli
    Amaro M.
Mag
    AP M.
magdalena
Magendie
    foramen of M.
Magentonikum
    Klosterfrau M.
maggi plant
maggot
    botfly m.
    m. debridement therapy (MDT)
    surgical m.
magistral
magna
    chorda m.
    coxa m.
    vertebra m.
magnesium
    m. deficiency
    ionized m.
    m. sulfate
    white blood cell m.
magnesium-containing laxative
magnet
    ear m.
    m. therapy
    water m.

M

239

magnetic
   m. field
   m. healing
   m. insoles
   m. jewelry
   m. mat pad
   m. microcapsule
   m. resonance imaging (MRI)
   m. support belt
   m. therapy
   m. wrap
magnetically influenced homeopathic remedy (MIHR)
magnetism
magnetoresonance spectroscopy
Magnolia
   M. lilliflora
   M. officinalis
magnolia vine berry
magnum
   foramen m.
   os m.
magnus
   musculus adductor m.
   musculus serratus m.
   raphe m.
Magrain
mahad
Maharishi
   M. Amrit Kalash-4 (MAK-4)
   M. Amrit Kalash-5 (MAK-5)
   M. ayurveda
mahonia
   trailing m.
Mahonia aquifolium
mahuuanggen root
mai
   chin ch'iao m.
   chong m.
   confluent point of dai m.
   dai m.
   du m.
   du m.
   fu xiao m.
   han zhi gan m.
   jenn m.
   m. men dung
   qi jing ba m.
   qi jingba m.
   ren m.
   renn m.
   yangqiao m.
   yangwei m.
   yinqiao m.
   yinwei m.
maid
   old m.
maiden's ruin
Maigne
   M. manipulation
   M. syndrome
main
   m. chakra
   m. channel
   m. d'accoucheur
   m. en crochet
   m. energy center
   m. en griffe
   m. en lorgnette
   m. fourchée
mainstream medicine
maintenance
   Metabolic M.
   Monthly M.
   m. therapy
Maissiat band
maitake
   m. mushroom
   m. tea
Maitland mobilization
maiy
   farasyon m.
maize pollen
majalis
   Convallaria m.
majja
Majocarmin
major
   m. amputation
   m. energy center
   fossa scarpae m.
   happy m.
   incisura ischiadica m.
   m. mineral
   m. motion loss
   musculus helicis m.
   musculus pectoralis m.
   musculus psoas m.
   musculus rectus capitis anticus m.
   musculus rhomboideus m.
   rectus capitis posterior m.
   rhomboid m.
   trochanter m.
   m. yang channel axis
   m. yin channel axis

majorana
  Origanum m.
majoranae
  oleum m.
majoris
  crista tuberculi m.
  pars clavicularis musculi
    pectoralis m.
  pars sternocostalis musculi
    pectoralis m.
majus
  Ammi m.
  Chelidonium m.
MAK-4
  Maharishi Amrit Kalash-4
MAK-5
  Maharishi Amrit Kalash-5
mala
Malabar cardamom
malabsorption
maladaptive response
malaise
malare
  os m.
malaria
malaxation
maldigestion
male
  m. fern
  m. fern oleoresin
  m. lily
malformation
  Arnold-Chiari m.
  arteriovenous m.
  cerebral arteriovenous m.
  mermaid m.
malignancy
malignant
  m. effusion
  m. hyperthermia
  m. illness
  m. lymphoma
mallei
  caput m.
  collum m.

malleolar
  m. articular surface of fibula
  m. articular surface of tibia
malleolus
  external m.
  fibular m.
  fossa of lateral m.
  inner m.
  internal m.
  lateral m.
  m. lateralis
  medial m.
  m. medialis
  outer m.
  tibial m.
malleotomy
mallet finger
malleus
  axis ligament of m.
  hallux m.
  head of m.
  lateral ligament of m.
  neck of m.
mallow
  blue m.
  field m.
  high m.
malpighian glomerulus
malposition
  static m.
malum
  m. coxae
  m. coxae senile
  m. vertebrale suboccipitale
malva
  m. flower
  M. parviflora
  M. sylvestris
malve
Malvedrin
Malveol
mamelonation
mammillary process
mammoplasty
  reduction m.
mamsa

M

NOTES

241

man
    medicine m.
    old m.
managed service organization (MSO)
management
    cognitive behavioral stress m.
    home m. (HM)
    stress m.
    time m.
mandala
    m. drawing
mandible
    angle of m.
    m. condyle
    condyloid process of m.
    m. fossa
    head of m.
    inferior border of m.
    interradicular septa of maxilla and m.
    oblique line of m.
    ramus of m.
    temporal articulation of m.
    m. torsion
mandibulae
    angulus m.
    linea obliqua m.
    symphysis m.
mandibular
    m. drainage
    m. fossa
    m. joint
    m. ramus
mandibularis
    fossa m.
    m. (V3)
mandibuloacral dysostosis
mandibulofacial
    m. dysostosis
    m. dysotosis syndrome
    m. dysplasia
Mandragora officinalis
mandrake
    American m.
    European m.
    m. root
maneuver
    bilateral shoulder abduction m.
    load-and-shift m.
    locking m.
    Spurling m.
    unwinding m.

manganese
mangiant
    Easter m.
mania
    mental m.
manifesta
    spina bifida m.
manifestation
    level of m.
    musculoskeletal m.
Manihot esculenta
maniphalanx
manipulable lesion
manipulation
    chiropractic m.
    cranial m.
    Cyriax m.
    dietary m.
    eclectic m.
    gentle m.
    intensive m.
    long-lever m.
    Maigne m.
    muscle energy m.
    musculoskeletal m.
    needle m.
    nonspecific osteopathic m.
    osteopathic m.
    short-lever m.
    soft tissue m.
    spinal m.
    m. therapy
    m. under anesthesia
    visceral m.
manipulative
    m. medicine
    m. medicine prescription
    m. physiotherapy
    m. procedure
    m. therapeutics
    m. therapeutic technique
    m. treatment
Manipura
mannan
    konjac m.
manometer
    aneroid m.
mansa
manshuriensis
    Aristolochia m.
mantle
    field lady's m.
    lady's m.

Mantoux
  M. test
  M. test skin reaction
mantra
  m. yoga
manual
  m. healing
  m. medicine
  m. medicine armamentarium
  m. medicine therapy
  m. needle acupuncture
  m. needle twirling
  m. organ stimulation technique
    (MOST)
  m. palpation
  m. stimulation
  m. stretching
  m. treatment
  m. trigger point therapy
  m. twirling
**manubrioglodiolar sternal
dysfunction**
manubriosternal
  m. joint
  m. junction
  m. symphysis
manubriosternalis
  symphysis m.
  synchondrosis m.
manubrium
  m. sterni
  m. of sternum
manus
  articulationes m.
  articulationes
    interphalangeae m.
  m. cava
  digitus m.
  dorsum m.
  m. extensa
  fascia dorsalis m.
  m. flexa
  musculi interossei dorsalis m.
  musculus abductor digiti
    minimi m.
  musculus extensor digitorum
    brevis m.

musculus flexor digiti minimi
  brevis m.
musculus lumbricalis m.
os naviculare m.
palma m.
m. plana
rete venosum dorsale m.
m. superextensa
torus m.
vagina communis tendinum
  musculorum flexorum m.
vaginae fibrosae digitorum m.
vaginae synoviales
  digitorum m.
m. valga
m. vara
vinculum breve digitorum m.
vinculum longum digitorum m.
manzanita
MAO
  monoamine oxidase
  MAO inhibitor
mao
  hsien m.
map
  acupoint m.
mapato
mapped acupuncture point
mapping
  dermatome m.
maraschino cherry
marble
  m. bone
  m. bone disease
march
  m. everlasting
  m. fracture
Marcille triangle
marfanoid hypermobility syndrome
Marfan syndrome
Margarite Acne Pills
margas
margin
  m. of acetabulum
  anterior m.
  articular m.
  free m.

M

NOTES

margin *(continued)*
   frontal m.
   inferior m.
   interosseous m.
   lateral m.
   medial m.
   m. of safety
marginal
margo, pl. **margines**
   m. acetabularis
   m. anterior fibulae
   m. anterior radii
   m. anterior tibiae
   m. anterior ulna
   m. falciformis hiatus sapheni
   m. fibularis pedis
   m. frontalis
   m. frontalis ossis parietalis
   m. inferior
   m. interosseus
   m. interosseus fibulae
   m. interosseus radii
   m. interosseus tibiae
   m. interosseus ulna
   m. lateralis
   m. lateralis antebrachii
   m. lateralis humeri
   m. lateralis pedis
   m. lateralis scapulae
   m. liber
   m. mastoideus squamae
   occipitalis
   m. medialis
   m. medialis antebrachii
   m. medialis humeri
   m. medialis pedis
   m. medialis scapulae
   m. medialis tibiae
   m. posterior fibulae
   m. posterior radii
   m. posterior ulna
   m. radialis antebrachii
   m. superior scapulae
   m. tibialis pedis
   m. ulnaris antebrachii
margosa
Maria
   Santa M.
Marian thistle
marianum
   Silybum m.
marianus
   Carduus m.

marigold
   burr m.
   French m.
   garden m.
   pot m.
marijuana, marihuana
   medical m.
marina
   Quercus m.
maritima
   Cineraria m.
   Urginea m.
Marjolin ulcer
marjoram
   common m.
   knotted m.
   sweet m.
   wild m.
marker
Mark Seem needling
markweed
Marlow-Crown
   M.-C. score
   M.-C. Social Desirability scale
marma therapy
marron
   oseille m.
marrow
   bone m.
   influential point of the m.
   spinal m.
   vegetable m.
   m. washing qigong
marrubium
Marrubium vulgare
Marsdenia condurango
marsh
   m. apple
   m. cudweed
   m. herb
   m. parsley
   m. rosemary
   m. trefoil
   m. woundwort
marshaling point
marshmallow root
martial art
Maruyama vaccine
marvel
marvelous channel
masala
   garam m.
   pan m.

MASc
Master of Ayurvedic Science
maschale
mask
laryngeal m.
mass
erector spinae m.
lateral m.
lean muscle m.
mucilaginous m.
massage
abhyanga m.
biodynamic m.
chua ka m.
craniosacral m.
cross-fiber friction m.
European m.
friction m.
gentle soft tissue m.
geriatric m.
holistic m.
ice m.
integrative m.
lomilomi m.
lymphatic m.
neuromuscular m.
nonoriental m.
oil m.
perineal m.
pu tong an mo m.
qigong meridian m. (QMM)
Swedish m.
Swedish-Esalen m.
Thai m.
therapeutic m.
m. therapy
vibratory m.
masseter muscle
masseur
masseuse
massotherapy
mastalgia
mastectomy
master
M. of Ayurvedic Science
(MASc)
m. herbalist

m. meridian
qigong m.
m. spice
m. of the wood
mastery task
mastoid
m. foramen
m. notch
m. part of temporal bone
m. portion of temporal
m. process
mastoiditis
mat
yoga m.
maté
m. bulk loose tea
yerba m.
mater
dura m.
filum of spinal dura m.
pia m.
material
karaya self-adhesive
conductive m.
synovial m.
materia medica
mato
arruda do m.
Matonia
Matricaria
M. capensis
M. chamomilla
M. recutita
matrix
bone m.
cartilage m.
crests of nail m.
matsu-cha
matter
gray m.
white m.
Matteuccia struthiopteris
mauve
blue m.
max
glycine m.

M

NOTES

Maxa
Terra M.
MaxEPA
maxilla, pl. **maxillae**
septa interradicularia
mandibulae et maxillae
maxillaris (V2)
maxillary
m. bone
m. nerve
m. sinus
m. sinusitis
maxillofrontal suture
maxillonasal suture
maxima
Cucurbita m.
Spirulina m.
maximus
gluteus m.
musculus gluteus m.
Max Nutrition System
may
m. blob
M. lily
mayapple
maybush
maydis
stigmata m.
mayflower
maypop
mays
Zea m.
McGill scale
McKee line
McMurray
M. meniscal test
M. test
MD
muscular dystrophy
M'Dowel
frenulum of M.
MDT
maggot debridement therapy
ME
muscle energy
ME treatment
meadow
m. anemone
m. cabbage
m. clover
m. eyebright
queen of the m.
m. saffron

m. sage
m. windflower
meadowsweet
m. flower
m. herb
meadwort
measure
psychotherapeutic m.
therapeutic m.
measurement
Cobb method of scoliosis
curve m.
cun m.
hypnotic depth m.
proportional cun m.
whole-blood serotonin m.
measuring wire
meat
dried rattlesnake m.
rattlesnake m.
meate
cuckoo's m.
meatus
auditory m.
external acoustic m.
external auditory m.
Mecca senna
mechanical
m. analysis
m. link
mechanics
body m.
cranial m.
neutral m.
nonneutral m.
talotibial m.
type III m.
mechanism
bioelectric m.
body m.
central neurohumoral m.
craniosacral m.
defense m.
endorphin m.
gate m.
homeostatic m.
involuntary m.
neural m.
neuropeptide m.
primary respiratory m.
proprioceptive m.
respiratory m.
segmental m.

self-regulatory m.
tracking m.
whiplash injury m.
mechanoreceptor
cardiac m.
cutaneous m.
dynamic m.
static m.
Meckel cave
meconium
meda
mede-sweet
media
linea axillaris m.
otitis m.
Stellaria m.
medial
m. anesthesia
m. arch of foot
m. arcuate ligament
m. bicipital groove
m. border
m. border of foot
m. border of forearm
m. border of humerus
m. border of scapula
m. border of tibia
m. branch
m. cartilaginous plate
m. collateral ligament of elbow
m. condyle
m. condyle of femur
m. condyle of tibia
m. cord of brachial plexus
m. crest of fibula
m. crus
m. cuneiform
m. cuneiform bone
m. direction
m. epicondylar crest
m. epicondylar ridge
m. epicondyle of femur
m. epicondyle of humerus
m. femoral condyle
m. femoral tuberosity
m. great muscle

m. groove
m. head
m. lacunar node
m. and lateral meniscus technique
m. and lateral rotation
m. ligament of knee
m. ligament of talocrural joint
m. ligament of wrist
m. limb
m. lip of linea aspera
m. longitudinal arch of foot
m. longitudinal fasciculus
m. lumbar intertransversarii muscle
m. lumbar intertransverse muscle
m. lumbocostal arch
m. malleolar facet of talus
m. malleolar network
m. malleolus
m. margin
m. meniscal tracking
m. meniscus
m. meniscus technique
m. midpalmar space
m. part of longitudinal arch of foot
m. patellar retinaculum
m. pectoral nerve
m. plantar artery
m. plantar nerve
m. popliteal nerve
m. process of calcaneal tuberosity
m. pterygoid muscle
m. rotator
m. scapular area
m. segment
m. spring arch
m. supracondylar crest
m. supracondylar ridge
m. surface
m. surface of fibula
m. surface of tibia
m. surface of toe
m. surface of ulna

M

NOTES

medial *(continued)*
    m. talocalcaneal ligament
    m. tubercle of posterior
      process of talus
    m. vastus muscle
mediale
    caput m.
    crus m.
    os cuneiforme m.
    rete malleolare m.
    retinaculum patellae m.
    segmentum m.
medialis
    arcus lumbocostalis m.
    arcus pedis longitudinalis
      pars m.
    condylus m.
    crista supracondylaris m.
    facies m.
    malleolus m.
    margo m.
    meniscus m.
    musculus vastus m.
    sulcus bicipitalis m.
    vastus m.
medially
    iliosacral rotated m.
median
    m. atlantoaxial joint
    m. line
    m. nerve
    m. nerve distribution
    m. nerve entrapment
    m. nerve motor
    m. plane
    m. sacral crest
    m. section
mediana
    articulatio atlantoaxialis m.
    crista sacralis m.
medianae
    membrana tectoria articulationis
      atlantoaxialis m.
mediastinalis
    pleura m.
mediastinum
mediation
medica
    materia m.
    Smilax m.
    traditional Chinese materia m.
    (TCMM)
Medicago sativa

medical
    m. divination
    m. herbalist
    m. hypnosis
    m. marijuana
medicament
medicate
medicated bath
medication
    antimicrobial m.
    blood-thinning m.
    injectable m.
    oral m.
    preanesthetic m.
    prescription m.
    Red Cross Toothache M.
medicephalic
medicinal
    dried m.
    m. herb
    m. leech
medicinalis
    Hirudo m.
medicine
    Academy of Traditional
      Chinese M.
    allopathic m.
    alternative m. (AM)
    American Association of
      Colleges of Osteopathic M.
      (AACOM)
    anthroposophic m.
    anthroposophically extended m.
    antiaging m.
    Ayurvedic m.
    behavioral m.
    bioelectromagnetic m.
    bioenergetic m.
    botanical m.
    Chinese m.
    Chinese herbal m.
    chiropractic m.
    complementary and
      alternative m. (CAM)
    craniosacral manual m.
    doctor of Oriental m. (DOM)
    Eastern m.
    energy m.
    environmental m.
    folk m.
    herbal m.
    homeovitic m.
    Indian m.

integral traditional Chinese m. (ITCM)
integrative m.
internal m.
mainstream m.
m. man
manipulative m.
manual m.
mind-body m.
molecular m.
National Accreditation Commission for Schools and Colleges of Acupuncture and Oriental M. (NACSCAOM)
National Center for Complementary and Alternative M. (NCCAM)
National Certification Committee for Acupuncture and Oriental M. (NCCAOM)
Native American m.
naturopathic m.
North American Academy of Manipulative M. (NAAMM)
nutritional m.
nutritional functional m.
Office of Alternative M. (OAM)
Office of Cancer Complementary and Alternative M. (OCCAM)
Oriental m.
orthodox m.
orthomolecular m.
osteopathic m.
osteopathic manipulative m. (OM)
patent m.
physical m.
m. plant
podiatric m.
preventive m.
proprietary m.
psychosomatic m.
quantum m.
m. rattle
Tibetan m.

traditional m.
traditional Chinese m. (TCM)
transpersonal m.
Unani m.
Vedic m.
vibrational m.
Western m.
Western botanical m.
m. wheel
Yellow Emperor's textbook of physical m.
medio-axillaris
linea m.-a.
mediocarpal
mediocarpalis
articulatio m.
medioclavicularis
linea m.
mediodorsal
mediolateral
m. episiotomy
mediotarsal
meditation
m. bench
Buddhist m.
concentrative m.
healing m.
mindfulness m.
m. qigong
Tibetan Buddhist m.
TM-Siddhi m.
transcendental m. (TM)
meditation-oriented qigong
meditative yoga
Mediterranean squill
medium
ganglion cervicale m.
medius
digitus manus m.
lacertus m.
m. muscle
musculus gluteus m.
musculus scalenus m.
medulla
m. oblongata
spinal m.

M

NOTES

medullare
    cavum m.
    osteoma m.
medullaris
    cavitas m.
    conus m.
medullary
    m. callus
    m. cavity
    m. spinal arteries
medullization
medulloarthritis
medullovasculosa
    zona m.
meeting point
mega
    Glucosamine M.
    M. Juice
    M. Men Men's Vitapak
    M. Primrose oil
megadactyly
megadose vitamin
megamineral sideroblastic anemia
meganutrient therapy
Megavital Forte
megavitamin therapy
meibomian gland
meichong
    ub 3 m.
Meissner
    M. corpuscle
    M. plexus
mel
melagra
Melaleuca
    M. alternifolia
    M. leucadendron
melaleuca oil
melalgia
melamine
    m. formaldehyde
    m. resin
melampode
melancholy
melanocyte-stimulating hormone
melanoma
    metastatic m.
melanosis coli
melatonin
    m. rhythm
    m. with vitamin B_6
Meleney ulcer
Melilotus officinalis

Melisana
Melissa officinalis
mellifera
    Apis m.
mellitus
    insulin-dependent diabetes m.
    (IDDM)
melon
    bitter m.
    m. tree
melon-seed body
melorheostosis
melosalgia
Melzack pain questionnaire
member
membra
membrana
    m. atlantooccipitalis anterior
    m. atlantooccipitalis posterior
    m. intercostalis externa
    m. intercostalis interna
    m. interossea antebrachii
    m. interossea cruris
    m. obturatoria
    m. suprapleuralis
    m. tectoria articulationis
        atlantoaxialis medianae
membranaceus
    Astragalus m.
membranae intercostales
membrane
    atlantooccipital m.
    m. bone
    craniosacral reciprocal
        tension m.
    dural m.
    external intercostal m.
    glial limiting m.
    intercostal m.
    internal intercostal m.
    intracranial m.
    keratogenous m.
    m. motility
    mucous m.
    obturator m.
    pial-glial m.
    pleuroperitoneal m.
    posterior atlantooccipital m.
    postsynaptic m.
    presynaptic m.
    reciprocal tension m. (RTM)
    synovial m.

tympanic m.
virginal m.
membranocartilaginous
membranous
    m. ossification
    m. tension restriction
membrum
    m. inferius
    m. muliebre
    m. superius
    m. virile
memory
    M. 2000
    cellular m.
    implicit to explicit m.
    repressed m.
    short-term m.
men
    Formula 600 Plus for M.
menadione
menaquinone
mend
    Fem M.
mengkoedoe
meningeal
    m. branch
    m. hernia
    m. layer
meninges (*pl. of* meninx)
meningoencephalomyelitis
meningomyelitis
meningomyelocele
meningo-osteophlebitis
meningosis
meningovascular
meninx, pl. **meninges**
    arachnoid layer of meninges
    cranial meninges
    dura layer of meninges
    pia layer of meninges
meniscal
    m. tear
    m. tracking
menisci (*pl. of* meniscus)
meniscitis
meniscofemoral ligament

meniscoid
    synovial m.
meniscus, pl. **menisci**
    articular m.
    m. articularis
    m. entrapment theory
    m. extrapment theory
    lateral m.
    m. lateralis
    medial m.
    m. medialis
Menispermum canadense
Mennell
    M. diagnostic and therapeutic
      joint play technique
    M. rules
Menodoron
Meno-Fem
menopause
menor
    consuelda m.
menorrhagia
Men's Multiple Formula
Menstrim
menstrual
    m. cramp
    m. disorder
Mensuosedyl
mensuration
    radiographic m.
menta de lobo
mental
    m. activity
    m. depression
    m. distraction
    m. function
    m. healing
    m. imagery
    m. mania
    m. protuberance
    m. receptivity
    m. stress
    m. symphysis
    m. tubercle
mentalis
    symphysis m.
mentally relaxing effect

M

NOTES

Mentastics
    Trager M.
Mentat
Mentha
    M. aquatica
    M. haplocalyx
    M. piperata
    M. piperita
    M. pulegium
    M. spicata
menthol
menti
    symphysis m.
mentoring
    spiritual m.
meralgia paresthetica
mercury
meridian
    m. acupoint
    acupuncture m.
    bladder m.
    conception m.
    curious m.
    distinct m.
    energy m.
    m. energy
    extraordinary m. (EM)
    m. function
    gallbladder m.
    governing m.
    heart m.
    homeostatic m.
    kidney m.
    kidney and bladder
      tendinomuscular m.
    kidney-heart m.
    large intestine m.
    m. level
    liver m.
    lung m.
    master m.
    pericardium m.
    principal m.
    propagated sensation along
      the m. (PSM)
    sanjiao m.
    small intestine m.
    small intestine-bladder m.
    spleen m.
    stomach m.
    m. subcircuit
    tendinomuscular m.
    m. theory

    m. therapy
    urinary bladder m.
Merkel disk
mermaid malformation
meromelia
merorachischisis
Mesc
mescal button
mescaline
mesenchyme
    interzonal m.
    synovial m.
mesenteric
    m. artery
    m. ganglion
    m. lift
    m. plexus
    m. release
mesentery
    m. of esophagus
    esophagus dorsal m.
mesocarpal
mesocuneiform
mesogluteal
mesogluteus
mesoscapulae
    delta m.
mesotarsal
mesotendineum
mesotendon
message
    pain m.
meta-analysis
Meta-Balance
metabolic
    m. acidosis
    m. alkalosis
    m. bone disease
    m. dysfunction
    m. energy
    m. imbalance
    M. Maintenance
    m. rate
    m. therapy
metabolism
    androgen m.
    body fluid m.
    bone m.
    cellular m.
    fatty acid m.
    glucose m.
    zinc m.

metabolite
cholesterol m.
non-end product m.
metacarpal
base of m.
m. bones [I–V]
head of m.
m. index
m. joint
m. joint dorsal tilt
metacarpal-carpal
first m.-c.
m.-c. joint
metacarpalis
basis ossis m.
caput ossis m.
corpus ossis m.
metacarpi
ossa m.
spatia interossea m.
metacarpophalangeae
articulationes m.
metacarpophalangeal
m. articulation
m. joint
metacarpus
Meta-Fem
Metaform
Metagenics
metal
m. element
m. point
metallicum
Aurum m.
metamorphic technique
Metamucil
metaphysial, metaphyseal
m. dysostosis
m. dysplasia
m. fibrous cortical defect
metaphysical
metaphysician
metaphysis
metaphysitis
metastases
pulsating m.

metastatic
m. abscess
m. bone disease
m. breast cancer
m. calcification
m. melanoma
m. pneumonia
metasternum
metatarsal
m. arch
m. artery
base of m.
m. bone dysfunction
m. bones [I–V]
head of m.
m. head
metatarsalgia
metatarsalis
basis ossis m.
caput ossis m.
metatarsea
syndesmitis m.
metatarsi
ossa m.
spatia interossea m.
metatarsophalangeae
articulationes m.
metatarsophalangeal
m. articulation
m. joint
metatarsus
m. adductovarus
m. adductus
m. atavicus
m. latus
m. varus
metathesis
metel
Datura m.
meter
galvanic skin response m.
GSR m.
methacholine
methadone
methanol
methicillin-resistant *Staphylococcus aureus* (MRSA)

M

NOTES

methionine
method
  Bier m.
  bu m.
  combined m.
  direct m.
  dispersing m.
  draining m.
  Egoscue m.
  exaggeration m.
  Feldenkrais m.
  four diagnostic m.'s
  indirect m.
  intrinsic chi m.
  Japanese m.
  LeShan M.
  m. of moxibustion
  needling m.
  m. of needling
  oblique needling m.
  Ortho-Bionomy m.
  perpendicular needling m.
  physiological response m.
  Pilates m.
  qigong meridian
    examination m.
  reducing m.
  Rosen m.
  Rubenfield Synergy M.
  Ryodoraku m.
  sedating m.
  sedative m.
  self-applied health
    enhancement m. (SAHEM)
  Simonton m.
  six-word m.
  Skeffington m.
  strengthening m.
  symptothermal m.
  tangential needling m.
  tonifying m.
  traditional m.
  xie m.
methodology
  biophysical m.
methotrexate
methylation
methyl salicylate
methylsulfonylmethane (MSM)
methysticum
  Piper m.
metoclopramide
metopic suture

Metrecom device
Metrin
Metrophyt-V
Mexican
  M. arnica
  M. damiana
  M. flame leaf
  M. sarsaparilla
  M. scammony
  M. tea
  M. vanilla
  M. wild yam
  M. yam
mexicana
  Larrea m.
Mexico weed
Meyers Briggs Inventory
MFR
  myofascial release
  MFR treatment
MI
  myocardial infarction
miasm
micosolle
microaerosol
microampere current
microamps TENS unit
microbe
microbial
microbic
microbicidal
microbicide
microbiologic
microbiologist
microbiology
microbiotic
microbrachia
microcapsule
  magnetic m.
microcheiria
microcirculation
microcosmic
  m. energy system
  m. orbit circulation
microcoulomb
microdactyly
microglia
microinjection
micromelica
  rachitis fetalis m.
micrometer
micro mineral
microneurography

micronodular cirrhosis
micronutrient
microphage
micropodia
microscope
    infrared m.
    laser m.
    ultraviolet m.
MicroStim 100 TENS device
microtrauma
microwave
    m. radiation
    m. resonance therapy
micturition
midaxillary line
midbrain monoamine
midcarpal joint
midclavicular line
middle
    m. atlantoepistrophic joint
    m. axillary line
    m. burner
    m. carpal joint
    m. cervical fascia
    m. cervical ganglion
    m. comfrey
    m. costotransverse ligament
    m. cuneiform bone
    m. dan tian
    m. finger
    m. jiao
    m. jiao deficiency
    m. to lower thoracic spine
    m. palmar space
    m. qi
    m. radioulnar joint
    m. scalene muscle
    m. talar articular surface of
      calcaneus
    m. transverse axis
midheel line
midline sphenobasilar movement
midmalleolar line
midpalmar space
midsagittal
    m. plane
    m. section

midsternum
midsummer daisy
midtarsal joint
midwife
midwifery
migraine
    classical m.
    full-blown m.
    m. headache
    m. prophylaxis
migrating abscess
migration
    ionic m.
MIHR
    magnetically influenced
      homeopathic remedy
mild
milfoil
milieu
    cellular m.
    internal m.
military-bearing posture
milk
    acidophilus m.
    cow's m.
    goat's m.
    soy m.
    m. thistle
    m. thistle extract
    m. thistle fluid extract
    M. Thistle Phytosol
    M. Thistle Power
    m. thistle seed whole
    m. thistle tablet
milk-alkali syndrome
milking
    m. of maxillary sinus
    nasal m.
milkweed
milkwort
millefolium
    Achillea m.
millepertuis
milliamp (mA)

NOTES

M

255

millibar
millijoule (mJ)
millisecond (ms)
milliwatt (mW)
   m. intensity
miltiorrhiza
   Salvia m.
Minadex Mix Ginseng
mind-body
   m.-b. approach
   m.-b. connection
   m.-b. exercise
   m.-b. interaction
   m.-b. medicine
   m.-b. skills
   m.-b. technique
   m.-b. therapy
mindfulness meditation
mindful qigong
mindless qigong
mineral
   chelated m.
   m. concentration
   major m.
   micro m.
   minor m.
   trace m.
mineralization
miner's elbow
ming
   m. men huo
   m. men xu
mingmen
   du 4 m.
minimal
   m. lethal dose
   m. motion loss
minimi
   musculus extensor digiti m.
   musculus opponens digiti m.
   vagina tendinis musculi
     extensoris digiti m.
minimus
   digitus manus m.
   gluteus m.
   m. muscle
   musculus adductor m.
   musculus gluteus m.
   musculus scalenus m.
ministerial fire
ministroke
Minnesota Multiphasic Personality
  Inventory (MMPI)

minor
   m. amputation
   m. centaury
   M. Construct the Middle
   Decoction
   m. energy center
   fossa supraclavicularis m.
   incisura ischiadica m.
   m. intervertebral derangement
   m. mineral
   musculus complexus m.
   musculus helicis m.
   musculus iliacus m.
   musculus pectoralis m.
   musculus psoas m.
   musculus rectus capitis
     anticus m.
   musculus rhomboideus m.
   musculus teres m.
   m. operation
   rectus capitis posterior m.
   rhomboid m.
   Sanguisorba m.
   m. surgery
   trochanter m.
   m. yang channel axis
   m. yin channel axis
minoris
   crista tuberculi m.
mint
   balm m.
   brandy m.
   m. family
   green m.
   lamb m.
   mountain m.
   Our Lady's m.
   m. tea
   tea with m.
minus
   os multangulum m.
miodidymus
miraa
miracle plant
mirtil
misalignment
miso
Missouri
   M. milk vetch
   M. snakeroot
mist
   catnip m.
   Feverfew Nasal M.

floral water m.
herbal water m.
mistletoe
American m.
juniper m.
Mitchella
M. repens
M. undulata
Mitchell lumbosacral angle
mitella
mitochondria
m. energy support
m.l function
mitogen
pokeweed m. (PWM)
mitoquinone
mitral valve prolapse (MVP)
mittelschmerz
mix
trail m.
mixed
m. nerve
m. tocopherol concentrate
mixer approach
mixture
Atkinson & Barker's Gripe M.
Catarrh M.
Indigestion M.
Neo Baby M.
Nurse Harvey's Gripe M.
Spanish Tummy M.
mJ
millijoule
MK-639
MMPI
Minnesota Multiphasic Personality
Inventory
mo
jenn m.
m. point
renn m.
tou m.
m. ya
mobile point
mobility
articular m.
m. of brain

central nervous system
inherent m.
cranial bone articular m.
decreased m.
dura mater m.
head m.
m. of head and neck
inherent m.
intracranial m.
intraspinal membrane m.
joint m.
muscle-tissue m.
sacral involuntary m.
spinal m.
sternoclavicular joint m.
m. testing
mobilization
cervical m.
combined method joint m.
direct method joint m.
exaggeration method joint m.
high-velocity low-amplitude
joint m.
iliosacral joint m.
indirect method joint m.
joint m.
Maitland m.
physiological response method
joint m.
sacrococcygeal joint m.
soft tissue m.
m. technique
m. with impulse direct action
technique
m. with impulse and muscle
energy technique
m. with impulse technique
m. without impulse
m. without impulse
(articulatory) treatment
m. without impulse technique
mobilize
mobilizing technique
moccasin flower
modality
caring-healing m.'s

M

NOTES

mode
  diagnostic m.
  therapeutic m.
model
  bioenergy m.
  neuroendocrine m.
  neurological m.
  pain m.
  postural-structural m.
  psychobehavioral m.
  respiratory circulatory m.
  Smith drug treatment m.
modeling
moderate
  m. hypnotic ability
  m. hypothermia
moderator band
modification
  behavior m.
  neural reflex m.
  work site m.
modify reflex
modiolus
  plate of m.
modulate muscle action
modulation
  neuroimmune m.
  steroid secretory m.
Moerman anticancer diet
Mohrenheim
  M. fossa
  M. space
moist-dry
moist heat
moksha
  rakta m.
molasses
  blackstrap m.
mold
  Aspergillus m.
  common m.
molding technique
molecular
  m. biology
  m. iodine
  m. medicine
molecule
  endorphin m.
molmol
  Commiphora m.
moluccana
  Aleurites m.
molybdenum

moment
  m. arm
  m. of force
momentum
  gait m.
Momordica charantia
monarthric
monarthritis
monarticular
monascus
Monascus purpureus
Mongolian ephedra
mongolicum
  Taraxacum m.
monitoring
  gastroscopic m.
  somatic m.
  therapeutic m.
monkey hand
monkey-paw
monkey's bench
monkshood
monk's pepper
monnieri
  Cnidium m.
monoamine
  midbrain m.
  m. oxidase (MAO)
  m. oxidase inhibitor
monoamine-dependent system
monocyte
monodactyly
monoethyl fumarate
monogyna
  Crataegus m.
monohydrate
  creatine m.
monohydrochloride
  L-lysine m.
monolocular
monomelic
monomelica
  osteosis eburnisans m.
mononucleosis
monoorotate
  L-lysine m.
monophosphate
  cyclic 3',5' adenosine m.
  (cAMP)
monopodia
monopus
  sympus m.
monoscelous

monostotic fibrous dysplasia
monoterpene
monotherapy
monounsaturated fat
Monro line
Monro-Richter line
montana
    Arnica m.
    Calamintha m.
    Satureja m.
Montana Naturals
Monthly Maintenance
monticulus
mood
    dysphoric m.
    One-A-Day Tension and M.
    M. Support
moon
    m. grass
    m. weed
Moor Mud
moose elm
mora de la India
morado
    lapacho m.
Morand foot
morbid obesity
MoreDophilus
Morgagni cartilage
morifolium
    Chrysanthemum m.
Morinda
    M. citrifolia
    M. citrifolia capsule
Mormon tea
mormuscone
morning
    m. glory
    m. sickness
    M. Wellness
Moro reflex
morphine
morphogenesis
morphogen gradient
morphology
Morquio syndrome
Morter Health System

mortification root
mortise
    m. joint
    talotibiofibular m.
Morton
    M. foot
    M. neuroma
    M. syndrome
    M. toe
morus
    M. alba
    m. fruit
Mosaro
moscada
    noz m.
    nuez m.
moschata
    Cucurbita m.
    Nux m.
moschiferus
    Moschus m.
Moschus moschiferus
mosquito plant
moss
    consumption m.
    Iceland m.
    Irish m.
    lung m.
    lungwort m.
    muskeag m.
    peat m.
    sphagnum m.
    tongue m.
Mosso ergograph
MOST
    manual organ stimulation technique
mother
    m. cell
    m. element
    m. essence
    m. point
    m. tonifying point
mother's
    m. die
    m. heart
mother-son law

M

NOTES

motherwort
  Chinese m.
  Siberian m.
motility
  inherent bone m.
  intestine m.
  membrane m.
motion
  active m.
  active range of m.
  alteration of m.
  m. analysis
  asymmetric m.
  m. available
  axis of rib m.
  axis of sacral m.
  backward-bending vertebral m.
  m. barrier
  barrier to m.
  bucket-handle rib m.
  calcaneal m.
  caliper m.
  caliper rib m.
  capitulum m.
  chest wall m.
  coiling m.
  continuous passive m.
  coupled m.
  cranial m.
  dynamic m.
  ease and bind concept in m.
  extension test for C2–7 m.
  forward-bending vertebral m.
  Happy M.
  ice tongs m.
  ilial m.
  iliosacral m.
  induced m.
  inherent m.
  inherent tissue m.
  intersegmental m.
  intervertebral m.
  intestinal m.
  involuntary m.
  joint m.
  knee joint m.
  laws of m.
  m. loss
  lumbar m.
  lumbar spine m.
  lumbosacral junction m.
  musculoskeletal system
    inherent m.

musculoskeletal system
  involuntary m.
neutral vertebral m.
nonneutral vertebral m.
normal m.
normal active range of m.
normal passive range of m.
m. palpation
passive m.
passive range of m.
physiologic m.
postural m.
principles of thoracic and
  lumbar spinal m. I–III
pump-handle rib m.
quality of m.
m. of radial head
radioulnar joint m.
range of m. (ROM)
repetitive m.
restriction of m.
m. restriction
restriction of intervertebral m.
restrictive barrier to m.
rib m.
rib head m.
rotation vertebral m.
sacral postural m.
sacroiliac joint m.
sacroiliac joint four-point m.
scapulohumeral joint m.
secondary joint m.
segmental m.
m. sense
m. sickness
sidebending vertebral m.
skin m.
skull bone m.
m. spectrum
spinal m.
m. test
m. testing
thoracic spine m.
tibiofibular joint m.
translatory m.
trochlea m.
type I vertebral m.
type II vertebral m.
type III vertebral m.
ulna m.
uncoiling m.
vertebral m.
vertebral column m.

voluntary m.
wringing m.
motivation
neuromuscular m.
patient m.
motor
m. cell
m. control
m. cortex pathway
m. fibers
m. impersistence
median nerve m.
m. nerve
m. neuron
m. neuron pool
plastic m.
m. system
m. unit
m. vehicle accident
mottling
mountain
m. arnica
m. balm
m. box
m. cranberry
m. daisy
m. flax
m. grape
m. hydrangea
m. mint
m. tea
m. tobacco
mouse ear
mouse-ear
m.-e. hawkweed
mouth
m. balancing
dry m.
mouth-to-mouth
m.-t.-m. respiration
m.-t.-m. resuscitation
movable joint
movement
accessory m.
accordion-type m.
active m.
anteroposterior m.

m. arc
assistive m.
Awareness Through M. (ATM)
body m.
chi m.
circus m.
counternutational m.
coupled m.
difficult m.
easy m.
m. education
eye m.
Feldenkrais Awareness
Through M.
flexion-extension m.
m. of fluid
free m.
iliosacral joint m.
inherent m.
m. integration technique
involuntary m.
involuntary nutation-
counternutation m.
limit of m.
midline sphenobasilar m.
muscular m.
nodding m.
nutational m.
passive m.
m. qigong
quality of m.
range of active m.
range of passive m.
resistive m.
respiratory m.
restricted m.
restricted coupled m.
separation-type m.
m. therapy
torsional m.
m. training
translatory m.
voluntary m.
movement-oriented qigong
mover
prime m.

M

NOTES

moxa
  m. cigar
  m. cone
  m. herb
  m. leaf
  m. roll
  m. wand
  m. wool
moxibustion
  m. by heating acupuncture
    needle
  indirect m.
  infrared m.
  method of m.
  m. with ginger slice isolation
  m. with moxa cigar
MPS
  myofascial pain syndrome
MRFIT
  Multiple Risk Factor Intervention
    Trial
MRI
  magnetic resonance imaging
MRSA
  methicillin-resistant *Staphylococcus*
    aureus
Mr. Steam
MS
  multiple sclerosis
ms
  millisecond
MSM
  methylsulfonylmethane
MSO
  managed service organization
MT
  muscle testing
mu
  m. front point
  m. point
  m. tong
  zhi m.
mucara
mucilage
mucilaginous mass
mucociliary clearance
Mucolytic Drainage Formula
mucoprotein
mucosa
  m. of colon
  intestinal m.
  tunica m.

mucositis
  oral m.
mucous
  m. membrane
  m. sheath of tendon
mucro sterni
mucus
mud
  m. bath
  Moor M.
mugo
  Pinus m.
muguet
mugwort
  burning m.
  dragon's m.
  smoldering m.
mukul
  Commiphora m.
Muladhara
mulata
  la m.
mulberry
  Indian m.
muliebre
  membrum m.
mullein
  American m.
  m. compress
  European m.
  m. flower oil
  great m.
  m. leaf
  orange m.
  petty m.
multangular bone
multiarticular
multiaxial joint
multicausal etiology
multidisciplinary
multifactorial problem
multifidi
  m. muscle
  m. musculi
multifidus
  m. muscle
  musculus m.
multiflorum
  Polygonum m.
multifocal osteitis fibrosa
Multigenics
  M. Chewable
  M. Intensive Care Formula

M. Maintenance Formula
M. Powders
M. Prenatal
M. Without Beta Carotene
Multi-Gland
Neonatal M.-G.
multi-infarct dementia
multimodal treatment
multinutrient supplement
multiple
m. amputation
m. epiphyseal dysplasia
m. exostoses
m. fracture
m. myeloma
M. Risk Factor Intervention
Trial (MRFIT)
m. sclerosis (MS)
multiple-plane thrust technique
multiplex
dysostosis m.
dysplasia epiphysealis m.
MultiPro table
multivitamin
Munich Quality of Life Dimensions List
muriaticum
Ammonium m.
Natrum m.
murillo bark
muroctasin
muscade
muscadier
muscaria
Amanita *m.*
muscatel sage
muscipula
Dionaea *m.*
muscle
m.'s of abdomen
abdominal m.
abdominal external oblique m.
abdominal internal oblique m.
abductor brevis m.
abductor digiti minimi m.
abductor digiti quinti m.
abductor hallucis m.

abductor longus m.
abductor magnus m.
abductor pollicis brevis m.
abductor pollicis longus m.
adductor m.
adductor brevis m.
adductor hallucis m.
adductor longus m.
adductor magnus m.
adductor minimus m.
adductor pollicis m.
adductor pollicis longus m.
agonist m.
agonistic m.
m. analysis
anconeus m.
antagonist m.
antagonistic m.
anterior scalene m.
anterior serratus m.
anterior tibial m.
antigravity m.
antitragicus m.
m. of antitragus
aponeurosis of vastus m.'s
appendicular m.
articular m.
articularis cubiti m.
articularis genus m.
m. atrophy
axial m.
axillary arch m.
m.'s of back
banding of m.
m. belly
biceps brachii m.
biceps femoris m.
m. biomechanics
bipennate m.
brachial m.
brachialis m.
brachioradial m.
brachioradialis m.
buccinator m.
bulge of m.
Casser perforated m.
cervical flexor m.

M

NOTES

263

muscle *(continued)*
cervical iliocostal m.
cervical interspinal m.
cervical longissimus m.
cervical rotator m.
clavicular head of pectoralis
  major m.
clavicular part of pectoralis
  major m.
coccygeus m.
common tendinous ring of
  extraocular m.'s
contracted m.
contractility of m.
m. contractility
m. contraction
m. contracture
contractured m.
m. cooperation
coracobrachial m.
coracobrachialis m.
cowl m.
cricopharyngeal sphincter m.
cruciate m.
cucullaris m.
m. curve
cutaneous m.
deepithelialized rectus
  abdominis m.
deep part of masseter m.
deep transverse perineal m.
deltoid m.
detrusor m.
digastric m.
digitorum longus m.
m. disorder
dorsal m.
dorsal interosseous m.
dorsal sacrococcygeal m.
dorsal sacrococcygeus m.
Dupré m.
dynamic phasic m.
ECRB m.
ECRL m.
EDB m.
m. elasticity
elasticity of m.
m. energy (ME)
m. energy manipulation
m. energy technique
m. energy technique for ribs
m. energy treatment
epicranial m.

epicranius m.
erector spinae m.
m. extensibility
extensibility of m.
extensor back m.
extensor carpi radialis
  brevis m.
extensor carpi radialis
  longus m.
extensor carpi ulnaris m.
extensor comminicus m.
extensor digiti minimi m.
extensor digiti quinti m.
extensor digitorum m.
extensor digitorum brevis m.
extensor digitorum
  communis m.
extensor digitorum longus m.
extensor hallucis brevis m.
extensor hallucis longus m.
extensor indicis m.
extensor indicis proprius m.
extensor pollicis brevis m.
extensor pollicis longus m.
external intercostal m.
external oblique m.
external obturator m.
external rotator m.
extrinsic m.
m. fascicle
m. fatigue
femoral m.
m. fiber
m. fiber action potential
m. fiber conduction velocity
m. fiber type
finger flexor m.
m. firing pattern
fixator m.
m. flap
flexor m.
flexor carpi radialis m.
flexor carpi ulnaris m.
flexor digiti quinti m.
flexor digitorum brevis m.
flexor digitorum longus m.
flexor digitorum profundus m.
flexor digitorum
  superficialis m.
flexor hallucis brevis m.
flexor hallucis longus m.
flexor pollicis brevis m.
flexor pollicis longus m.

fourth-layer m.
fourth-layer spinal m.
m. function
fusiform m.
Gantzer m.
gastrocnemius m.
gastrocsoleus m.
gemellus m.
gemellus inferior m.
gemellus superior m.
gluteal m.
gluteus m.
gluteus maximus m.
gluteus medius m.
gluteus minimus m.
gracilis m.
gracilis m.
great adductor m.
greater pectoral m.
greater psoas m.
greater rhomboid m.
m. guarding
hamstring m.
handbag m.
helicis major m.
helicis minor m.
m. hernia
hip adductor m.
hypertonic m.
m. hypertonicity
hypothenar m.
iliac m.
iliacus m.
iliacus minor m.
iliococcygeal m.
iliococcygeus m.
iliocostal m.
iliocostalis m.
iliocostalis cervicis m.
iliocostalis lumborum m.
iliocostalis thoracis m.
iliopsoas m.
m. imbalance
index extensor m.
indicator m.
inferior gemellus m.
inferior posterior serratus m.

inferior retinaculum of
   extensor m.'s
inferior tarsal m.
infraspinatus m.
inhibited gluteus m.
inhibited rectus abdominis m.
inhibited tibialis anterior m.
innermost intercostal m.
m. insufficiency
intercostal m.
intermediate great m.
intermediate vastus m.
intermedius m.
internal intercostal m.
internal oblique m.
internal obturator m.
internal rotator m.
interosseous m.
interspinal m.
interspinales lumborum m.
intertransversarii m.
intertransverse m.
intervening m.
intraoral m.
intraspinous m.
intrinsic m.
intrinsic m.
m. ischemia
ischiococcygeus m.
m. knot
Langer m.
lateral great m.
lateral lumbar
   intertransversarii m.
lateral lumbar
   intertransverse m.
lateral pterygoid m.
lateral vastus m.
latissimus dorsi m.
layered m.'s
lesser rhomboid m.
levator costales m.
levatores costarum m.
levator scapulae m.
line for soleus m.
long adductor m.
long fibular m.

M

NOTES

muscle *(continued)*
   longissimus m.
   longissimus capitis m.
   longissimus cervicis m.
   longissimus thoracis m.
   long levatores costarum m.
   long palmar m.
   long peroneal m.
   longus capitis m.
   longus cervicis m.
   longus colli m.
   lumbar erector spinae m.
   lumbar iliocostal m.
   lumbar interspinal m.
   lumbar quadrate m.
   lumbar rotator m.
   lumbrical m.
   lumbricalis m.
   masseter m.
   medial great m.
   medial lumbar
     intertransversarii m.
   medial lumbar
     intertransverse m.
   medial pterygoid m.
   medial vastus m.
   medius m.
   middle scalene m.
   minimus m.
   m. mobilizing technique
   multifidi m.
   multifidus m.
   m.'s of neck
   nerve to stapedius m.
   m. and neurological stimulation
     electrotherapy device
   oblique m.
   obliquus abdominis m.
   obliquus capitis inferior m.
   obliquus capitis superior m.
   obturator m.
   obturator externus m.
   obturator femoris m.
   obturator internus m.
   M. Octane
   omohyoid m.
   OP m.
   opponens digiti minimi m.
   opponens digiti quinti m.
   opponens pollicis m.
   palmar interossei
     interosseous m.
   palmar interosseous m.

palmaris brevis m.
palmaris longus m.
m. palpation
papillary m.
paraspinal m.
paravertebral m.
m. pathology
m. patterning sequence
pectinate m.
pectineal m.
pectineus m.
pectoral m.
pectoralis m.
pectoralis major m.
pectoralis minor m.
pectorodorsal m.
pectorodorsalis m.
m. pedicle bone graft
pelvic floor m.
pennate m.
perineal m.
peroneal m.
peroneus m.
peroneus brevis m.
peroneus longus m.
peroneus tertius m.
phasic m.
physical elasticity of m.
physiologic elasticity of m.
piriform m.
piriformis m.
plantar m.
plantar interossei
   interosseous m.
plantaris m.
plantar quadrate m.
plantar tendon sheath of
   peroneus longus m.
platysma m.
m. play
pollicis longus m.
popliteal m.
popliteus m.
posterior cervical
   intertransversarii m.
posterior cervical
   intertransverse m.
posterior deltoid m.
posterior scalene m.
posterior serratus m.
posterior tibial m.
postural m.
Pozzi m.

profundus m.
pronator quadratus m.
pronator teres m.
psoas m.
psoas major m.
psoas minor m.
pterygoid m.
pubococcygeal m.
pubococcygeus m.
pyramidalis m.
quadrate m.
quadrate pronator m.
quadratus m.
quadratus femoris m.
quadratus lumborum m.
quadratus planta m.
quadratus plantae m.
quadriceps femoris m.
rectus abdominis m.
rectus capitis anterior m.
rectus capitis lateralis m.
rectus capitis posterior
  major m.
rectus capitis posterior
  minor m.
rectus femoris m.
red m.
m. relaxant
m. relaxation
released ulnar intrinsic m.
m. repositioning
retinacula of extensor m.'s
retinacula of peroneal m.'s
retinaculum of flexor m.'s
m. retraining
rhomboid m.
rhomboid major m.
rhomboid minor m.
rider's m.'s
rotator m.
rotatores m.
rotatores cervicis m.'s
rotatores lumborum m.'s
rotatores thoracis m.'s
round pronator m.
salpingopharyngeal m.
salpingopharyngeus m.

Santorini m.
sartorius m.
satellite cell of skeletal m.
scalene m.
scalenus anterior m.
scalenus anticus m.
scalenus medius m.
scalenus minimus m.
scalenus posterior m.
scalp m.
scapulohumeral m.
scapulothoracic m.
Sebileau m.
second tibial m.
semimembranosus m.
semimembranous m.
semispinal m.
semispinalis m.
semispinalis cervicis m.
semitendinosus m.
semitendinous m.
serratus m.
serratus anterior m.
serratus posterior inferior m.
serratus posterior superior m.
shawl m.
m. sheath
short adductor m.
shortened psoas m.
short fibular m.
short levatores costarum m.
short palmar m.
short peroneal m.
shunt m.
Sibson m.
skeletal m.
m. slide
smaller pectoral m.
smaller psoas m.
smallest scalene m.
soleus m.
m. spasm
spastic m.
spastic hamstring m.
spastic quadratus lumborum m.
sphincter urethrae m.
spinal m.

M

NOTES

muscle *(continued)*
spinalis m.
spinalis capitis m.
spinalis cervicis m.
spinalis thoracis m.
m. spindle
m. spindle reflex
spindle-shaped m.
splenius m.
splenius capitis m.
splenius cervicis m.
spurt m.
spurt and shunt action of m.
static m.
sternal m.
sternalis m.
sternochondroscapular m.
sternoclavicular m.
sternocleidomastoid m.
sternocostal head of pectoralis
major m.
sternocostalis m.
sternocostal part of pectoralis
major m.
sternohyoid m.
sternomastoid m.
sternothyroid m.
m. strain
strap m.
m. strength testing
m. stretch reflex
striated m.
subanconeus m.
subclavian m.
subclavius m.
subcostal m.
subcrural m.
subquadricipital m.
subscapular m.
subscapularis m.
superficial back m.
superior belly of omohyoid m.
superior gemellus m.
superior pharyngeal
constrictor m.
superior posterior serratus m.
superior retinaculum of
extensor m.
superior tarsal m.
supinator m.
supraclavicular m.
supraspinalis m.
supraspinatus m.

supraspinous m.
syndrome of psoas m.
synergistic m.
synergistic m.
tailor's m.
temporalis m.
tendinous arch of soleus m.
tendinous sheath of extensor
carpi radialis m.
tendinous sheath of extensor
carpi ulnaris m.
tendinous sheath of extensor
digiti minimi m.
tendinous sheath of extensor
hallucis longus m.
tendinous sheath of extensor
pollicis longus m.
tendinous sheath of flexor
carpi radialis m.
tendinous sheath of flexor
hallucis longus m.
tendinous sheath of flexor
pollicis longus m.
tendinous sheath of superior
oblique m.
tendinous sheath of tibialis
anterior m.
tendinous sheath of tibialis
posterior m.
m. tension
tensor fasciae latae m.
teres m.
teres major m.
teres minor m.
test of hamstring m.
m. testing (MT)
thenar m.
m. therapy
third peroneal m.
thoracic interspinal m.
thoracic interspinales m.
thoracic intertransversarii m.
thoracic intertransverse m.
thoracic longissimus m.
thoracic rotator m.
m.'s of thorax
thyroarytenoid m.
thyroepiglottic m.
tibial m.
tibialis anterior m.
tibialis posterior m.
m. tissue
m. toe

toe extensor m.
toe flexor m.
m. tone
tonic m.
total elasticity of m.
trachealis m.
tracheloclavicular m.
m. transfer
transversospinal m.
transversospinales m.
transversus abdominis m.
transversus nuchae m.
transversus thoracis m.
trapezius m.
triangular m.
M. Tribe
triceps brachii m.
triceps coxae m.
triceps sura m.
triceps surae m.
trigone m.
tubercle of anterior scalene m.
tuberosity for serratus
  anterior m.
unequal length of
  hamstring m.
unequal length of psoas m.
unipennate m.
upper trapezius m.
uptight m.
vastus intermedius m.
vastus lateralis m.
vastus medialis m.
vastus medialis obliquus m.
ventral sacrococcygeal m.
ventral sacrococcygeus m.
vertebral column m.
vestigial m.
vocal m.
vocalis m.
voluntary m.
m. wasting
white m.
muscle-balancing procedure
muscle-bound
muscle-contraction headache
muscle-setting exercise

muscle-tendon attachment
muscle-tissue mobility
muscone
muscular
  m. artery
  m. atrophy
  m. attachment
  m. branch
  m. coat
  m. coat of pharynx
  m. contraction
  m. coordination
  m. cramp
  m. dysfunction
  m. dystrophy (MD)
  m. lacuna
  m. lesion
  m. movement
  m. neurofibromatosis
  m. palpation
  m. point
  m. pulley
  m. reeducation
  m. response
  m. sense
  m. system
  m. tissue
  m. torticollis
  m. triangle of neck
  m. trophoneurosis
muscularis
  trochlea m.
  tunica m.
muscularity
musculature
  paraspinal m.
musculi (*pl. of* musculus)
musculocutaneous
musculomembranous
musculorum
  lacuna m.
musculoskeletal
  m. manifestation
  m. manipulation
  m. system
  m. system diaphragm
    attachment

M

NOTES

musculoskeletal *(continued)*
  m. system energy expenditure
  m. system evaluation
  m. system inherent motion
  m. system involuntary motion
musculospiral groove
musculotendinous
  m. cuff
  m. junction
musculotubarii
  septum canalis m.
musculotubarius
  canalis m.
musculus, pl. **musculi**
  musculi abdominis
  abductor digiti minimi
    magnus m.
  m. abductor digiti minimi
    manus
  m. abductor digiti minimi
    pedis
  abductor digiti minimi
    pedis m.
  m. abductor digiti quinti
  m. abductor hallucis
  m. abductor pollicis brevis
  m. abductor pollicis longus
  m. adductor brevis
  m. adductor hallucis
  m. adductor longus
  m. adductor magnus
  m. adductor minimus
  m. adductor pollicis
  m. anconeus
  m. antitragicus
  m. articularis
  m. articularis cubiti
  m. articularis genus
  m. biceps brachii
  m. biceps femoris
  m. biceps flexor cruris
  m. bipennatus
  m. brachialis
  m. brachioradialis
  m. buccopharyngeus
  m. cephalopharyngeus
  m. cervicalis ascendens
  m. cleidoepitrochlearis
  m. cleidomastoideus
  musculi colli
  m. complexus
  m. complexus minor
  m. coracobrachialis

m. cruciatus
m. cutaneus
m. deltoideus
musculi dorsi
m. epicranius
m. epitrochleoanconeus
m. erector spinae
m. extensor brevis digitorum
m. extensor brevis pollicis
m. extensor carpi radialis
  brevis
m. extensor carpi radialis
  longus
m. extensor carpi ulnaris
m. extensor coccygis
m. extensor digiti minimi
m. extensor digiti quinti
  proprius
m. extensor digitorum
m. extensor digitorum brevis
m. extensor digitorum brevis
  manus
m. extensor digitorum
  communis
m. extensor digitorum longus
m. extensor hallucis brevis
m. extensor hallucis longus
m. extensor indicis
extensor indicis proprius m.
m. extensor indicis proprius
m. extensor longus digitorum
m. extensor longus pollicis
m. extensor minimi digiti
m. extensor ossis metacarpi
  pollicis
m. extensor pollicis brevis
m. extensor pollicis longus
m. fibularis brevis
m. fibularis longus
m. fibularis tertius
m. flexor accessorius
m. flexor brevis digitorum
m. flexor brevis hallucis
m. flexor carpi radialis
m. flexor carpi ulnaris
m. flexor digiti minimi brevis
  manus
m. flexor digiti minimi brevis
  pedis
m. flexor digitorum brevis
m. flexor digitorum longus
m. flexor digitorum profundus
m. flexor digitorum sublimis

m. flexor digitorum
  superficialis
m. flexor hallucis brevis
m. flexor hallucis longus
m. flexor longus digitorum
m. flexor longus hallucis
m. flexor longus pollicis
m. flexor pollicis brevis
m. flexor pollicis longus
m. flexor profundus
m. flexor sublimis
m. fusiformis
m. gastrocnemius
m. gemellus inferior
m. gemellus superior
m. glossopharyngeus
m. gluteus maximus
m. gluteus medius
m. gluteus minimus
m. gracilis
m. helicis major
m. helicis minor
m. iliacus
m. iliacus minor
m. iliocapsularis
m. iliocostalis
m. iliocostalis cervicis
m. iliocostalis dorsi
m. iliocostalis lumborum
m. iliocostalis thoracis
m. iliopsoas
m. infracostalis
m. infraspinatus
m. intercostalis externi
m. intercostalis internus
m. intercostalis intimus
musculi interossei
musculi interossei dorsalis
  manus
musculi interossei dorsalis
  pedis
m. interosseus palmaris
musculi interosseus plantaris
m. interosseus volaris
musculi interspinales
m. interspinalis cervicis
m. interspinalis lumborum

m. interspinalis thoracis
musculi intertransversarii
musculi intertransversarii
  anteriores cervicis
intertransversarii laterales
  musculi
musculi intertransversarii
  laterales lumborum
intertransversarii mediales
  lumborum musculi
musculi intertransversarii
  mediales lumborum
musculi intertransversarii
  posteriores cervicis
musculi intertransversarii
  thoracis
m. latissimus dorsi
m. levator anguli scapulae
m. levator costae
musculi levatores costarum
musculi levatores costarum
  breves
musculi levatores costarum
  longi
m. levator glandulae thyroideae
m. levator scapulae
m. longissimus
m. longissimus capitis
longissimus capitis m.
longissimus cervicis m.
m. longissimus cervicis
m. longissimus dorsi
m. longissimus thoracis
longus capitis m.
m. longus capitis
m. longus colli
m. lumbricalis manus
m. lumbricalis pedis
multifidi musculi
m. multifidus
m. multifidus spinae
m. mylopharyngeus
obliquus capitis inferior m.
m. obliquus capitis inferior
obliquus capitis superior m.
m. obliquus capitis superior
m. obliquus externus abdominis

NOTES

musculus *(continued)*
m. obliquus internus abdominis
m. obliquus superior
m. obturator externus
m. obturator internus
m. opponens digiti minimi
m. opponens digiti quinti
m. opponens minimi digiti
m. opponens pollicis
m. palmaris brevis
m. palmaris longus
m. papillaris
musculi pectinati
m. pectineus
m. pectoralis major
m. pectoralis minor
m. peroneocalcaneus
m. peroneus brevis
m. peroneus longus
m. peroneus tertius
m. piriformis
m. plantaris
m. platysma
m. platysma myoides
m. popliteus
m. pronator pedis
m. pronator quadratus
m. pronator radii teres
m. pronator teres
m. psoas major
m. psoas minor
m. pterygospinosus
m. quadratus
m. quadratus femoris
m. quadratus lumborum
m. quadratus plantae
m. quadriceps extensor femoris
m. quadriceps femoris
m. rectus capitis anticus major
m. rectus capitis anticus minor
m. rectus femoris
m. rectus thoracis
m. rhomboatloideus
rhomboideus major m.
m. rhomboideus major
m. rhomboideus minor
musculi rotatores
rotatores breves musculi
musculi rotatores cervicis
rotatores longi musculi
musculi rotatores lumborum
rotatores thoracis musculi
musculi rotatores thoracis

m. sacrococcygeus anterior
m. sacrococcygeus dorsalis
m. sacrococcygeus posterior
m. sacrococcygeus ventralis
m. sacrolumbalis
m. sacrospinalis
sacrospinalis m.
m. salpingopharyngeus
m. sartorius
m. scalenus anterior
m. scalenus anticus
m. scalenus medius
m. scalenus minimus
m. scalenus posterior
m. scalenus posticus
m. semimembranosus
m. semispinalis
m. semispinalis capitis
m. semispinalis cervicis
m. semispinalis colli
m. semispinalis dorsi
m. semispinalis thoracis
m. semitendinosus
m. serratus anterior
m. serratus magnus
m. serratus posterior inferior
m. serratus posterior superior
m. soleus
m. spinalis
m. spinalis capitis
m. spinalis cervicis
m. spinalis colli
m. spinalis dorsi
m. spinalis thoracis
m. splenius capitis
m. splenius cervicis
m. splenius colli
m. sternalis
m. sternochondroscapularis
m. sternoclavicularis
m. sternocleidomastoideus
m. sternofascialis
m. sternothyroideus
m. subclavius
m. subcostalis
m. subscapularis
m. supinator radii brevis
m. supraclavicularis
m. supraspinalis
m. supraspinatus
m. tarsalis inferior
m. tarsalis superior
m. tensor fasciae femoris

m. tensor fasciae latae
m. tensor tarsi
m. teres minor
m. tetragonus
musculi thoracis
m. thyroarytenoideus
m. thyroarytenoideus externus
m. thyroarytenoideus internus
m. tibialis gracilis
m. tibialis posterior
m. tibialis posticus
m. tibialis secundus
m. tibiofascialis anterior
m. tracheloclavicularis
m. transversalis capitis
m. transversalis cervicis
m. transversus nuchae
m. transversus thoracis
m. trapezius
m. triangularis sterni
m. triceps brachii
m. triceps coxae
m. triceps surae
m. unipennatus
m. vastus externus
m. vastus intermedius
m. vastus internus
m. vastus lateralis
m. vastus medialis
mushroom
  dancing m.
  forest m.
  immunotonic m.
  m. intoxication
  kawaratake m.
  king of m.'s
  kombucha m.
  maitake m.
  shiitake m.
music therapy
musk
  m. deer
  Tonquin m.
muskat
muskatbaum
muskeag moss

mussel
  m. extract
  freeze-dried m.
  New Zealand green-lipped m.
    (NZGLM)
  sea m.
mustard
  black m.
  brown m.
  Indian m.
  white m.
  wild m.
  yellow m.
Musterole
mutilans
  arthritis m.
mutong
mutra
mutterkraut
mutual resistance
muzei mu huang
MVP
  mitral valve prolapse
mW
  milliwatt
  mW intensity
my
  M. Favorite Evening Primrose
    oil
  m. li
myalgia
myasthenia
  m. angiosclerotica
  m. gravis
myasthenic syndrome
myatonia congenita
myatrophy
mycelium
Mycobacterium
  M. intracellulare
  M. tuberculosis
mycological
mycologist
mycosis fungoides
mycotic aneurysm
mycturia
mydriatic

M

NOTES

myectopy
myelauxe
myelinated nerve fiber
myelination
myelitis
  acute necrotizing m.
  acute transverse m.
  ascending m.
  funicular m.
  postinfectious m.
  postvaccinal m.
  radiation m.
  subacute necrotizing m.
  systemic m.
  transverse m.
myelocyte
myelodiastasis
myelodysplasia
myelogram
  cervical m.
  CT m.
  lumbar m.
myelography
  pantopaque m.
myeloma
  endothelial m.
  multiple m.
myelomalacia
myelomeningocele
myelonic
myelopathy
  carcinomatous m.
  paracarcinomatous m.
  radiation m.
  transverse m.
myelophthisic
myelophthisis
myelopoiesis
myelopoietic
myeloradiculodysplasia
myelorrhagia
myelorrhaphy
myelosis
  funicular m.
myelosuppression
myenteric plexus
Myers cocktail
myesthesia
Mylabris
mylopharyngeus
  musculus m.
myoarchitectonic

myocardial
  m. contractility
  m. infarction (MI)
myocardium
  ischemic m.
myochronoscope
myoclonus
myocrismus
myocutaneous
myodermal
myodiastasis
myodynamics
myodynamometer
myodynia
myodystony
myodystrophy
myoedema
myoelectric
myoesthesis
myofascial
  m. connection
  m. continuity
  m. pain
  m. pain syndrome (MPS)
  m. passive technique
  m. release (MFR)
  m. release technique
  m. release therapy
  m. release treatment
  m. shortening
  m. structure
  m. syndrome
  m. technique
  m. technique for pelvic
    diaphragm
  m. tender point
  m. tension
  m. tight-loose concept
  m. trigger point
myofibrositis
myofunctional
myogenic
  m. potential
  m. tonus
myoglobinuria
myoglobulin
myograph
myography
myoidema
myoides
  musculus platysma m.
myokinematics
  laws of m.

myokinesimeter
myologia
myologist
myology
    descriptive m.
myoma
myometer
myoneural blockade
myonosus
myonymy
myopathic
    m. atrophy
    m. scoliosis
myopathy
    carcinomatous m.
myositis
    proliferative m.
myosthenometer
myotactic
myotasis
myotatic
    m. contraction
    m. irritability
myotendinous junction
myotenositis
myotherapy
    Bonnie Prudden m.
myothermic
myotomal
    m. distribution
    m. pain pattern
    m. pattern
myotome
myotomy
myotone
myotonia
    m. atrophica
    m. dystrophica
myotonica
    dystrophia m.

myotonic dystrophy
myotonoid
myotony
Myrica
    M. cerifera
    M. pensylvanica
myrica
myristica
    M. fragrans
    m. oil
myristicin
Myroxylon
    M. balsamum
    M. pereirae
myroxylon
myrrh, myrrha
    African m.
    Arabian m.
    British m.
    gum m.
    m. gum
    m. gum-resin
    Somali m.
    Yemen m.
myrrha
    Commiphora m.
myrtillus
    Vaccinium m.
myrtle
    bridal m.
    common m.
    Dutch m.
    Jew's m.
    Roman m.
    southern wax m.
    sweet m.
mysticism
myxoid cyst

M

NOTES

na
    tui n.
NAAMM
    North American Academy of
    Manipulative Medicine
Nac
    Cellguard Co-Q10 N.
N-acetyl C-cysteine
N-acetylglucosamine
N-acetyl-5-methoxytryptamine
NACSCAOM
    National Accreditation Commission
    for Schools and Colleges of
    Acupuncture and Oriental
    Medicine
Nada yoga
NADH
    nicotinamide adenine dinucleotide
nadi
Naeser laser home treatment
  program for the hand
Naffziger sign
nail
    body of n.
    brittle n.'s
    n. extension
    free border of n.
    ingrown n.
    lateral border of n.
    occult border of n.
    n. plate
    proximal border of n.
    retinacula of n.
    root of n.
    Ultra N.'s
nailing
nail-patella syndrome
naja
naloxone
naltrexone
Nambudripad
name
    generic n.
Nana yoga
NANDA
    North American Nursing Diagnosis
    Association
nanism
    renal n.
    symptomatic n.

nanny
    stinking n.
nannyberry
nanometer (nm)
naohu
    du 17 n.
naoshu
    si 10 n.
nape
    transverse muscle of n.
napellus
    Aconitum n.
naprapathic
naprapathy
naproxen
Narcissus
narcosis
narcotic
    n. hunger
    n. reversal
narcotism
nardo
naringenin
narrow dock
narrowing
narrowleaf plantain
narrow-leaved purple coneflower
nasal
    n. antiseptic
    n. bone
    n. drainage
    n. milking
    n. sinus drainage technique
    n. sinus innervation
    n. turbinate
nasion
nasotracheal intubation
nasturtium
Nasturtium officinale
nasya
nata
    pro re n.
Natchez Mobil-Trac system
nates
National
    N. Accreditation Commission
    for Schools and Colleges of
    Acupuncture and Oriental
    Medicine (NACSCAOM)

N.

National *(continued)*
    N. Acupuncture Detoxification Association
    N. Board of Chiropractic Examiners (NBCE)
    N. Center for Complementary and Alternative Medicine (NCCAM)
    N. Certification Committee for Acupuncture and Oriental Medicine (NCCAOM)
    N. College of Chiropractic
    N. Heart, Lung, and Blood Institute (NHLBI)
    N. Institute for Healthcare Research (NIHR)
    N. Nutritional Foods Association (NNFA)
    N. Osteopathic Foundation
Nationally Certified Therapeutic Massage and Bodywork (NCTMB)
native
    N. American ethnobotany
    N. American medicine
Natren
Natrum
    N. muriaticum
    N. sulfuricum
naturae
    vis medicatrix n.
natural
    n. alternative
    Anabol N.'s
    N. Arthro-Rx
    N. Brand Shark Cartilage
    n. ecstasy
    n. foods diet
    n. killer (NK)
    n. killer cell
    Montana N.'s
    N. Nite
    n. opiate
    n. perfusion
    Source N.'s
Naturalax 2
Naturalvite
Nature's
    N. Answer
    N. Best
    N. Chi
    N. Secret

    N. Three
    N. Way
Natureworks Marigold ointment
naturopath
naturopathic
    n. doctor (ND, NMD)
    n. medicine
    n. physician
    N. Physicians Licensing Examination (NPLEx)
    n. remedy
naturopathy
nausea
    anticipatory n.
NAVEL
    nerve, artery, vein, empty space, lymphatics
navel
Navelbine
navelwort
    Indian water n.
navicular
    n. articular surface of talus
    n. bone
    n. bone dysfunction
    n. bone of hand
    n. bone internally rotated
    n. bone tender point
naviculare
    os n.
navicularis
    tuberositas ossis n.
navy bean
NBCE
    National Board of Chiropractic Examiners
NCCAM
    National Center for Complementary and Alternative Medicine
NCCAOM
    National Certification Committee for Acupuncture and Oriental Medicine
NCTMB
    Nationally Certified Therapeutic Massage and Bodywork
NCV
    nerve conduction velocity
ND
    naturopathic doctor
NDA
    new drug application
nearthrosis

nebulizer
 jet n.
 spinning disk n.
 ultrasonic n.
necessary cause
neck
 buffalo n.
 deep fascia of n.
 n. disability index
 n. extensor
 extra point on the head
  and n. (Ex-HN)
 n. of femur
 n. of fibula
 n. flexion curl
 n. flexor
 n. of humerus
 lateral region of n.
 long muscle of n.
 n. of malleus
 mobility of head and n.
 muscles of n.
 muscular triangle of n.
 posterior region of n.
 posterior triangle of n.
 n. of radius
 n. reflexes
 regions of n.
 n. of rib
 n. roll
 n. of scapula
 semispinal muscle of n.
 spinal muscle of n.
 splenius muscle of n.
 n. of talus
 tension n.
 n. of thigh bone
 wry n.
neck-shaft angle
necrosis
 aseptic n.
 epiphysial aseptic n.
 renal tubular n.
 subcutaneous fat n.
necrosteon
necrotic tissue
necrotizing enterocolitis

nectar of the gods
needle
 acupuncture n.
 Adam's n.
 bleeding n.
 blunt n.
 disposable n.
 disposable acupuncture n.
 double-webbed n.
 dragonhead n.
 energy-moving n.
 face n.
 filiform n.
 filiform steel n.
 gold n.
 n. grab
 hooked n.
 Ito n.
 long retention of the n.
 n. manipulation
 moxibustion by heating
  acupuncture n.
 permanent n.
 pine n.
 n. resistance
 Seirin acupuncture n.
 seven star n.
 sham n.
 shepherd's n.
 silver n.
 n. stimulation
 subcutaneous n.
 thin n.
 thin acupuncture n.
 n. treatment
 n. twirling
needled
needling
 deep n.
 distal nonsegmental n.
 dry n.
 even method of n.
 high-frequency low-intensity n.
 local segmental n.
 low-frequency, high-intensity n.
 Mark Seem n.
 n. method

N

NOTES

needling *(continued)*
    method of n.
    pain-free n.
    plain n.
    n. of point
    sham-point n.
    subcutaneous n.
    therapeutic n.
    tonifying n.
    true-point n.
neem
    n. oil
    N. Plus
negative
    n. affectivity
    n. correlation
    false n.
    n. feedback loop
    n. flavor affinity
    n. intrathoracic pressure
    n. pulse
nei
    n. dan qigong
    n. guan point
neiguan
    n. anti-emetic acupuncture
      point
    n. point
neima
    extrapoint n.
    n. point
neiting
    st 44 n.
Nélaton line
nematicidal
NEO
    Neuroticism, Extroversion, and
      Openness
    NEO Personality Inventory
neo
    N. Baby Mixture
    N. Ginsana
neoarthrosis
Neo-Ballistol
Neo-Cleanse
neoformans
    Cryptococcus n.
Neo-Lax
Neoloid
neonatal
    N. Multi-Gland
    n. tetanus
neoplasia

neoplasm
neoplastic disease
Nepeta cataria
nephrolithiasis
nephropathy
    IgA n.
nephrosis
nephrotic syndrome
nephrotoxic
Nephrubin
Nerium indicum
neroli oil
nerve
    abdominopelvic plexus of n.
    abducens n.
    accessory n. [CN XI]
    afferent n.
    afferent fibers of vagus n.
    anococcygeal n.
    n., artery, vein, empty space,
      lymphatics (NAVEL)
    articular n.
    augmentor n.
    Bell respiratory n.
    n. block
    n. block anesthesia
    carotid n.
    C1–C8 n.'s
    cervical n.'s [C1–C8]
    cervical splanchnic n.'s
    coccygeal n. [Co]
    cochlear n.
    n. conduction study
    n. conduction velocity (NCV)
    n. conduction velocity study
    cranial n.
    cranial n.'s II–XII
    efferent n.
    efferent fibers of vagus n.
    n. entrapment
    esodic n.
    exodic n.
    facial n.
    femoral n.
    n. fiber
    fourth lumbar n. [L4]
    n. ganglion
    genitofemoral n.
    glossopharyngeal n.
    great sciatic n.
    hypoglossal n.
    iliohypogastric n.
    n. impingement

internal carotid n.
lateral cutaneous femoral n.
loops of spinal n.'s
lumbar n.'s [L1–L5]
maxillary n.
medial pectoral n.
medial plantar n.
medial popliteal n.
median n.
mixed n.
motor n.
obturator n.
oculomotor n.
olfactory n.
parasympathetic n.
peripheral n.
peripheral motor n.
peroneal n.
phrenic n.
n. plexus
n. plexus entrapment
posterior cutaneous femoral n.
preganglionic sympathetic n.
presacral n.
proprioception n.
pudendal n.
radial n.
n. regeneration
n. to rhomboid
n. root
n. root sleeve
rule of the n.
sacral n.'s [S1–S5]
sciatic n.
sensory n.
sinovertebral n.
small sciatic n.
spinal n.
spinal accessory n.
splanchnic n.
n. to stapedius muscle
n. stimulation
superficial n.
sympathetic n.
third cranial n. [CN III]
thoracic n.'s [T1–T12]
tibial n.

trigeminal n.
trochlear n.
ulnar n.
vagus n.
vertebral n.
vestibulocochlear n.
Wrisberg n.
nerveroot
nervi (*pl. of* nervus)
nervine
Nervonocton N
nervosa
  anorexia n.
Nervospur
nervous
  n. system
  n. system facilitation
  n. system segmentalization
  n. tissue
nervousness
nervus, pl. **nervi**
  n. articularis
nest
  bird's n.
nettle
  n.'s capsule
  common n.
  freeze-dried n.
  greater n.
  n. leaf
  n.'s liquid extract
  stinging n.
network
  articular n.
  articular vascular n.
  capillary n.
  n. chiropractic
  dorsal carpal n.
  energy circulation n.
  lateral malleolar n.
  medial malleolar n.
  patellar n.
  psychosomatic n.
  trabecular n.
Neuquinone
neural
  n. element

N

NOTES

neural *(continued)*
n. entrapment
n. limb tension test
n. mechanism
n. organization therapy
n. reflex modification
n. restriction
n. spine
n. therapist
n. therapy
n. traffic
n. tube
n. tube defect
neuralgia
intercostal n.
postherpetic n.
stump n.
trigeminal n.
trigeminal nerve n.
neuralgic amyotrophy
neurapophysis
neuritis
brachial n.
neuroanatomic
neuroanatomical activity
neuroarthropathy
neurobehavioral reaction
neuroblastoma
neurocellular repatterning
neurocentral
n. joint
n. synchondrosis
neurochemical
Neurochol
neurocompression
neurodegeneration
neurodermatitis
neuroemotional technique
neuroendocrine
n. control
n. function
n. model
n. system
neurofibroma
plexiform n.
neurofibromatosis
muscular n.
neurogenic
n. atrophy
n. claudication
neurohormone
neuroimmune modulation
neuroleptanalgesia

neuroleptanesthesia
neuroleptic agent
neurolinguistic programming
neurologic
n. deficit
n. dysfunction
neurological
n. complication
n. disease
n. disorder
n. effect
n. function
n. hypothesis
n. model
neurolymphatic reflex
neuroma
fibrillary n.
Morton n.
plexiform n.
neuromagnetic stimulation
Neuromins DHA
neuromuscular
n. anatomy
n. blocking agent
n. disorder
n. integration
n. massage
n. motivation
n. reeducation
n. reflex
n. rehabilitation
n. relaxant
n. system
neuromusculoskeletal system
neuromyelitis
neuron
alpha motor n.
gamma motor n.
motor n.
preganglionic n.
spinal cord transmission n.
ventral motor n.
neuronal pathway
neuropathic
n. arthritis
n. arthropathy
n. joint
n. pain
neuropathy
brachial plexus n.
carcinomatous n.
cranial nerve n.
diabetic n.

entrapment n.
peripheral n.
sensory n.
uremic n.
neuropeptide mechanism
neurophysiological
　n. balance
　n. test
neurophysiologic pathway
neurophysiologist
neurophysiology
neuroreflexive
　n. change
　n. response
neurosis
　cardiac n.
　torsion n.
neurosurgeon
neurotendinous
neurotensin
neuroticism
　N., Extroversion, and Openness
　　(NEO)
　N., Extroversion, and Openness
　　Personality Inventory
neurotome
neurotransmitter
neurotrophic atrophy
neurotrophicity
neurotrophy
neurovascular
　n. bundle
　n. entrapment
　n. side effect
Neutracalm
neutral
　n. dysfunction
　n. extension
　n. external rotation
　n. flexion
　n. internal rotation
　n. internal rotation stage 1
　n. internal rotation stage 2
　n. lumbar spine
　n. mechanics
　pathological n.
　n. position

n. spinal position
n. vertebral motion
neutralization plate
neutral, sidebent right, rotated left
　(NSRRL)
neutropenia
neutrophil
　n. leukocytosis
　polymorphonuclear n.
nevadensis
　Ephedra n.
new
　n. drug application (NDA)
　N. York Heart Association
　　(NYHA)
　N. York Heart Association
　　functional class
　N. Zealand green-lipped mussel
　　(NZGLM)
Newcastle disease
Newton laws of lever
NHLBI
　National Heart, Lung, and Blood
　　Institute
niacin
　crystalline n.
　sustained-release n.
niacinamide
nian
　zheng ti guan n. (ZTGN)
NIC
　Nursing Interventions Classification
nicotinamide adenine dinucleotide
　(NADH)
nicotinate
　inositol n.
nicotine addiction
nicotinic acid
nidus
nieguan
　pe 6 n.
niger
　Hyoscyamus n.
　Sambucus n.
night
　queen of the n.
　Silent N.

NOTES

N

night *(continued)*
    n. sweat
    n. sweating
night-blooming cereus
nightcap
    old maid's n.
nightshade
    bittersweet n.
    black n.
    deadly n.
    n. poisoning
    woody n.
nigra
    Brassica n.
    Juglans n.
    Pinus n.
    Populus n.
nigricans
    acanthosis n.
    Pulsatilla n.
nigrum
    Piper n.
    Ribes n.
    Solanum n.
NIHR
    National Institute for Healthcare
    Research
nim
nimba
nimodipine
nine hooks
nine-point scale
ninjin
nip
nippon
    Cervus n.
Nite
    Natural N.
nitida
    Cola n.
nitric oxide
nitricum
    Argentum n.
nitrogen
    blood urea n. (BUN)
nitrosamine
nitrous oxide (NO)
nituri
    Phyllanthus n.
niu she t'ou
Nivalin

NK
    natural killer
    NK cell
nm
    nanometer
NMD
    naturopathic doctor
N,N+1
NNFA
    National Nutritional Foods
    Association
NO
    nitrous oxide
No.
    N. 2040 Headache Remedy
    N. 2090 Indigestion Remedy
Noah's ark
nobile
    Chamaemelum n.
nobilis
    Laurelis n.
    Laurus n.
nobleza gaucha
nocebo
    n. effect
    n. response
nociception
nociceptive
    n. pain
    n. pathway stimulation
    n. reflex
nociceptor
n-octacosanol
nocturia
nocturnal
    n. emission
    n. enuresis
nodal
nodding movement
node
    apical axillary lymph n.
    atrioventricular n.
    axillary lymph n.
    brachial lymph n.
    central axillary lymph n.
    cervical lymph n.
    coronary n.
    cubital lymph n.
    deep lateral cervical lymph n.
    fibular n.
    fibular lymph n.
    gluteal lymph n.
    Heberden n.

intermediate lacunar n.
interpectoral lymph n.
juguloomohyoid n.
lateral lacunar n.
lateral lacunar lymph n.
lumbar lymph n.
lymph n.
medial lacunar n.
occipital lymph n.
parotid lymph n.
popliteal lymph n.
postauricular lymph n.
preauricular lymph n.
promontorial common iliac n.
retroauricular lymph n.
right lumbar lymph n.
Rosenmüller n.
submandibular lymph n.
superficial parotid lymph n.
supraclavicular lymph n.
Tawara n.
nodi (*pl. of* nodus)
nodosa
arthritis n.
nodose rheumatism
nodosum
Ascophyllum n.
nodular lesion
nodule
rheumatoid n.
subcutaneous n.
tender n.
nodulus
nodus, pl. **nodi**
noetic science
noi
phi n.
noise
white n.
noiseless restoration
nomogram
nonacupoint
nonacupuncture point
nonadaptive lumbar response
noncompliance
noncontact therapeutic touch
noncontained disk herniation

nondepolarizing
n. block
n. relaxant
nondirected prayer
non-end product metabolite
noni
noninvasive procedure
nonlamellar bone
nonlinear logic
nonneutral
n. dysfunction
n. lumbar spine
n. mechanics
n. vertebral motion
nonoperative cranioplasty
nonordinary state of consciousness
nonoriental massage
nonossifying fibroma
nonosteogenic fibroma
nonphototoxic
nonphysical stressor
nonpoint
nonreductionistic phenomenology
nonresting energy expenditure
nonrigid skull
nonsegmental effect
nonspecific
n. hypnotherapy
n. osteopathic manipulation
nonsteroidal
n. antiinflammatory agent
n. antiinflammatory drug
(NSAID)
nonsynchronous
nontoxic
nonunion
nonvascular
nonvolitional response
No Pain HP
nor-binaltorphimine
norepinephrine
nori
normal
n. active range of motion
n. barrier
easy n. (EN)
n. feel

N

NOTES

285

normal *(continued)*
    n. function
    n. motion
    n. muscle firing pattern
    n. passive range of motion
normotonic
North
    N. American Academy of
      Manipulative Medicine
      (NAAMM)
    N. American Nursing
      Diagnosis Association
      (NANDA)
northern
    n. prickly ash
    n. senega
Norwegian
    N. exercise
    N. Kelp
nosebleed plant
nose inflammation pill
nosode
nosology
    functional n.
nostrum
notal
notch
    acetabular n.
    costal n.
    cotyloid n.
    fibular n.
    greater sciatic n.
    iliosciatic n.
    interclavicular n.
    intercondyloid n.
    intertragic n.
    intervertebral n.
    ischiatic n.
    lesser sciatic n.
    mastoid n.
    popliteal n.
    presternal n.
    radial n.
    sacrosciatic n.
    scapular n.
    sternal n.
    supraorbital n.
    suprasternal n.
    tentorial n.
    ulnar n.
    vertebral n.
notha
    sutura n.

notoginseng
    Panax n.
Now Foods
noxious
noxious stimulus
noz moscada
NPLEx
    Naturopathic Physicians Licensing
      Examination
NSAID
    nonsteroidal antiinflammatory drug
NSRRL
    neutral, sidebent right, rotated left
Nu
    N. Veg goldenseal herb
    N. Veg goldenseal root
    N. Veg Milk Thistle Power
Nubian senna
nucha
nuchae
    fascia n.
    musculus transversus n.
nuchal
    n. fascia
    n. ligament
    n. plane
    n. region
nuchalis
    regio n.
nucifera
    Cocos n.
Nuck diverticulum
nuclear
    n. bag
    n. bag fiber
    n. chain fiber
nucleus
    accessory cuneate n.
    n. accumbens
    n. accumbens septi
    arcuate n.
    cuneate n.
    gracile n.
    paraventricular n.
    n. pulposus
    raphe n.
    supraoptic n.
nuez moscada
number
    Avogadro n.
numbness
numerology
Nurse Harvey's Gripe Mixture

nursemaid's elbow
nursing
    holistic n.
    N. Interventions Classification
      (NIC)
nut
    areca n.
    betel n.
    Brazil n.
    chop n.
    esere n.
    kola n.
nutation
nutational movement
nutgall
nutmeg
    n. seed
    n. toxicity
Nutrajoint
NutraPack
Nutri-Calm
nutricium
    foramen n.
nutricius
    canalis n.
nutrient
    N. 950
    brain n.
    n. canal
    n. foramen
    n. qi
    Ultra N.
nutrient-dependency syndrome
Nutri-Fem

Nutri-Joint
nutrition
    Chinese n.
    clinical n.
    ISP N.
    Oriental n.
    therapeutic n.
    Universal N.
nutritional
    Bio N.
    n. biochemistry
    n. evaluation
    n. functional medicine
    n. medicine
    n. rickets
    n. status
nutritionist
nutritive perfusion
Nutri Zac
Nux
    N. moschata
    N. vomica
    N. vomica seed
nux-vomica
    Strychnos n.-v.
NYHA
    New York Heart Association
nystagmus
Nytol Herbal
nyug
    txiu kub n.
NZ glandular
NZGLM
    New Zealand green-lipped mussel

NOTES

N

oak

o. apple
o. bark
British o.
brown o.
common o.
Eastern poison o.
English o.
o. gall
o. lung
lungs of o.
poison o.
stone o.
sweet o.
white o.

OAM

Office of Alternative Medicine

oat

o. bran
o. extract
green o.'s
O.'s and Honey
o. straw
o. straw tea
whole o.'s

oat-herb tea
oatmeal bath
Ober test
obesity

exogenous o.
morbid o.

object

power o.

objective

enabling o.
terminal o.

obligate parasite
obliqua

diameter o.
linea o.

oblique

o. amputation
o. axis
o. axis of the sacrum
o. bandage
o. cord of interosseous
  membrane of forearm
o. diameter
o. fracture
o. head

o. insertion
o. ligament of elbow joint
o. line
o. line of mandible
o. line of thyroid cartilage
o. muscle
o. needling method
o. popliteal ligament
o. projection
o. ridge of trapezium
o. section

obliquum

caput o.

obliquus

o. abdominis muscle
o. capitis inferior muscle
o. capitis inferior musculus
o. capitis superior muscle
o. capitis superior musculus

obliterans

bronchiolitis o.

obliteration

sutural o.

oblongata

medulla o.

observer attitude
obsessive-compulsive disorder (OCD)
obstetric

o. back pain
o. hand

obstipation
obstruction

bladder outlet o.
lymphatic o.

obtecta

pelvis o.

obturation
obturator

o. artery
o. canal
o. crest
o. externus muscle
o. fascia
o. femoris muscle
o. foramen
o. groove
o. internus muscle
o. membrane
o. muscle

O

obturator *(continued)*
  o. nerve
  o. tubercle
obturatoria
  crista o.
  membrana o.
obturatorium
  tuberculum o.
obturatorius
  canalis o.
obturatum
  foramen o.
OCCAM
  Office of Cancer Complementary
  and Alternative Medicine
occidentalis
  Rubus o.
occipital
  o. articulation
  o. condyle
  o. crest
  o. lymph node
  o. mastoid suture
  o. protuberance
  o. squama
occipitalis
  craniopagus o.
  margo mastoideus squamae o.
occipitoatlantal
  o. cervical spine
  o. joint
  o. junction functional technique
  o. region linear stretch
  o. vertebra
occipitomastoid suture
occiput
  o. articulation
  basilar portion of o.
  o. bone
  condylar portion of o.
  o. motion testing
  o. torsion
occult
  o. border of nail
  o. fracture
occulta
  spina bifida o.
occupational
  o. asthma
  o. therapist
  o. therapy
  o. therapy assessment

OCD
  obsessive-compulsive disorder
OCF
  osteopathy in the cranial field
ochronotic arthritis
Ocimum basilicum
octacosanol
  o. capsule
  Super O.
octacosonol
octacosyl alcohol
octane
  Muscle O.
Ocu-Care
OcuGuard
ocular
  o. anaphylaxis
  o. inflammation
  o. scoliosis
oculoauriculovertebral dysplasia
oculocephalogyric reflex
oculomandibulofacial syndrome
oculomotor nerve
oculovertebral
  o. dysplasia
  o. syndrome
Odara
oderwort
O'Donaghue triad
odontoid process
odor
  acid o.
  putrid o.
  sour o.
odorata
  Asperula o.
  Cananga o.
  Dipteryx o.
  Hierochloe o.
  Viola o.
odoratism
odoratum
  Anthoxanthum o.
  Galium o.
Odorless Garlic Tablets
Oenothera biennis
OEP
  oil of evening primrose
off
  back o.
  toe o.

Office
    O. of Alternative Medicine
      (OAM)
    O. of Cancer Complementary
     and Alternative Medicine
     (OCCAM)
officinale
    Cynoglossum o.
    Guaiacum o.
    Levisticum o.
    Lithospermum o.
    Nasturtium o.
    Symphytum o.
    Taraxacum o.
    Zingiber o.
officinalis
    Althaea o.
    Anchusa o.
    Asparagus o.
    Betonica o.
    Borago o.
    Calendula o.
    Euphrasia o.
    Hyssopus o.
    Lavandula o.
    Magnolia o.
    Mandragora o.
    Melilotus o.
    Melissa o.
    Parietaria o.
    Pimenta o.
    Rosmarinus o.
    Salvia o.
    Sanguisorba o.
    Saponaria o.
    Sassafras o.
    Smilax o.
    Stachys o.
    Valeriana o.
    Verbena o.
officinalus
    Cornus o.
officinarum
    Alpinia o.
    Pilosella o.
Ohashiatsu technique
Ohm law

ohmmeter
oil
    Actualize o.
    anise o.
    Aromatic Castor O.
    Australian tea tree o.
    Balance o.
    Barlean's Flax O.
    Begin o.
    bhringraj o.
    birch tar o.
    birch wood o.
    bitter orange o.
    black currant seed o.
    black pepper essential o.
    borage seed o.
    botanical essential o.
    o. of carrot
    castor o.
    o. of cedar
    Celebrate o.
    celery seed o.
    Change o.
    chaulmogra o.
    chenopodium o.
    China-wood o.
    o. of citronella
    clary o.
    clove o.
    o. of cloves
    cold-pressed olive o.
    Complete o.
    cottonseed o.
    croton o.
    Emerge o.
    o. enema
    enteric-coated fish o.
    essential o.
    o. of eucalyptus
    eucalyptus o.
    o. of evening primrose (OEP)
    evening primrose o. (EPO)
    Experience o.
    extra-virgin olive o.
    fish o.
    flaxseed o.
    o. from seed

O

NOTES

oil (*continued*)
    gaultheria o.
    grapeseed o.
    gynocardia o.
    Harvest o.
    hydnocarpus o.
    Jason Winter's Tea Tree O.
    joint o.
    Koong Yick Hung Fa O.
    lavender o.
    lavender essential o.
    lemon essential o.
    Lorenzo's O.
    o. massage
    Mega Primrose O.
    melaleuca o.
    mullein flower o.
    My Favorite Evening
      Primrose O.
    myristica o.
    neem o.
    neroli o.
    olive o.
    orange o.
    o. of oregano
    parsley o.
    o. of pennyroyal
    pennyroyal o.
    pennyroyal essential o.
    peppermint o.
    perilla o.
    Prepare O.
    primrose o.
    pumpkin seed o.
    rose o.
    rosemary o.
    o. of rosemary
    o. of rue
    rue o.
    safflower o.
    salmon o.
    santal o.
    sesame o.
    shark liver o.
    Swanson Ultra Tea Tree O.
    sweet birch o.
    sweet marjoram essential o.
    tansy o.
    o. of tea
    tea tree o. (TTO)
    Thursday Plantation Tea
      Tree O.
    turpentine o.
    ultimate o.
    unrefined canola o.
    virgin o.
    wheat germ o.
    white sandalwood o.
    o. of wintergreen
    wintergreen o.
    yellow sandalwood o.

ointment
    aloe vera o.
    BF&C O.
    BF&S O.
    Black o.
    comfrey o.
    Natureworks Marigold O.
    podophyllum o.
    Traumeel o.

oja
olacoides
    Ptychopetalum o.

Olbas

old
    o. maid
    o. maid's nightcap
    o. man
    o. man's pepper
    o. woman's broom

old-maid's pink

oleander
    o. bush
    o. toxicity

olecrani
    fossa o.

olecranon
    o. bursitis
    o. fossa
    o. process

oleic acid

oleoresin
    aspidium o.
    male fern o.

oleum
    o. cari
    o. carvi
    o. caryophylli
    o. majoranae

olfaction

olfactory nerve

oligodactyly

oligomer
    procyanidol o. (PCO)

oligomeric proanthocyanidin (OPC)

oligospermia

oligo therapy
oliguria
olive oil
olivospinal tract
Ollier
    O. disease
    O. theory
OM
    osteopathic manipulative medicine
omega-3
    o. essential fatty acid
    o. family
    o. polyunsaturated fatty acid
Omega-Plex
omicha
omoclaviculare
    trigonum o.
omoclavicular triangle
omohyoid muscle
omothyroid
omotracheal triangle
OMT
    osteopathic manipulative technique
    osteopathic manipulative treatment
    indirect OMT
oncologist
oncology
Onconase
oncostatic
one
    balance testing level o.
One-A-Day
    O.-A.-D. Bone Strength
    O.-A.-D. Cholesterol Health
    O.-A.-D. Cold Season
    O.-A.-D. Energy Formula
    O.-A.-D. Garlic
    O.-A.-D. Memory and
      Concentration
    O.-A.-D. Menopause Health
    O.-A.-D. Prostate Health
    O.-A.-D. Tension and Mood
one-berry
one-legged
    o.-l. stander
    o.-l. stork test
oneness

onion
    o. poultice
    sea o.
onlay
Onosma bracteatum
onychocryptosis
onychoid
onychomycosis
onychostroma
onyx
onyxis
OP
    opponens pollicis
    OP muscle
OPC
    oligomeric proanthocyanidin
OPC-85
open
    o. dislocation
    o. drop anesthesia
    o. facet
    o. fracture
    o. reduction of fracture
opening
    o. of the chakra
    esophageal o.
    o. facet
    femoral o.
    horns of saphenous o.
    tendinous o.
    vaginal o.
Openness
    Neuroticism, Extroversion,
      and O. (NEO)
opera-glass hand
operant conditioning
operate
operation
    flap o.
    minor o.
    subcutaneous o.
operator guiding technique
opercular fold
operculum
Ophiopogon japonicus
ophryospinal angle
ophthalmia

O

NOTES

ophthalmicus (V1)
opiate
    o. addiction
    natural o.
    o. receptor blocking
opioid
opisthenar
opium
    gum o.
    lettuce o.
    o. poppy
Oplopanax horridus
opobalsam
opponens
    o. digiti minimi muscle
    o. digiti quinti muscle
    o. pollicis (OP)
    o. pollicis muscle
opposer
    o. muscle of little finger
    o. muscle of thumb
opposita
    Dioscorea o.
opposite
    dialectic o.
optometry
    syntonic o.
opulus
    Viburnum o.
oral
    o. acupuncture
    o. cancer
    o. flora
    o. leukoplakia
    o. medication
    o. mucositis
    o. steroid
    o. therapy
orange
    o. carotenoid
    o. juice
    o. mullein
    o. oil
Orange-Chew
Orbeli effect
orbicular
    o. ligament
    o. ligament of radius
orbit torsion
orchialgia
ordeal bean
ordinate
Oregamax

oregano
    oil of o.
Oregon
    O. grape
    O. grape root
    O. yew
organ
    o. association
    o. axis
    Chinese o.
    corresponding o.
    deficient o.
    delicate o.
    disorder of the sense o.'s
    o. energy
    energy-producing o.
    followup o.
    fu o.
    Golgi tendon o.
    hollow o.
    o. level
    paired o.'s
    parenchymal o.
    sensory o.
    solid o.
    storage o.
    substance-transporting o.
    urogenital o.
    visceral o.
    yang o.
    yin o.
    zang o.
organa
organic
    o. chamomile
    o. compound
    o. disease
    o. impotence
    o. symptom
organically grown food
organization
    Joint Commission on
      Accreditation of
      Healthcare O.'s (JCAHO)
    managed service o. (MSO)
    World Health O. (WHO)
organoleptic
organon
organ-specific
organum
orgonomy
orgotein
    intraarticular o.

Oriental
O. bodywork therapy
O. ginseng
O. medicine
O. nutrition
orientalis
Biota o.
Liquidambar o.
Thuja o.
orientation
facet o.
spine o.
vertebral o.
orifice
orificial
orificium
origanum
Origanum majorana
origin
aponeurosis of o.
sternal o.
original
o. essence
o. qi
ornamental yew
ornata
Smilax o.
ornithine
orofaciodigital syndrome
oropharynx verde
orotracheal intubation
orphan
o. drug
o. product
orthesis
orthetics
Ortho-Bionomy method
orthodigita
orthodox medicine
orthogonal risk factor
orthokinetics
orthomechanical
orthomechanotherapy
orthomelic
orthomolecular
o. medicine

o. psychiatry
o. therapy
orthopaedist
orthopedic
orthopedics
orthosis
ankle-foot o.
cervical o.
cervicothoracic o.
knee-ankle-foot o.
thoracolumbosacral o.
wrist-hand o.
orthostatic
orthothanasia
orthotic
o. device
foot o.
Levitor o.
orthotics
orthotist
orvale
oryzae
Aspergillus o.
Oryza sativa
os
o. acromiale
o. basilare
o. breve
o. calcis
o. capitatum
o. centrale
o. centrale tarsi
o. coccygis
o. costale
o. coxae
o. cuboideum
o. cuneiforme intermedium
o. cuneiforme laterale
o. cuneiforme mediale
o. femoris
o. frontale
o. hamatum
o. hyoideum
o. iliacum
o. ilium
o. innominatum
o. intermedium

O

NOTES

os *(continued)*
  o. intermetatarseum
  o. irregulare
  o. ischii
  o. lacrimale
  o. longum
  o. lunatum
  o. magnum
  o. malare
  o. multangulum minus
  o. naviculare
  o. naviculare manus
  o. planum
  o. pneumaticum
  o. pterygoideum
  o. pyramidale
  o. sacrum
  o. scaphoideum
  o. sesamoideum
  o. sphenoidale
  o. subtibiale
  o. tibiale posterius
  o. trapezium
  o. trapezoideum
  o. triangulare
  o. trigonum
  o. triquetrum
  o. vesalianum
oscillation
  to-and-fro o.
oscillator
oscillatory circuit
Oscillococcinum
oseille marron
Osgood-Schlatter disease
osmosis
osmotic diarrhea
ossa
  o. carpi
  o. digitorum
  o. membri inferioris
  o. membri superioris
  o. metacarpi
  o. metatarsi
  o. suprasternalia
  o. tarsi
osseous
  o. change
  o. cranium
  o. hydatid cyst
  o. part of skeletal system
  o. pelvis

ossificans
  pelvospondylitis o.
ossification
  o. center
  center of o.
  endochondral o.
  membranous o.
  point of o.
  primary center of o.
  primary point of o.
  secondary center of o.
  secondary point of o.
ossificationis
  punctum o.
ossium
  juncturae o.
ostealgia
ostealgic
osteitic
osteitis
  caseous o.
  central o.
  o. condensans ilii
  condensing o.
  cortical o.
  o. deformans
  o. fibrosa circumscripta
  o. fibrosa cystica
  o. fibrosa disseminata
  hematogenous o.
  o. pubis
  sclerosing o.
  o. tuberculosa multiplex cystica
ostemia
ostempyesis
osteoanagenesis
osteoarthritis
  o. gait
  hyperplastic o.
osteoarthropathy
  hypertrophic pulmonary o.
  idiopathic hypertrophic o.
  pneumogenic o.
  pulmonary o.
osteoarthrosis
osteoblast
osteoblastic
osteoblastoma
Osteo-B-plus
osteochondritis
  o. deformans juvenilis
  o. dissecans
  syphilitic o.

osteochondrodystrophia deformans
osteochondrodystrophy
osteochondrogenic cell
osteochondroma
osteochondrosarcoma
osteochondrosis
osteoclasis
osteoclast activating factor
osteoclastoma
osteocollagenous fibers
osteocystoma
osteodermatopoikilosis
osteodiastasis
osteodynia
osteodysplasty
osteodystrophy
   renal o.
osteoepiphysis
osteofibroma
osteofibrosis
osteogenesis
   distraction o.
   o. imperfecta
osteogenetic
   o. fibers
   o. layer
osteogenic
   o. cell
   o. sarcoma
osteoid osteoma
osteologia
osteologist
osteology
   lumbar spine o.
   thoracic spine o.
osteolysis
osteolytic
osteoma
   o. medullare
   osteoid o.
   o. spongiosum
osteomalacia
   senile o.
osteomalacic pelvis
osteomatoid
osteomere
osteometry

osteomyelitis
   recalcitrant o.
osteomyelodysplasia
osteoncus
osteonecrosis
osteonectin
osteopath
osteopathia
   o. condensans
   o. striata
osteopathic
   o. lesion
   o. lesion complex
   o. manipulation
   o. manipulative medicine (OM)
   o. manipulative technique (OMT)
   o. manipulative treatment (OMT)
   o. medicine
   o. philosophy
   o. postural examination
   o. scoliosis
   o. structural examination
osteopathology
osteopathy
   alimentary o.
   American Academy of O.
   cranial o.
   o. in the cranial field (OCF)
   doctor of o. (DO)
   total lesion o.
osteopenia
osteoperiostitis
osteopetrosis
osteopetrotic
osteophyma
osteophyte
osteopoikilosis
osteoporosis
   juvenile o.
   posttraumatic o.
osteoporotic
osteoprogenitor cell
osteoprotegerin
osteopuncture
osteorrhaphy

NOTES

O

297

osteosarcoma
    periosteal o.
osteosclerosis
osteosclerotic anemia
osteosis
    o. eburnisans monomelica
    parathyroid o.
osteospongioma
osteosuture
osteosynthesis
osteothrombosis
osteotribe
osteotrite
osterick
ostia (*pl. of* ostium)
ostial
ostitic
ostitis
ostium, pl. ostia
ostrich fern
Ostrin plus GTZ 611
Oswestry scale
otaheite walnut
OTC
    over the counter
otitis media
Oto-Plex
ouabain
our
    O. Lady's keys
    O. Lady's mint
    O. Lady's tears
    O. Lord's candle
ousia aromatherapy
out
    o. of place
    toeing o.
outcome criteria
outer
    o. malleolus
    o. yin point
outflare
    iliosacral o.
    o. of ilium
    left innominate o.
outlet
    o. syndrome
    thoracic o.
outpatient anesthesia
ovale
    foramen o.
ovarian plexus

ovary
    polycystic o.
ovata
    Liriosma o.
    Plantago o.
over the counter (OTC)
overdose
    intravenous o.
    procedure o.
overextension
overlay
    spinal o.
overproduction theory
overriding
overtraumatization
overventilation
ovoidalis
    articulatio o.
ovolacteal vegetarian
oxalate
    calcium o.
    potassium o.
    o. stone
    urinary o.
oxalic acid
ox balm
oxidase
    enzyme monoamine o.
    monoamine o. (MAO)
oxidation
oxidative
    o. stress
    o. therapy
oxide
    nitric o.
    nitrous o. (NO)
oxidized cellulose
oxidizing agent
ox's tongue
Oxy-5000 Forte
Oxy C-2 Gel
oxycoccos
    Vaccinium o.
OxyFresh
oxygen
    hyperbaric o.
    o. poisoning
    o. therapy
    o. toxicity
    o. uptake
oxygenation
    apneic o.
    hyperbaric o.

oxylate
    sodium o.
oxymedicine
oxyphenisatin acetate
oxytocic
oyster extract

ozonating aliquot
ozone
    o. gas
    o. therapy
ozone-enriched blood

NOTES

O

P6

P6 acupressure point
P6 acupuncture
P6 point

P-14

Target P-14

P₄₅₀

cytochrome P₄₅₀

PA

phenylacetate

paan

PABA

paraaminobenzoic acid

pacchionian bodies

pacemaker

circadian p.
demand cardiac p.
gastric p.

pacho

la p.

pachydactylia

pachydactylous

pachydactyly

pachydermoperiostosis syndrome

pachyperiostitis

pachypoda

Actaea p.

pachypodous

Pacific

P. kelp
P. yew

pacinian corpuscle

pack

castor oil p.
hot p.
hot castor oil p.
hot moist p.
hydrocollator p.
ice p.
loose p.

Packera candidissima

paclitaxel

pad

anterior fat p.
articular fat p.
BDP p.
electrode p.
heat p.
heel p.
magnetic mat p.

table heating p.
TENS p.
witch hazel p.

Padang cassia

paddock pipe

padma 28

Padma-Lax

pads

knuckle p.

PAE

Pygeum africanum extract

Paecilomyces

Paeonia lactiflora

PAF

platelet-activating factor

PAG

periaqueductal gray
phenylacetylglutamine

Paget disease

paigle

pain

Achilles p.
acute p.
acute back p.
back p.
p. behavior
bone p.
chronic p.
chronically recurrent low
   back p.
chronically recurring back p.
chronic back p.
chronic musculoskeletal p.
chronic pelvic p. (CPP)
p. condition
p. control
cramp-type p.
diffuse p.
P. Disability Index (PDI)
p. drawing
dull p.
p. fiber
gate-control theory of p.
gate theory of p.
p. generator
heel p.
hypochondriac p.
idiopathic low back p.
intractable p.
ischemic p.

P

pain *(continued)*
    kidney stone p.
    p. killer
    location of p.
    low back p.
    p. message
    p. model
    myofascial p.
    neuropathic p.
    nociceptive p.
    obstetric back p.
    p. perception
    peripheral neuropathic p.
    phantom limb p.
    radiating p.
    radiation of p.
    radicular p.
    p. restrictive barrier
    rheumatic p.
    sacroiliac joint p.
    sclerotomal p.
    p. score
    p. syndrome
    temporomandibular joint p.
    tension back p.
    p. therapy
    thigh p.
    p. threshold
    p. transmission
    p. treatment
pain-free
    p.-f. laxity
    p.-f. needling
painful
    p. anesthesia
    p. arc sign
    p. arc syndrome
    p. disorder of the locomotor system
    p. heel
    p. toe
painful-nonpainful
painkiller
painless restoration
pain-looseness-pain
paint
    Indian p.
    yellow p.
painting
    sand p.
pair of channels

paired
    p. organs,
    p. skull bone
Pak
    Detox P.
    PostDetox P.
    ProDetox P.
    Protocol P.
palatine bone
pale
    p. gentian
    p. tongue
paleopathology
palidiflora
    Glycyrrhiza p.
palliation
    p., quality, radiation, severity, time (PQRST)
pallida
    Echinacea p.
pallidum
    Sargassum p.
pallor
palm
    betel p.
    cabbage p.
    cup of p.
    dwarf p.
palma
    p. Christi
    p. manus
palmar
    p. aponeurosis
    p. carpal ligament
    p. carpometacarpal ligament
    carpometacarpal ligaments dorsal and p.
    p. crease
    p. fascia
    p. fibromatosis
    p. flexion
    p. interossei interosseous muscle
    p. interosseous muscle
    p. ligament
    p. metacarpal ligament
    p. radiocarpal ligament
    p. surface
    p. surfaces of fingers
    p. tunnel
    p. ulnocarpal ligament
palmar-dorsiflexion

palmaris
    aponeurosis p.
    p. brevis muscle
    p. longus
    p. longus muscle
    musculus interosseus p.
palmatum
    Rheum p.
palmatus
    Cocculus p.
palmetto
    saw p.
palming
Palmitol
palpable finding
palpation
    anterior p.
    articular p.
    carotid artery p.
    diagnostic p.
    layer p.
    ligament p.
    manual p.
    motion p.
    muscle p.
    muscular p.
    posterior p.
    radial artery p.
    static p.
    subcutaneous tissue p.
    suture p.
    tendon p.
    vein p.
palpatory
    p. change
    p. diagnosis
    p. procedure
    p. sensation
    p. test
palpitation
palsy
    Bell p.
    cerebral p.
    crutch p.
    long thoracic nerve p.
    paresis after cerebral p.
palsywort

palustre
    Equisetum p.
    Ledum p.
palustris
    Pinus p.
pan
    p. masala
    p. parag
    p. peyote
panacea
Panama bark
Panang cinnamon
panarthritis
panax
    p. complex
    P. ginseng
    P. notoginseng
    P. pseudo-ginseng
    P. quinquefolius
panchakarma
Panch Phoron
pancreatic enzyme
pancreatin
pancreatitis
pancytopenia
pangamic acid
pangguangshu
    p. point
    ub 28 p.
panic disorder
paniculata
    Dioscorea p.
    Eugenia p.
    Pfaffia p.
paniculatum
    Syzygium p.
panmyelophthisis
panniculus carnosus
pannus
Panoderm I
pansy
    field p.
    wild p.
pantopaque myelography
pantothenic acid
PAOD
    peripheral arterial occlusive disease

NOTES

P

papagallo
papain
Papaver
    P. rhoeas
    P. somniferum
papaveretum
papaverine
papaya
    Carica p.
    p. enzyme
    P. Enzyme with Chlorophyll
    p. tablet
papilla, pl. papillae
    dermal papillae
    papillae dermis
papillaris
    musculus p.
papillary muscle
papillula
papoose root
paprika
paraaminobenzoic acid (PABA)
paracarcinomatous myelopathy
paracervical block anesthesia
paracervix
parachordal cartilage
paradigm
paraffin
    p. bath
    p. wax
parag
    pan p.
Paragar
paragigantocellularis
    reticularis p.
paraguariensis
    Ilex p.
Paraguay tea
parallel stretch
paralysis
    chronic facial nerve p.
    facial nerve p.
    hypokalemic p.
paralytic scoliosis
parameter
    functional p.
parametric
parametrics
paranalgesia
paranasal sinus
paranesthesia
paranoid
paranormal healing

paraparesis
paraphysiological space
parapsychology
pararama
parasacral
parasagittal
    p. plane
    p. section
parasite
    autistic p.
    autochthonous p.
    commensal p.
    facultative p.
    incidental p.
    inquiline p.
    obligate p.
parasiticus
    craniopagus p.
paraspinal
    p. muscle
    p. musculature
parasternalis
    linea p.
parasternal line
parasympathetic
    p. activity
    p. effect
    p. ganglion
    p. nerve
    p. nervous system
    p. self-regulation
parasympatholytic
parasympathomimetic
parasynaptic system
parathyroid
    p. gland
    p. hormone
    p. osteosis
parathyroidea
    glandula p.
paraventricular nucleus
paravertebral
    p. anesthesia
    p. ganglion
    p. gutter
    p. line
    p. muscle
paravertebralis
    linea p.
Paraway Plus
pareira
    p. brava

p. complex
p. radix
parenchymal organ
parenteral
paresis
  p. after cerebral palsy
  p. after poliomyelitis
  facial p.
  long-standing p.
  spastic p.
paresthesia
paresthetica
  brachialgia statica p.
  meralgia p.
parietal
  p. bone
  p. bone articulation
  p. foramen
  p. layer
  p. pelvic fascia
  p. peritoneum
  p. pleura
  p. squama
parietalis
  fascia pelvis p.
  margo frontalis ossis p.
  pleura p.
Parietaria officinalis
parietomastoid suture
Paris
  plaster of P.
Parkinson disease
parkinsonism
Parodontax
Parona space
parosteal
parosteitis
parostitis
parotid lymph node
paroxysmal nocturnal dyspnea (PND)
parry fracture
pars, pl. **partes**
  p. abdominalis ductus thoracici
  p. anterior
  p. autonomica systematis nervosi peripherici

p. cartilaginea systematis skeletalis
p. cervicalis ductus thoracici
p. cervicalis esophagi
p. cervicalis medullae spinalis
p. clavicularis musculi pectoralis majoris
p. coccygea medullae spinalis
p. inferior
p. infraclavicularis plexus brachialis
p. interarticularis
p. intermedia
p. intracranialis arteriae vertebralis
p. lateralis arcus pedis longitudinalis
p. lateralis ossis sacri
p. lumbalis medullae spinalis
p. medialis arcus pedis longitudinalis
p. ossea systematis skeletalis
p. perpendicularis
p. recta musculi cricothyroidei
p. sacralis medullae spinalis
p. spinalis nervi accessorii
p. sternalis diaphragmatis
p. sternocostalis musculi pectoralis majoris
p. supraclavicularis plexus brachialis
p. sympathica divisionis autonomicae systematis nervosei peripherici
p. thoracica aortae
p. thoracica ductus thoracici
p. thoracica esophagi
p. thoracica medullae spinalis
p. tibiocalcanea ligamenti collateralis medialis articulationis talocruralis
p. tibionavicularis ligamenti collateralis medialis articulationis talocrucalis
p. tibiotalaris anterior ligamenti collateralis medialis articulationis talocruralis

NOTES

P

305

pars *(continued)*
    p. tibiotalaris posterior
      ligamenti collateralis medialis
      articulationis talocruralis
    p. vagalis nervi accessorii
parsley
    p. breakstone
    Chinese p.
    common p.
    p. fern
    garden p.
    p. herb
    p. leaf
    marsh p.
    p. oil
    p. piercestone
    p. piert
    rock p.
    sea p.
parsley-leaved yellow root
part
    aerial p.
    anterior p.
    inferior p.
    intermediate p.
    ischiocondylar p.
    lower p.
    tympanic p.
    upper p.
partes *(pl. of* pars)
parthenium
    Tanacetum p.
Parthenium integrifolium
partial
    p. hip flexion
    p. prothrombin time (PTT)
partially flexed hip muscle energy technique
particulate wear debris
partner
    contralateral p.
partridgeberry, partridge berry
parts
    soft p.
parviflora
    Malva p.
parvum
    phu p.
pas diane
pasiania fungus
pasque flower
Passiflora incarnata

passion
    p. fruit
passionflower, passion flower
passive
    p. hip abduction
    p. length-tension curve
    p. motion
    p. movement
    p. myofascial technique
    p. range of motion
    p. relaxation
    p. technique
    p. treatment
password
pasta
    dry p.
paste
    fruit p.
    guarana p.
    lime p.
    tumeric p.
past life therapy
pastora
    herba de la p.
patagium
patch
    acupuncture point skin p.
    electrode p.
    Peyer p.
patchouli leaf
patella, pl. patellae
    p. alta
    apex patellae
    apex of p.
    articular surface of p.
    p. baja
    base of p.
    basis patellae
    chondromalacia patellae
    floating p.
    slipping p.
patellalgia
patellar
    p. apprehension sign
    p. crease
    p. deep tendon reflex
    p. ligament
    p. network
    p. retinaculum
    p. surface of femur
    p. tendinitis
    p. tendon

p. tendon reflex
p. tracking
patellare
rete p.
patellaris
plica synovialis p.
patelliform
patellofemoral
p. grinding test
p. stress syndrome
p. syndrome
patent
p. medicine
p. suture
path
fire p.
water p.
pathogenesis
pathogenic
p. cold
p. damp
p. factor
p. force
p. influence
p. internal wind disturbance
p. qi
p. wind influence
pathognomic
pathologic
p. amputation
p. barrier
p. diagnosis
p. fracture
pathological
p. health problem
p. neutral
pathologist
pathology
disk p.
functional p.
muscle p.
spinal p.
surgical p.
pathophysiology
pathotropism
pathway
brainstem p.

cortical p.
corticobulbar p.
corticospinal p.
descending brainstem p.
descending cortical p.
descending neural p.
dorsolateral p.
drainage p.
glycolytic metabolic p.
homocysteine p.
motor cortex p.
neuronal p.
neurophysiologic p.
reflex p.
somaticosomatic reflex p.
sympathetic reflex p.
ventral medial p.
ventral medial brainstem p.
patience
p. dock
garden p.
patient
p. activity
comatose p.
p. motivation
p. muscle force
p. response
spinalized p.
stroke rehabilitation control p.
patient-active muscle contraction
patient-controlled
p.-c. analgesia (PCA)
p.-c. anesthesia (PCA)
pa ting fen zhu tang
patrem
filius ante p.
Patrick
P. FABERE test
P. test
pattern
abnormal muscle firing p.
autonomic innervation p.
common compensatory p.
compensatory p.
compensatory fascial p.
dermatomal p.
dialectic p.

NOTES

P

pattern *(continued)*
  p. of disharmony
  emptiness p.
  energy p.
  fascial p.
  firing p.
  fullness/emptiness p.
  hip capsular p.
  hip joint capsular p.
  hip joint firing p.
  holistic p.
  hot/cold p.
  human response p.
  interior/exterior p.
  muscle firing p.
  myotomal p.
  myotomal pain p.
  normal muscle firing p.
  reflex p.
  restoration of symmetrical movement p.
  sclerotomal p.
  p. of strain
  universal p.
  wispy p.
  yin/yang p.
patterning
  Aston p.
  spine p.
  uncompensated fascial p.
patula
  Tagetes p.
pau
  p. d'arco
  p. d'arco inner bark
  p. d'arco lotion
  p. d'arco tea
pauciarticular
Paullinia
  P. cupana
  P. yoco
Paul's betony
Pausinystalia
  P. yohimbe
Pavlik harness
paw
  bear's p.
pawpaw
payadito
PCA
  patient-controlled analgesia
  patient-controlled anesthesia

PCO
  procyanidol oligomer
p-coumaric acid
PCP
  Pneumocystis carinii pneumonia
PDI
  Pain Disability Index
pe
  pericardium channel
    pe 7 daling
    pe 5 jianshe
    pe 8 laogong
    pe 6 nieguan
    pe 3 quze
    pe 1 tianchi
    pe 4 ximen
    pe 9 zhongchong
pea
  rosary p.
Peace of Mind gumballs
peach
peagle
peak
  p. current
  p. flow
pearl-worker's disease
peat moss
Pecquet
  P. cistern
  P. duct
pectin
  apple p.
pectinate muscle
pectinati
  musculi p.
pectineal
  p. ligament
  p. line of femur
  p. muscle
pectineus
  p. muscle
  musculus p.
pectinic acid
pectoral
  p. fascia
  p. girdle
  p. gland
  p. muscle
  p. pull
  p. region
  p. release
  p. ridge
  p. traction technique

pectoralis
    fascia p.
    p. major muscle
    p. minor muscle
    p. minor tendon
    p. muscle
    regio p.
pectoris
    angina p.
pectorodorsalis muscle
pectorodorsal muscle
pectus
    p. carinatum
    p. excavatum
    p. recurvatum
pedal
    p. lymphatic pump
    p. pump
pedestal massage table
pediatric ecology
pedicle of arch of vertebra
pediculi
pediculus arcus vertebrae
pedicure
pediphalanx
pedis
    arcus venosus dorsalis p.
    articulationes p.
    articulationes interphalangeae p.
    calcar p.
    digitus p.
    dorsum p.
    fascia dorsalis p.
    margo fibularis p.
    margo lateralis p.
    margo medialis p.
    margo tibialis p.
    musculi interossei dorsalis p.
    musculus abductor digiti
      minimi p.
    musculus flexor digiti minimi
      brevis p.
    musculus lumbricalis p.
    musculus pronator p.
    planta p.
    pollex p.
    rete venosum dorsale p.

    tinea p.
    trochlea phalangis manus et p.
    tuberositas phalangis distalis
      manus et p.
    vaginae fibrosae digitorum p.
    vaginae tendinum digitorum p.
pedodynamometer
pedogram
pedograph
pedography
pedometer
pedorthist
Peerless Composition Essence
peg-and-socket
    p.-a.-s. articulation
    p.-a.-s. joint
pegu katechu
pegwood
PEITC
    phenethyl isothiocyanate
Pektan N
Pelargonium graveolens
pelican flower
pellagroid dermopathy
pellitory of the wall
pelma
pelmatic
pelmatogram
peltatum
    podophyllum p.
pelvic
    p. articulatory technique
    p. bone
    p. clock
    p. control
    p. declination
    p. diaphragm
    p. fascia
    p. floor dysfunction
    p. floor muscle
    p. girdle dysfunction
    p. index
    p. ligament
    p. limb
    p. motion testing
    p. plexus
    p. rotation

NOTES

P

pelvic *(continued)*
    p. and sacral tender points
    p. seesaw
    p. sideshift
    p. somatic dysfunction
    p. surface of sacrum
    p. tilt
    p. tilt functional curve
    p. tilt and heel slide
    p. tilt syndrome
    p. traction
    p. unleveling
pelvis
    aditus p.
    assimilation p.
    beaked p.
    caoutchouc p.
    cavitas p.
    cavum p.
    p. compression functional technique
    fascia p.
    inclinatio p.
    inclination of p.
    innervation of female p.
    kyphoscoliotic p.
    kyphotic p.
    level of p.
    linea terminalis of p.
    lordotic p.
    p. obtecta
    osseous p.
    osteomalacic p.
    pseudoosteomalacic p.
    rachitic p.
    rostrate p.
    rubber p.
    scoliotic p.
    spondylolisthetic p.
    p. tilt
    tilting of p.
pelvisacral
pelvivertebral angle
pelvofemoral muscular dystrophy
pelvospondylitis ossificans
pen
    ITO laser p.
    red-beam laser p.
pendulum
    p. exercise
    trillium p.
penguin walk
penile wart

penis
pennate muscle
pennyroyal
    American p.
    p. essential oil
    European p.
    p. herb tea
    oil of p.
    p. oil
pennywort
    Indian p.
    wall p.
PENS
    percutaneous electrical nerve stimulation
pensylvanica
    Myrica p.
pentadactyl
pentatonic scale
people
    elastic p.
PEP
    P. Formula
Pep
    P. Products
    Ultra Diet P.
pepe
peper
pepo
    Cucurbita p.
pepper
    bell p.
    black p.
    cayenne p.
    chili p.
    clove p.
    P. Defense
    hot p.
    Jamaica p.
    monk's p.
    old man's p.
    red p.
    Tabasco p.
peppermint oil
pepperridge bush
pepperroot
peptic
    p. ulcer
    p. ulcer disease
peptide
    calcitonin gene-related p.
    endorphin p.
    vasoactive intestinal p.

perarticulation
peraxillary
perception
  autonomic p.
  high-risk model of threat p.
  (HRMTP)
  pain p.
  threat p.
perceptual field
percolate
percussing
percussion
  p. hammer technique
  p. hammer work
  spinal p.
percutaneous
  p. absorption
  p. electrical nerve stimulation
  (PENS)
  p. transluminal angioplasty
Perdiem
pereirae
  Myroxylon p.
perfoliatum
  Eupatorium p.
perforans
perforating
  p. abscess
  p. branch
  p. fiber
  p. vein
perforatum
  Hypericum p.
performance
  hypnotic p.
performer
  circus p.
perfusion
  natural p.
  nutritive p.
periaqueductal gray (PAG)
periarterial
periarthritis humeroscapularis
periarticular
  p. abscess
  p. structure
  p. tissue reaction

periaxial
periaxillary
peribursal
pericardial channel
pericarditis
  constrictive p.
pericardium
  p. channel (pe)
  p. meridian
  p. meridian of hand
perichondral bone
perichondrium
perichoroidal
pericoronitis
pericranium
peridesmitis
peridesmium
peridural anesthesia
Perika
periligamentous
perilla
  P. frutescens
  p. oil
perillyl alcohol
perilunar dislocation
perimyelitis
perimyositis
perimysial
perimysiitis
perimysium internum
perineal
  p. massage
  p. muscle
perinealis
  luxatio p.
perineometer
perineum
perineural semiconduction
period
  effective refractory p.
  functional refractory p.
  refractory p.
periodic arthralgia
periodontal abscess
perionychium
perionyx
periost

NOTES

P

periostea
periosteal
p. bud
p. chondroma
p. elevator
p. ganglion
p. implantation
p. osteosarcoma
p. reaction
p. sarcoma
periosteitis
periosteoma
periosteomedullitis
periosteomyelitis
periosteopathy
periosteophyte
periosteosis
periosteous
periosteum
periostitis
periostoma
periostosis
periostosteitis
peripapillary
peripheral
p. afferent transmission
p. aneurysm
p. arterial occlusive disease (PAOD)
p. awareness
p. blood flow
p. bloody supply
p. circulation
p. and core temperature
p. edema
p. motor nerve
p. nerve
p. nervous system
p. neuropathic pain
p. neuropathy
p. occlusive arterial disease (POAD)
p. skin temperature
p. stimulation
p. stimulation therapy
p. vascular disease
p. vasodilator
peripheralis
peripherici
pars autonomica systematis nervosi p.

pars sympathica divisionis autonomicae systematis nervosei p.
peripherocentral
periphery
Periploca sepium
perisplanchnic
perispondylic
perispondylitis
peritendineum
peritendinitis
p. calcarea
p. serosa
peritenon
peritenonitis
perithoracic
peritoneal cavity
peritonei
cavum p.
peritoneum
distention of visceral p.
parietal p.
visceral p.
peritonitis
peritrochanteric
periungual
perivascular
p. interstitial fluid circulation
p. sympathetic fiber conduction
perivenous leukoencephalitis
perivertebral
perivisceral
periwinkle
Cape p.
Madagascar p.
red p.
permanent
p. callus
p. cartilage
p. needle
permanganate
potassium p.
Permixon
pernambuco Jaborandi
pernicious anemia
perobrachius
perochirus
perodactyly
peromelia
perone
peroneal
p. anastomotic ramus
p. artery

p. bone
p. communicating branch
p. muscle
p. muscular atrophy
p. nerve
p. nerve entrapment
p. pulley
p. retinaculum
p. trochlea of calcaneus
peronealis
spina p.
trochlea p.
peroneocalcaneus
musculus p.
peroneorum
retinaculum musculorum p.
peroneotibial
peroneus
p. brevis muscle
p. longus muscle
p. muscle
p. tertius
p. tertius muscle
peropus
peroxidase
glutathione p.
peroxidation
lipid p.
peroxide
benzoyl p.
hydrogen p.
perpendicular
p. insertion
p. needling method
p. plate of ethmoid
p. stretch
p. thoracic spine traction
p. traction
perpendicularis
lamina p.
pars p.
Persian licorice
Persica
persimmon
personality
borderline p.
placebo p.

personal will
personata
perspiration
pertrochanteric fracture
Pertussin N
Peru
apple of P.
P. balsam
balsam of P.
life-giving vine of P.
Peruvian
P. balsam
P. bark
P. rhatany
pes
p. abductus
p. adductus
p. anserinus bursitis
p. cavus
p. equinovalgus
p. equinovarus
p. planus
p. pronatus
p. valgus
p. varus
pestroot
European p.
Petadolex
Petaforce
petal
calendula p.
lavender p.
Petasites
petechia, pl. **petechiae**
Peter
herb P.
petiolus
Petit lumbar triangle
pétrissage
p. massage technique
p. procedure
petroleum jelly
petrosal sinus
Petroselinum
P. crispum
P. sativum
petrosquamous fissure

NOTES

P

petrous
p. bone
p. portion of temporal
p. ridge
pet therapy
pettigree
petty mullein
Peumus boldus
pewterwort
Peyer patch
peyote
p. button
grandfather p.
pan p.
Pfaffia paniculata
Pfaundler-Hurler syndrome
pfeffer
Pfeiffer's Cold Sore Preparation
Pfrimmer
P. deep muscle therapy
P. technique
PGE_1
prostaglandin E_1
PGE_2
prostaglandin E_2
phagocyte
phagocytosis
phalangeal joint
phalangis
basis p.
phalanx, pl. **phalanges**
base of p.
tufted p.
ungual p.
Phalen
P. sign
P. test
phalloides
Amanita p.
phantom
p. limb
p. limb pain
pharmaceutical agent
pharmacists
American Association of
Homeopathic P. (AAHP)
pharmacodynamic
pharmacognosy
pharmacokinetic
pharmacologics
pharmacology
pharmacopeia
United States P. (USP)

pharyngitis
pharyngobasilar fascia
pharyngobasilaris
fascia p.
pharynx
cavity of p.
muscular coat of p.
phase
exhalation p.
five p.'s
flexion p.
p. gradient
p. I block
p. II block
P. III trial
P. II trial
inhalation p.
P. I trial
P. IV trial
return p.
separation p.
transition p.
phase-response curve (PRC)
phases: metal, water, wood, fire, and earth
phasic muscle
pheasant's eye
phenacetin
phenethyl isothiocyanate (PEITC)
phenol
phenolic estrogen
phenomenology
nonreductionistic p.
phenomenon
adaptation p.
adjustment p.
blush p.
cavitation p.
ease and bind p.
Huneke p.
release p.
Ritter-Rollet p.
vacuum p.
vacuum disk p.
wind-up p.
phenothiazine
phenotype
phenylacetate (PA)
phenylacetylglutamine (PAG)
phenylacetylisoglutamine (isoPAG)
phenylalanine
phenylketonuria
phenylpropanoid

phenytoin
pheresis
pheromone
philanthropos
philosophy
  osteopathic p.
phi noi
phlebitis
  septic p.
phlegm
  p. affecting the head
  deficiency of the gallbladder
    and stagnation of p.
  p. disturbance
  hot p.
  p. obstructs the lung
phlegmonous abscess
phlomoides
  Verbascum p.
phobia
  clinical p.
  dental p.
phobic behavior
phocomelia
Phoenix
  P. BioLabs
  P. Rising yoga therapy
Phoradendron
  P. flavescens
  P. leucarpum
  P. macrophyllum
  P. serotinum
  P. tomentosum
Phoron
  Panch P.
phosphatidylcholine
phosphatidylserine
phospholipid
phosphonecrosis
phosphorica
  Calcarea p.
phosphoric acid
phosphoricum
  ferrum p.
  ferrum phos
phosphorus

photocurrent deficit
photodermatitis
photodynamic therapy
photography
  Kirlian p.
photosensitivity
phototherapy
  topical p.
phototoxic
phrase
  autogenic training p.
phrenic nerve
phrenicopleural fascia
phrenicopleuralis
  fascia p.
phrenology
phthinoid chest
phu
  p. germanicum
  p. parvum
Phyllanthus
  P. amarus
  P. emblica
  P. nituri
phyllanthus
physaliphorous cell
physeal
physiatrics
physiatrist
physiatry
physic
  Culver's p.
  p. root
physical
  P. Activity Recall Scale
  p. elasticity of muscle
  p. excessive stress
  p. exercise
  p. exhaustion
  p. medicine
  p. medicine and rehabilitation
    (PM&R)
  p. stressor
  p. therapist
  p. therapy
  p. trauma

NOTES

P

315

physician
American Association of Naturopathic P.'s (AANP)
integrative p.
naturopathic p.
Physician's Choice
physiologic
p. anatomy
p. barrier
p. elasticity of muscle
p. hypermobility
p. hypertrophy
p. incompatibility
p. motion
p. saline
p. therapeutics
physiological
p. response method
p. response method joint mobilization
p. therapeutics
physiologics
physiology
physiotherapeutic
physiotherapist
physiotherapy
manipulative p.
physique
physis
Physostigma venenosum
phytobezoar
phytochemical
phytochemistry
phytoestrogen
phytoestrogenic
phytohemagglutinin
Phytolacca
P. *americana*
P. *decandra*
P. *dodecandra*
P. *rigida*
Phytolyn
phytomedicine
Phytomin
phytonadione
phytonutrient supplement
phytonutrition
phytopharmacology
PhytoQuest
PhytoShield
Phytosol
Milk Thistle P.

Phytosome
Ginkgo P.
Hawthorne P.
phytosterol
phytotherapy
pi
han shi kun p.
p. qi xu
wu jia p.
p. xia
p. xie feng qing yin
p. yang xu
p. yun shi re
pia
p. layer
p. layer of meninges
p. mater
pial-glial membrane
pianli
picolinate
chromium p.
picrotoxin
picture-frame vertebra
piercestone
parsley p.
piercing energy
piert
parsley p.
pigeon
p. breast
p. grass
pigeonberry
pigmented
p. villonodular synovitis
p. villonodular tenosynovitis
pignut
pikkukarpalo
Pilates method
Piletabs
Potter's P.
pilewort
Pilexim
pill
birth control p. (BCP)
Carmichaeli Tea P.'s
Dendrobium Monilforme Night Sight P.'s
Hepatico Tonic P.'s
Kai Kit P.
Kai Yeung P.
Leukorrhea P.'s
Lung Tan Xie Gan P.
Margarite Acne P.'s

nose inflammation p.
Pinellia Expectorant P.'s
Pulmonary Tonic P.'s
Tso Tzu Otic P.'s
Women's Precious P.'s
pillar
anterior articular p.
articular p.
cervical segment articular p.
posterior articular p.
pill-bearing spurge
pillow
p. fulcrum
gypsum p.
herbal p.
lumbar p.
Pilocarpus jaborandi
pilomotor activity
pilon fracture
pilonidal sinus
pilosella
Pilosella officinarum
pilosula
Codonopsis p.
Pima Indian shamanism
Pimenta officinalis
pimento, pimenta
pimiento
pimpinella
P. anisum
p. sanguisorba
pin
pinang
pinaster
Pinus p.
pincement
pinch
pine
fir p.
p. needle
p. pollen
prince's p.
Scotch p.
Scot's p.
silver p.
wild p.
pineal gland

pineapple
smooth cayenne p.
pinebark
Pinellia
P. Expectorant Pills
P. tuber
ping-pong bone
ping wei san
pini
pollen p.
pink
p. aura
Indian p.
old-maid's p.
pinkroot
pinna, pl. pinnae
pinocytosis
reverse p.
pinprick sensation
Pinus
P. mugo
P. nigra
P. palustris
P. pinaster
P. sylvestris
pipe
p. bone
paddock p.
p. tree
water p.
Piper
P. betle
P. longum
P. methysticum
P. nigrum
piperata
Mentha p.
piperita
Mentha p.
Pippli
pipsissewa
piqured
piquring
piracetam
Pirie bone
piriformis, pyriformis
p. muscle

NOTES

piriformis *(continued)*
   p. muscle exercise
   p. muscle tender point
   musculus p.
   p. syndrome
piriform muscle
Pirogoff angle
pishu
   ub 20 p.
pisiform
   p. bone
   p. tone
pisohamate ligament
pisometacarpal ligament
pisotriquetral joint
pisounciform ligament
pisouncinate ligament
piston
pit
   p. of head of femur
   pterygoid p.
   superior costal p.
pitta
   p. dosha
   p. imbalance
pitta-kapha
pituitary
   p. adrenal axis
   p. stalk
pituitary-portal venous system
pituri
pivot
   p. area
   cranial p.
   p. joint
   p. shift test
   sphenosquamous p.
pjerets
place
   out of p.
placebo
   p. effect
   p. personality
   p. response
placebo-controlled trial
placement
   foot p.
plafond
plagiocephaly
plague
   devil's p.
plain
   p. film

   p. needling
   p. radiograph
   p. x-ray
plan
   birth p.
plana (*pl. of* planum)
plane
   anterior p.
   cardinal p.
   coronal p.
   coronary p.
   fascial p.
   frontal p.
   horizontal p.
   interspinal p.
   intertubercular p.
   p. joint
   p. of joint
   median p.
   midsagittal p.
   nuchal p.
   parasagittal p.
   posterior p.
   sagittal p.
   sternal p.
   subcostal p.
   supracrestal p.
   supracristal p.
   suprasternal p.
   transpyloric p.
   transverse p.
   xy p.
   xz p.
   yz p.
planetary disposition
planifolia
   Vanilla p.
planigraphy
planithorax
planography
planovalgus
plant
   beefsteak p.
   burn p.
   caper p.
   cart track p.
   castor oil p.
   compass p.
   dew p.
   entire p.
   p. extract
   febrifuge p.
   first-aid p.

God's wonder p.
grapple p.
gum p.
p. of immortality
lobster flower p.
maggi p.
medicine p.
miracle p.
mosquito p.
nosebleed p.
red ink p.
Roman p.
scrofula p.
p. stanols
p. sterol
sweating p.
tangantangan oil p.
tract p.
umbrella p.
wax myrtle p.

plantae
musculus quadratus p.

Plantago
P. *afra*
P. *lanceolata*
P. *ovata*
P. *psyllium*

plantago
blond p.
p. extract
Indian p.
p. seed

plantago-aquatica
Alisma p.-a.

plantagoside
plantain
broadleaf p.
common p.
English p.
greater p.
narrowleaf p.
wild p.

plantalgia
planta pedis
plantar
p. aponeurosis
p. arch

p. arterial arch
p. calcaneocuboid ligament
p. calcaneonavicular ligament
p. cuboideonavicular ligament
p. cuneocuboid ligament
p. cuneonavicular ligament
p. fascia
p. fasciitis
p. flexion
p. foot ulcer
p. interossei interosseous muscle
p. ligament
p. ligament
p. metatarsal ligament
p. muscle
p. quadrate muscle
p. space
p. surface of toe
p. tendon sheath of peroneus longus muscle

plantare
rete venosum p.

plantaris
aponeurosis p.
arcus venosus p.
p. muscle
musculi interosseus p.
musculus p.
regio p.
talipes p.
vagina tendinis musculi peronei longi p.

planum, pl. plana
articulatio plana
coxa plana
p. interspinale
p. intertuberculare
manus plana
os p.
p. popliteum
p. sternale
p. subcostale
p. supracristale
p. transpyloricum
vertebra plana

NOTES

P

planus
  pes p.
  talipes p.
plaque
  urticarial p.
plasma
  p. cell
  p. colloid osmotic pressure
  p. half-life
  p. homocysteine
  p. level
  p. lipid
  p. total homocysteine
  p. triglycerides
plasmacytoma
plasmapheresis
plaster
  p. bandage
  p. of Paris
  p. splint
plastic
  p. deformation
  p. motor
plasticity
  CNS p.
plastron
plate
  buttress p.
  compression p.
  energy circulation p.
  epiphysial p.
  foot p.
  Kühne p.
  lateral cartilaginous p.
  medial cartilaginous p.
  p. of modiolus
  nail p.
  neutralization p.
  sagittal p.
  tarsal p.'s
platelet
  p. aggregation
platelet-activating factor (PAF)
platicond
plating
  compression p.
platycnemia
platycnemic
platycnemism
Platycodon grandiflorum
platyhieric
platymeric

platyphyllos
  Tilia p.
platysma
  p. muscle
  musculus p.
platyspondylia
play
  cat's p.
  hip joint p.
  joint p.
  loss of joint p.
  muscle p.
playing
  role p.
pledget
plegma
pleura
  p. mediastinalis
  parietal p.
  p. parietalis
  posterior parietal p.
pleural cavity
pleurapophysis
pleurisy root
pleurocentrum
pleuroperitoneal membrane
plexal
plexiform
  p. neurofibroma
  p. neuroma
plexogenic
plexus
  Auerbach p.
  axillary p.
  Batson p.
  Batson venous p.
  brachial p.
  cardiac p.
  cervical p.
  coccygeal p.
  coccygeal nerve p.
  Frankenhäuser p.
  gonadal p.
  hypogastric p.
  iliac nervous p.
  inferior hypogastric p.
  inferior trunk of brachial p.
  ischiadic p.
  lateral cord of brachial p.
  lumbar p.
  lumbar nervous p.
  lumbosacral p.
  lumbosacral nervous p.

medial cord of brachial p.
Meissner p.
mesenteric p.
myenteric p.
nerve p.
ovarian p.
pelvic p.
popliteal p.
posterior cord of brachial p.
pulmonary p.
rectal venous p.
sacral p.
solar p.
spermatic p.
subclavian p.
superior hypogastric p.
vertebral p.
vertebral venous p.
vesical p.
pliability
plica
    p. axillaris
    p. interdigitalis
    p. synovialis
    p. synovialis infrapatellaris
    p. synovialis patellaris
plum
    black p.
    jambulon p.
    java p.
    umeboshi p.
plumb
    p. line
    p. line examination
plumrocks
plumule
    lotus p.
pluricaulis
    Convolvulus p.
pluriglandular
plus
    Action Super Saw Palmetto P.
    Activex 40 P.
    Astragalus 10 P.
    Bacopa P.
    Ephedra P.
    Fasting P.

    Femcal P.
    Fitness P.
    Guarana P.
    IsoProtein P.
    Macuna P.
    Neem P.
    Paraway P.
    Red Clover P.
    Saw Palmetto Pygeum P.
    Snuz P.
    Synergy P.
    Taurine P.
    Tylophora P.
PM&R
    physical medicine and rehabilitation
PMS
    premenstrual syndrome
    PMS Aid
    PMS Serene
PND
    paroxysmal nocturnal dyspnea
pneumarthrogram
pneumarthrography
pneumarthrosis
pneumatic
    p. bone
    p. device
    p. tire injury
pneumaticum
    os p.
pneumoarthrography
Pneumocystis carinii **pneumonia**
    (PCP)
pneumogenic osteoarthropathy
pneumomyelography
pneumonia
    lipid p.
    lipoid p.
    metastatic p.
    Pneumocystis carinii p. (PCP)
pneumonitis
pneumoperitoneum
pneumotaxic center in pons
pneumothermomassage
pneumothorax
PNF stretching

NOTES

P

POAD
 peripheral occlusive arterial disease
pocon
poculum diogenis
podalgia
podalic
Podalyria tinctoria
podarthritis
podedema
Podi
 Sambaar P.
podiatric medicine
podiatrist
podiatry
podismus
poditis
Podocon-25
pododynamometer
pododynia
Podofilm
podogram
podograph
podologist
podology
podomechanotherapy
podometer
podophyllin toxicity
podophyllotoxin
 topical p.
podophyllum
 p. hexandrum
 p. ointment
 p. peltatum
 p. resin
podospasm
POET2
 point of entry, traction and twist
POETZ
 point of entry, traction and twist
poikiloderma
 p. atrophicans and cataract
 p. congenitale
poinsettia
 Euphorbia p.
point
 acupuncture p.
 ah shi p.
 alarm p.
 analgesic p.
 ankle and foot tender p.
 ashi p.
 auriculotherapy p.
 back shu p.

bafeng p.
ba xie p.
beishu p.
beishuxue p.
calf's nose p.
p. category
cervical tender p.
chakra p.
Chapman reflex p.
classic acupuncture p.
cleft p.
confluent p.
connecting p.
contact p.
CRI still p.
cutanea-organ reflex p.
dachangshu p.
da ling p.
dangerous p.
distal p.
distal ba xie p.
ear p.
ear heart p.
ear kidney p.
ear liver p.
ear shenmen p.
ear sympathicus p.
eight influential p.'s
p. of elbow
elbow tender p.
p. of entry, traction and twist
 (POET2, POETZ)
extra p. (Ex)
feishu p.
p. finder
five shu p.
focal p.
p. of freedom
front-mu p.
ganshu p.
general tonification p.
ge shu p.
governing p.
H7 acupuncture p.
harmonizing p.
he p.
heart p.
he sea p.
hip tender p.
ho p.
homeostatic p.
hourly p.
hua toe jia jie p.

huatuo p.
huatuojiaji p.
hui xue p.
ileus tender p.
immune-enhancing p.
influential p.
inguinal ligament tender p.
injection therapy for
  trigger p.'s
intramuscular trigger p.
jing p.
jing well p.
Jones tender p.
jong p.
K3 acupuncture p.
king p.
knee tender p.
large intestine p.
lateral xiyan p.
latissimus dorsi tender p.
liver p.
lo p.
local p.
local acupuncture p.
locus dolendi p.
lumbar tender p.
luo p.
luo connecting p.
mapped acupuncture p.
marshaling p.
p. of maximum ease
meeting p.
metal p.
mo p.
mobile p.
mother p.
mother tonifying p.
mu p.
mu front p.
muscular p.
myofascial tender p.
myofascial trigger p.
navicular bone tender p.
needling of p.
neiguan p.
nei guan p.

neiguan anti-emetic
  acupuncture p.
neima p.
nonacupuncture p.
p. of ossification
outer yin p.
P6 p.
P6 acupressure p.
pangguangshu p.
pelvic and sacral tender p.'s
piriformis muscle tender p.
p. prescription
pressure p.
pressure sensitive p.
qimen p.
qi tonifying p.
p. of reference
reference p.
reflex p.
rib tender p.
riyue p.
rotation on a p.
rue p.
sacral urinary bladder p.
sedative p.
p. selection
shensu p.
shoulder tender p.
shu p.
shu p.'s: jing, ying,
  shu/yuan, jing, and he
shu-stream p.
son p.
son sedating p.
source p.
specific tonification p.
spinal p.
spontaneously sensitive p.
starting p.
still p.
subscapular muscle tender p.
supraspinatus muscle tender p.
tai-yang p.
tai-yin p.
tan zhong p.
tender p.
p. tenderness

NOTES

P

point *(continued)*
thoracic tender p.
tianshu p.
ting p.
tonification p.
traditionally chosen p.
transport p.
Travell myofascial trigger p.
Travell and Simons myofascial
trigger p.
Travell tender p.
Travell trigger p.
trigger p.
trunk p.
tsri p.
vibrational contact p.
xi p.
xi-cleft p.
xinshu p.
ying p.
yinmen acupuncture p.
yong p.
yu p.
yuan p.
yuan-source p.
yunn p.
zhongfu p.
zhongji p.
zhongwan p.
Pointer-Plus
pointes
torsades de p.
pointillage
poison
p. ash
p. dogwood
p. elder
p. flag
p. hemlock
p. ivy
P. Ivy/Oak Tablets
p. oak
p. plant dermatitis
p. sumac
poisonberry
poisoning
Amanita p.
blood p.
hyoscine p.
lead p.
nightshade p.
oxygen p.
Solanaceae p.

poivre
poke
p. greens
Indian p.
p. root
p. salad
p. salet
Virginia p.
pokeberry
poker
p. back
p. spine
pokeroot
powdered p.
pokeweed
p. mitogen (PWM)
p. root
polar extreme
polarity
p. balancing
p. chakra
p. squat
p. therapy
polarization
pole
inferior p.
superior p.
pole-cat cabbage
policosanol
poliomyelitis
paresis after p.
poliovirus
polish
Body P.
pollen
bee p.
buckwheat p.
CC P.
maize p.
pine p.
p. pini
typha p.
pollex pedis
pollicis
articulatio carpometacarpalis p.
caput obliquum musculi
adductoris p.
caput transversum musculi
adductoris p.
p. longus muscle
musculus adductor p.
musculus extensor brevis p.
musculus extensor longus p.

musculus extensor ossis
metacarpi p.
musculus flexor longus p.
musculus opponens p.
opponens p. (OP)
pollicization
polus
polyarthric
polyarthritis
p. chronica villosa
vertebral p.
polyarticular
polyaxial joint
polycephalum
Gnaphalium p.
polycheiria
polycystic ovary
polycythemia
polydactylism
polydipsia
polydrug abuse
polygala
p. root
P. senega
P. tenuifolia
polygalae radix
polyglycolic acid
Polygonum
P. bistoria
P. multiflorum
polyhalogenated biphenyl
polymelia
polymetacarpalia
polymetatarsalia
polymorpha
Angelica p.
polymorphonuclear
p. leukocyte
p. neutrophil
polymyositis
polyneuritis
polyneuropathy
sensory p.
polyostotic fibrous dysplasia
polypharmacy
polyphenol
polypodia

Polyporus Decoction
polysaccharide
complex p.
high molecular weight p.
polyscelia
polysymbrachydactyly
polysynaptic reflex
polysyndactyly
polyunsaturated fat
pomegranate
POMES
prospective outcomes monitoring
evaluation system
POMR
problem-oriented medical record
POMS
Profile of Mood States
ponderal index
ponograph
pons
apneustic center in p.
pneumotaxic center in p.
pontine-geniculate-occipital wave
pool
motor neuron p.
poor
camphor of the p.
poor-man's-treacle
pop
articulatory p.
cavitation p.
joint p.
poplar
black p.
p. bud
white p.
poples
poplitea
fossa p.
linea p.
popliteal
p. arch
p. artery
p. cyst
p. entrapment syndrome
p. fascia
p. fossa

NOTES

P

popliteal *(continued)*
    p. groove
    p. line
    p. lymph node
    p. muscle
    p. notch
    p. plane of femur
    p. plexus
    p. region
    p. space
    p. surface of femur
popliteum
    planum p.
popliteus
    p. muscle
    musculus p.
    sulcus p.
popotillo
popping sound
poppy
    California p.
    celandine p.
    corn p.
    field p.
    Flanders p.
    great scarlet p.
    opium p.
    poppyseed p.
    red p.
    rock p.
    p. seed
    thebaine p.
poppyseed poppy
Populus
    P. balsamifera
    P. nigra
    P. var. balsamifera candicans
Poria cocos
porillon
porphyria
Porter fascia
portio
portion
    condylar p.
    squama p.
position
    anatomic p.
    body p.
    p. of comfort
    constant rest p.
    controlled joint p.
    cun p.
    energy of p.

ERS p.
extended, rotated and side bent vertebral p.
flexed, rotated, and side bend vertebral p.
flexed, rotated, sidebent p.
Fowler p.
FRS p.
lateral recumbent p.
neutral p.
neutral spinal p.
prone p.
prone prop p.
p., quality, radiation, severity, time (PQRST)
reeducation p.
retraining in sitting p.
self-correction p.
self-stretch thoracic spine elongation p.
Sims p.
sitting p.
sphinx p.
standing p.
supine p.
unloaded p.
positional treatment
positive
    p. correlation
    false p.
    p. flavor affinity
    p. reinforcement
    p. transference
    p. transference reaction
positometric relaxation
postauricular lymph node
postaxial
postaxillaris
    linea p.
postaxillary line
postbrachial
postclavicular
postcostal
postcubital
PostDetox Pak
posterior
    p. antebrachial region
    p. articular pillar
    p. articular surface of dens
    p. aspect
    p. atlantooccipital membrane
    p. axillary fold
    p. axillary line

p. border of fibula
p. border of radius
p. border of ramus
p. border of ulna
p. brachial region
p. branch
p. capsule stretch
p. carpal region
p. cervical intertransversarii muscle
p. cervical intertransverse muscle
p. column
p. component
p. condyloid foramen
p. cord of brachial plexus
p. costotransverse ligament
p. cruciate ligament
p. crural region
p. crus of stapes
p. cubital region
p. curvature
p. cutaneous femoral nerve
p. deltoid muscle
p. diaphragm
p. diaphragm myofascial release technique
p. direction
p. drawer test of knee
duplicitas p.
p. facet joint syndrome
facies p.
p. fibular head
fibular head p.
p. funiculus
p. ilium
p. ilium functional technique
p. inferior iliac spine
p. innominate iliac rotation
p. intercondylar area of tibia
p. intraoccipital joint
p. intraoccipital synchondrosis
p. knee region
p. kyphosis
p. ligament of head of fibula
p. ligament of knee
p. limb of stapes

linea axillaris p.
linea glutea p.
linea mediana p.
p. longitudinal ligament
p. median line
membrana atlantooccipitalis p.
p. meniscofemoral ligament
musculus sacrococcygeus p.
musculus scalenus p.
musculus tibialis p.
p. neck region
p. occipitoaxial ligament
p. palpation
p. parietal pleura
p. plane
p. plane symmetry
p. pole of skull
p. postural deviation
p. pressure
p. primary division
p. process of septal cartilage
p. process of talus
radial head p.
regio antebrachialis p.
regio brachialis p.
regio carpalis p.
regio cervicalis p.
regio cruralis p.
regio cubitalis p.
regio femoralis p.
regio genus p.
p. region of arm
p. region of elbow
p. region of forearm
p. region of leg
p. region of neck
p. region of thigh
p. sacroiliac ligament
p. sacrosciatic ligament
p. sacrum
p. scalene muscle
p. sclerosis
p. segment
p. serratus muscle
p. spinal sclerosis
p. sternoclavicular ligament
p. subluxation

NOTES

P

posterior *(continued)*
p. superior iliac spine (PSIS)
p. superior iliac spine motion testing
p. superior iliac spine, sacral base, and L5 test
p. surface
p. surface of arm
p. surface of elbow
p. surface of fibula
p. surface of forearm
p. surface of leg
p. surface of lower limb
p. surface of radius
p. surface of shaft of humerus
p. surface of thigh
p. surface of tibia
p. surface of ulna
synchondrosis intraoccipitalis p.
p. talar articular surface of calcaneus
p. talofibular ligament
p. talotibial ligament
p. tibial muscle
p. tibiofibular ligament
p. tibiotalar ligament
p. tibiotalar part of deltoid ligament
p. translated sacrum
translation p.
p. triangle of neck
p. tubercle of cervical vertebrae
posterioris
vagina tendinis musculi tibialis p.
posteriorly
convex p.
p. rotated left innominate
sacroiliac bilaterally nutated p.
posterius
os tibiale p.
rete carpi p.
segmentum p.
trigonum cervicale p.
posteroanterior projection
posteroexternal
posterointernal
posterolateral protrusion
posteromedial
posteromedian
posterosuperior
postextraction alveolitis

postfracture ileus
postganglionic motor fiber
postglenoid tubercle
posthemorrhagic anemia
postherpetic neuralgia
posthyoid
posthypnotic
p. amnesia
p. attenuation
posticum
tibiale p.
posticus
musculus scalenus p.
musculus tibialis p.
postinfectious myelitis
postischial
postisometric relaxation
postmastectomy pain syndrome
postmedian
postmediastinal
postmediastinum
postmicturition residue
postoperative
p. complication
p. ileus
p. vomiting
postpartum
p. carpal tunnel syndrome
p. de Quervain tenosynovitis
P. Self-Evaluation Questionnaire (PPSEQ)
postsacral
postscapular
postsphenoid bone
postsynaptic
p. endorphin synapse
p. inhibition
p. membrane
posttarsal
posttibial
posttransverse
posttraumatic
p. hemiparesis
p. osteoporosis
p. stress disorder (PTSD)
p. stress syndrome
postural
p. analysis
p. axis
p. balance
p. compensation
p. contraction
p. decompensation

p. gravitational stress
p. imbalance
p. integration
p. ischemia
p. motion
p. muscle
p. therapy
postural-structural model
posture
   compensated p.
   decompensated p.
   dynamic p.
   flat back p.
   forward head p.
   good p.
   p. imbalance
   kypholordotic p.
   military-bearing p.
   sagittal plane p.
   static p.
   swayback p.
postvaccinal myelitis
postvoid residual (PVR)
potassium
   p. channel blocker
   p. dichromate
   p.-magnesium aspartate
   p. oxalate
   p. permanganate
   serum p.
potato
   p. broth
   p. peel tea
   white p.
potency
   homeopathic p.
potenization
Potensan
potential
   action p.
   active p.
   bioelectric p.
   dynamic p.
   p. energy
   event-related brain p.
   evoked p.
   functional p.

   muscle fiber action p.
   myogenic p.
   p. space
potentiate
potentiation
potentiator
Potentilla
potentization by dilution
potherb
potion
   remedy p.
pot marigold
Pott
   P. abscess
   P. aneurysm
Potter's
   P. Antigian tablet
   P. Piletabs
poultice
   onion p.
   raw potato p.
   sage p.
pounding
   sacral p.
Poupart line
powder
   borage p.
   elderberry p.
   Every Body's Protein P.
   garlic p.
   Multigenics P.'s
   seed p.
powdered
   p. pokeroot
   p. slippery elm bark
power
   Cranberry P.
   Feverfew P.
   Ginger P.
   Ginkgo P.
   goldenseal p.
   Hawthorne P.
   Milk Thistle P.
   Nu Veg Milk Thistle P.
   p. object
   Primrose P.
   P. Trim

NOTES

P

PowerTilt
 HiLo P.
Pozzi muscle
PPSEQ
 Postpartum Self-Evaluation
 Questionnaire
PQRST
 palliation, quality, radiation,
 severity, time
 position, quality, radiation, severity,
 time
prabonex
 inosine p.
practice
 acupuncture p.
 complementary medical p.
 (CMP)
practitioner
 alternative p.
 bodywork p.
 colonic p.
 yogic p.
prairie anemone
prakruti
prana
pranayama
prani
prashnam
pratense
 Trifolium p.
prayer
 p. beads
 intercessory p.
 nondirected p.
 p. stretch
 p. therapy
PRC
 phase-response curve
preanesthetic medication
preauricular lymph node
preaxial
preaxillaris
 linea p.
preaxillary line
precancerous condition
precatory bean
prechordal
preclinical trial
precontemplation
precordia
precordial
precordium
precostal

predictive value
predisposition
preeclampsia
preganglionic
 p. fiber
 p. neuron
 p. sympathetic nerve
pregnancy
prehallux
prehelicine
prehensile motion of hand
prehyoid
prelimbic
preload
Premantaid
premature birth
premenstrual
 p. dysphoric disorder
 p. syndrome (PMS)
premorbid
premotor cortex
Prenatal
 Basic P.
 Fem P.
 Multigenics P.
preparation
 bile p.
 Pfeiffer's Cold Sore P.
 Shankhapushpi herbal p.
Prepare oil
prepatellar bursitis
presacral
 p. anesthesia
 p. nerve
prescription (RX, Rx)
 manipulative medicine p.
 p. medication
 point p.
 shotgun p.
preservative
 BHA p.
 BHT p.
presphenoid bone
prespinal
prespondylolisthesis
pressor
press-up
 unilateral prone p.-u.
pressure
 p. anesthesia
 blood p. (BP)
 capillary p.
 deep p.

detrusor p.
diastolic blood p.
p. epiphysis
interstitial fluid p.
interstitial fluid colloid
  osmotic p.
intracranial p.
intraocular p.
negative intrathoracic p.
plasma colloid osmotic p.
p. point
p. point therapy
posterior p.
p. probe
p. reversal
p. sensation
p. sensitive point
p. sore
systolic blood p.
p. ulcer
pressure-point massage technique
pressurized leggings
presternal
  p. notch
  p. region
presternalis
  regio p.
presternum
presynaptic
  p. inhibition
  p. membrane
pretarsal
pretibial
pretracheal fascia
Prevail
prevalence
preventive
  p. medicine
  Ultra P. III
prevertebral
  p. fascia
  p. ganglion
  p. layer of cervical fascia
  p. part of vertebral artery
prickly
  p. ash
  p. ash bark

prickwood
priest's-crown
primarium
  punctum ossificationis p.
primary
  p. aim
  p. amputation
  p. anesthetic
  p. carnitine deficiency
  p. center of ossification
  p. dorsal ramus
  p. dysmenorrhea
  p. inflammatory disease
  p. joint disease
  p. line of light
  p. machinery of life
  p. malignant bone disease
  p. point of ossification
  p. respiratory mechanism
  p. sequestrum
  P. Source
  p. ventral ramus
prime mover
primi
  tuberositas ossis metatarsalis p.
  [I]
primrose
  evening p.
  p. flower
  p. oil
  oil of evening p. (OEP)
  P. Power
  p. root
Primula veris
primus
  digitus manus p.
prince's pine
principal
  p. meridian
  p. meridian subcircuit
principle
  active p.
  dynamic functional p.
  empirical p.
  folk p.
  Fryette p.'s I–III
  Hueter-Volkman p.

NOTES

P

331

principle *(continued)*
  similia p.
  p.'s of thoracic and lumbar
    spinal motion I–III
  p. of treatment
  water p.
Pritikin diet
Pro
  Innerfresh P.
  Sinustop P.
  Thisilyn P.
proanthocyanidin
  oligomeric p. (OPC)
probe
  p. device
  pressure p.
Probiata
Pro-Bionate
probiotic
problem
  functional health p.
  multifactorial p.
  pathological health p.
**problem-oriented medical record
(POMR)**
procedure
  afferent reduction p.
  articulatory p.
  balance and hold p.
  ceremonial p.
  craniosacral vault four p.
  CV4 p.
  detoxification p.
  diagnostic p.
  dynamic functional p.
  hypnotic p.
  imaging p.
  indirect balance p.
  invasive p.
  isolytic p.
  joint mobilization p.
  lymphatic pump p.
  manipulative p.
  muscle-balancing p.
  noninvasive p.
  p. overdose
  palpatory p.
  pétrissage p.
  reflex p.
  shelf p.
  soft tissue p.
  therapeutic p.
  V-spread p.

process
  acromial p.
  p. acupressure
  agenesis of odontoid p.
  articular p.
  bifid transverse p.
  Civinini p.
  conoid p.
  coracoid p.
  costal p.
  costal pit of transverse p.
  dislocation of articular p.'s
  ensiform p.
  foot p.
  foramen of transverse p.
  induction p.
  inflammatory p.
  life p.
  mammillary p.
  mastoid p.
  odontoid p.
  olecranon p.
  pterygoid p.
  sheath of styloid p.
  spinous p.
  Stieda p.
  styloid p.
  supraepicondylar p.
  transverse p.
  trochlear p.
  uncoiling p.
  xiphoid p.
processed garlic
processing
  hypnotic mode of
    information p.
  information p.
processus
prochordal
procumbens
  Gaultheria p.
  Harpagophytum p.
procyanidol oligomer (PCO)
ProDetox Pak
prodrome
prodrug
product
  advanced glycosylation end-p.
    (AGE)
  E'Ola P.'s
  orphan p.
  Pep P.'s

soured milk p.'s
VitaLife Sport P.'s
production
theta wave p.
Pro-Essence
profile
biochemical p.
Hypnotic Induction P. (HIP)
P. of Mood State instrument
P. of Mood States (POMS)
psychophysiological p.
Sickness Impact P. (SIP)
stress p.
test p.
proformiphen
profound hypothermia
profunda
p. brachii artery
fascia p.
fascia cervicalis p.
p. femoris artery
lamina p.
profundus
arcus palmaris p.
arcus venosus palmaris p.
arcus volaris p.
p. muscle
musculus flexor p.
musculus flexor digitorum p.
prognosis
prognostic value
program
exercise p.
relapse prevention p.
TM-Siddhi p.
programming
neurolinguistic p.
progressiva
dysbasia lordotica p.
fibrodysplasia ossificans p.
progressive
p. muscle relaxation
p. muscular atrophy
p. relaxation
p. relaxation therapy
p. relaxation training (PRT)
p. spinal amyotrophy

projection
anteroposterior p.
AP p.
frog-leg lateral p.
oblique p.
posteroanterior p.
spot lateral p.
projective technique
prolacit
prolapse
mitral valve p. (MVP)
prolapsed uterus
Proleve 40
proliferant
p. solution
p. therapy
proliferation
cellular p.
p. therapy
proliferative
p. arthritis
p. myositis
proline
prolotherapy
Promensil
prominence
hypothenar p.
styloid p.
thenar p.
prominens
vertebra p.
prominent heel
prominentia styloidea
promontorial common iliac node
promontorium ossis sacri
promontory
sacral p.
p. of the sacrum
pronate
pronated right foot
pronation
cuboid p.
p. of foot
foot p.
forearm p.
p. of forearm

NOTES

P

pronator
  p. quadratus muscle
  p. ridge
  p. teres muscle
  p. teres syndrome
pronatus
  pes p.
prone
  p. iliac crest height test
  p. lateral stretch
  p. mesenteric release
  p. myofascial release technique
  p. position
  p. prop position
  retraining position p.
  self-correction position p.
  self-stretch position p.
  p. thrust technique
pronograde
pronometer
pronounced
  p. acupressure
  p. symptom
propagated
  p. sensation along the channel (PSC)
  p. sensation along the meridian (PSM)
propagation
Propalmex
properitoneal
property
  antiallergic p.
  immune-enhancing p.
  thixotropic p.
  yang p.
prophylaxis
  lysine p.
  migraine p.
Propionibacterium acnes
propolis
  p. balsam
  bee p.
  p. mouth rinse
  p. resin
  p. wax
proportional cun measurement
proportionate dwarfism
propria
  lamina p.
proprietary medicine
proprioception nerve

proprioceptive
  p. function
  p. mechanism
proprioceptor
  p. neuromuscular facilitation
  p. neuromuscular facilitation stretching
propriospinal pathway reflex
proprius
  musculus extensor digiti quinti p.
  musculus extensor indicis p.
pro re nata
Proscar
prosect
prosector
prosectorium
prosepina
  flor de p.
prospective
  p. outcomes monitoring evaluation system (POMES)
  p. study
Prostagen
prostaglandin
  p. E_1 (PGE$_1$)
  p. E_2 (PGE$_2$)
ProstaKit
Prostane
Prost-Answer Alcohol Free
Prostata
prostate
  p. enlargement
  p. secretion
  transurethral resection of the p. (TURP)
prostate-specific antigen (PSA)
prostatic adenoma
prostatitis
prosternation
prosthesis
prosthetic
prosthetics
prosthetist
ProStool
protecting qi
protective
  p. force
  p. qi
protein
  bone Gla p.
  colloidal silver p.

p. glycation
  immune p.
protein-energy utilization
proteinosis
  lipoid p.
proteolytic enzyme
Proteus vulgaris
prothrombin time (PT)
Protocol Pak
protoveratrine
  p. A
  p. B
protovertebra
protraction stretch
protractor
protruded disk
protrusio acetabuli
protrusion
  posterolateral p.
protuberance
  external occipital p.
  mental p.
  occipital p.
protuberantia
provider
  touch p.
proving
  Law of P.
provisional callus
provitamin A
provitamin B₃
provocation
provocative test
proximad
proximal
  p. area
  p. border of nail
  p. direction
  p. femoral focal deficiency
  p. interphalangeal joint
  p. radioulnar articulation
  p. radioulnar joint
  p. region
  p. tibiofibular joint
  p. tibiofibular joint dysfunction
  p. tibiofibular joint muscle
    energy technique

proximalis
  articulatio radioulnaris p.
proximate
proximoataxia
Prozac
PRT
  progressive relaxation training
prune juice
prunifolium
  Viburnum p.
Prunus
  P. africana
  P. armeniaca
  P. persica vulgaris
  P. serotina
  P. virginiana
pruritus
PS 100
PSA
  prostate-specific antigen
PSC
  propagated sensation along the
    channel
pseudankylosis
pseudarthrosis
pseudoaneurysm
pseudoarthrosis
pseudoclaudication
pseudocoxalgia
pseudofracture
pseudo-ginseng
  Panax p.-g.
pseudogout
pseudohypericin
pseudohypoparathyroidism
pseudojoint
  ulnomeniscotriquetral p.
pseudometatarsal arch
Pseudomonas aeruginosa
pseudoosteomalacia
pseudoosteomalacic
  p.-o. pelvis
pseudoparalysis
  congenital atonic p.
pseudoparesis
Pseudophage
pseudopolydystrophy

NOTES

P

pseudorheumatism
PSIS
    posterior superior iliac spine
PSM
    propagated sensation along the
    meridian
psoas
    p. abscess
    p. major muscle
    p. minor muscle
    p. minor tendon
    p. muscle
    p. muscle dysfunction
    p. muscle exercise
    p. muscle tension test
psoralen plus ultraviolet light of A
wave length (PUVA)
psoriasis
psoriatica
    arthropathia p.
psoriatic arthritis
psyche
psychiatry
    orthomolecular p.
psychic
    p. effect
    p. harmony
    p. surgery
psychoactive
psychobehavioral model
psychobiological
psychobiology
psychodynamic
    p. psychotherapy
    p. therapy
psychogenic
    p. character
    p. impotence
    p. urological symptom
psychological
    p. correlate
    p. effect
    p. evaluation
psychology
    somatic p.
psychometric
psychomotor skills
psychoneuroendocrinology
psychoneuroimmunology
psychoneurologic
psychooncology
psychophysical regeneration

psychophysiological
    p. profile
    p. response
    p. therapy
psychophysiologic self regulation
psychophysiology
psychosis
psychosocial history
psychosomatic
    p. condition
    p. disorder
    p. heart disorder
    p. medicine
    p. network
    p. self-regulation
    p. technique
psychospiritual vitalization
psychosynthesis
psychotherapeutic measure
psychotherapy
    psychodynamic p.
psychotropic drug
psyllium
    black p.
    p. colloid
    French p.
    p. husk
    Plantago p.
    p. seed
    Spanish p.
psyllium-enriched food
PT
    prothrombin time
P/T
    Glandiet Powder P/T
pterion
pterygoid
    p. chest
    p. muscle
    p. pit
    p. process
pterygoideum
    os p.
pterygospinal ligament
pterygospinosus
    musculus p.
PTSD
    posttraumatic stress disorder
PTT
    partial prothrombin time
Ptychopetalum
    P. olacoides
    P. uncinatum

pu
  shi chang p.
  p. tong an mo massage
pubens
  Sambucus p.
pubes
  p. functional technique
  left superior p.
  right inferior p.
  somatic dysfunction of p.
pubic
  p. angle
  p. bone
  p. branch of obturator artery
  p. dysfunction
  p. muscle energy technique
  p. rami
  p. region
  p. shear
  p. spine
  p. symphysis
  p. symphysis compression
  p. symphysis dysfunction
  p. symphysis levelness test
  p. tubercle
pubicum
  tuberculum p.
pubis
  corpus ossis p.
  inferior p.
  osteitis p.
  spina p.
  superior p.
  symphysis p.
pubocapsular ligament
pubococcygeal muscle
pubococcygeus muscle
pubofemoral ligament
puboprostatic
puccoon
  red p.
  yellow p.
pudding grass
pudendal
  p. anesthesia
  p. nerve
Pueraria lobata

puhuang
pukeweed
pulcherrima
  Euphorbia p.
pulegium
  Mentha p.
pulegone
pull
  p. force
  pectoral p.
pulley
  p. of humerus
  muscular p.
  peroneal p.
  p. of talus
pulmonaria
  P. angustifolia
  Lobaria p.
pulmonary
  p. edema
  p. elastic recoil
  p. embolus
  p. emphysema
  p. hypertension
  p. osteoarthropathy
  p. plexus
  p. sarcoidosis
  P. Tonic Pills
  p. vasculitis
pulp
  aloe vera p.
  apple p.
  p. of finger
pulposus
  herniated nucleus p. (HNP)
  nucleus p.
pulsatile force
pulsatilla
  Anemone p.
  P. Med Complex
  P. nigricans
pulsating metastases
pulse
  p. amplitude
  antipolarization biphasic p.
  big p.
  biphasic p.

NOTES

P

337

pulse *(continued)*
    brachial p.
    p. characteristic
    choppy p.
    p. diagnosis
    p. duration
    electric p.
    p. of electricity
    empty p.
    p. frequency
    Life P.
    negative p.
    radial p.
    p. recording of amplitude
    slippery p.
    slow p.
    square p.
    square wave p.
    strong and rapid p.
    superficial p.
    surging p.
    tense p.
    thin p.
    thready p.
    tight p.
    p. touching
    train of p.
    weak p.
    p. width
pulsed electromagnetic field
pulvo de vibora
pumacuchu
pump
    Dalrymple p.
    lymph p.
    lymphatic p.
    pedal p.
    pedal lymphatic p.
    thoracic p.
    thoracic lymphatic p.
    unilateral thoracic lymphatic p.
    upper extremity lymphatic p.
pump-handle
    p.-h. motion of rib
    p.-h. rib motion
pumping
    lymphatic p.
    thoracic p.
pumpkin
    p. seed oil
    P. Seed Shield
punarnava

punctata
    dysplasia epiphysialis p.
punctum
    p. coxale
    p. ossificationis
    p. ossificationis primarium
    p. ossificationis secundarium
puncture
    lumbar p.
pure
    p. consciousness
    p. tree tea oil and water
      gargle
    p. vegetarian
purgative enema
purge
purging
    p. buckthorn
    p. ritual
purification
    blood p.
    p. lodge
    p. ritual
    seasonal p.
purified chondroitin sulfate
puriform
puromucous
purple
    p. clover
    p. coneflower
    p. Kansas coneflower
    p. lapacho
    p. tongue
    p. trillium
purpura
purpurea
    Claviceps p.
    Digitalis p.
    Echinacea p.
    Ipomoea p.
purpureum
    Eupatorium p.
purpureus
    Monascus p.
purse
    shepherd's p.
purshiana
    Rhamnus p.
purulence
purulent inflammation
Purush
purusha
purvain

pus
Puschkina scilloides libanotica
pustule
pustulosum
    Allium p.
putrid odor
PUVA
    psoralen plus ultraviolet light of A
    wave length
        PUVA therapy
PVR
    postvoid residual
PWM
    pokeweed mitogen
Pycnogenol
pyelonephritis
pyemia
pyesis
Pygeum
    P. africana
    P. africanum
    P. africanum extract (PAE)
pygeum
pyknic
pylon
pylori
    Helicobacter p.

pyogen
pyogenesis
pyogenic
    p. arthritis
    p. infection
pyopoiesis
pyorrhea
pyosepticemia
pyosis
pyramid
    Lallouette p.
    p. of thyroid
pyramidal desiccation
pyramidale
    os p.
pyramidalis muscle
pyramis
pyrethrum
pyridoxine
pyrifera
    Macrocystis p.
pyrosis
pyrrolizidine alkaloid
Pyrus
pythogenesis

NOTES

P

Q

Q10, Q-10, Q₁₀
   coenzyme Q. (CoQ₁₀)
Q angle
Q-Dent
QDS
   qigong deviation syndrome
QGM
   infratonic QGM
qi
   q. balance
   big q.
   q. branch
   chest q.
   q. circulation
   da cheng q.
   de q.
   defensive q.
   deficiency of heart q.
   deficiency of kidney q.
   deficiency of lung q.
   deficiency of spleen q.
   q. energy
   evil q.
   exhaustion of liver q.
   fire q.
   q. flow
   flow of q.
   gathering q.
   q. gong (var. of qigong)
   guardian q.
   q. hai
   heart q.
   hereditary q.
   jing q.
   q. jing ba mai
   q. jingba mai
   q. jingbamai
   liver q.
   lung q.
   middle q.
   nutrient q.
   original q.
   pathogenic q.
   protecting q.
   protective q.
   rebellious q.
   q. reservoir
   river of q.
   sea of q.
   q. shield

   q. sinking
   sinking q.
   sinking spleen q.
   source q.
   stagnation of q.
   q. stagnation
   stagnation of liver q.
   stasis of q.
   q. state
   q. tonifying point
   q. transfer
   q. vessel
   water q.
   wei q.
   q. xu
   yang q.
   yin q.
   ying q.
   yuan q.
   q. zhi zheng
   zong q.
qian
   q. shi
   q. wei qiang hua yin
qiang huo
q.i.d.
   four times a day
   quater in die
qigong, qi gong, QiGong
   breathing q.
   breathing exercise-oriented q.
   q. deviation syndrome (QDS)
   q. exercise
   external q.
   q. induction
   internal q.
   marrow washing q.
   q. master
   meditation q.
   meditation-oriented q.
   q. meridian examination
      method
   q. meridian massage (QMM)
   mindful q.
   mindless q.
   movement q.
   movement-oriented q.
   nei dan q.
   q. respiration
   self-healing style of q. (SHQ)

qigong *(continued)*
    soaring crane q.
    tendon changing q.
    wai dan q.
qigongology
qihai
    ren 6 q.
qihaishu
    ub 24 q.
qimen
    liv 14 q.
    q. point
qin
    huang q.
qing
    q. hao
    q. su yi qi tang
    q. wei tang
    q. zao jie fei tang
qingdai
qiuhou
    Ex-HN 4 q.
qiuxu
    gb 40 q.
qiu xu
QMM
    qigong meridian massage
QR
    quieting response
quack grass
quadrangular space
quadrant
quadrate
    q. ligament
    q. muscle
    q. muscle of loins
    q. muscle of sole
    q. muscle of thigh
    q. pronator muscle
quadratus
    q. femoris muscle
    q. lumborum
    q. lumborum muscle
    q. lumborum muscle exercise
    q. lumborum stretch
    q. muscle
    musculus q.
    musculus pronator q.
    q. plantae muscle
    q. planta muscle
quadriceps
    q. angle
    q. femoris

    q. femoris muscle
    q. group
    q. muscle of thigh
quadricepsplasty
quadrilateral space
quadripolar
quadruple amputation
quai
    dong q.
    FC with dong q.
Quaker Oat Bran
quaking aspen
quality
    burning q.
    healing q.
    q. of motion
    q. of movement
    yang q.
    yin q.
quan
quanliao
    si 18 q.
quantum
    q. medicine
    Q. ReleaseWork
quarter
    lamb's q.'s
    upper q.
quartz-glass container
quassia
    Jamaica q.
    q. wood
quater in die **(q.i.d.)**
Quatre Epices
quchi
    li 11 q.
quebrachine
queen
    Q. Anne's lace
    q. bee jelly
    q. of the meadow
    q. of the night
queen-of-the-meadow
queen's
    q. delight
    q. root
Queensland asthmaweed
quepen
    st 12 q.
quercetin
    activated q.
quercifolium
    Toxicodendron q.

quercus
    cortex q.
    Q. marina
quest
    vision q.
questionnaire
    Attributional Style Q. (ASQ)
    Cognitive-Somatic Anxiety Q.
    Everyday Life Q.
    Melzack pain q.
    Postpartum Self-Evaluation Q.
      (PPSEQ)
qugu
    ren 2 q.
quick
    q. thrust
    q. withdrawal
quid
    betel nut q.
quiet hip disease
quieting response (QR)
Quietude Homeopathic Formula
quillaja
Quillaja saponaria
quina-quin

quinata
    Akebia q.
quince
    common q.
Quincke edema
quinghao
quinine
    wild q.
quinolizidine alkaloid
quinone
quinquefolius
    Panax q.
quinti
    musculus abductor digiti q.
    musculus opponens digiti q.
    tuberositas ossis metatarsalis q.
    [V]
quintus
    digitus manus q. [V]
quitel
Quit Smoking
ququan
    liv 8 q.
quze
    pe 3 q.

NOTES

R
resistance
RA
rheumatoid arthritis
rabbeting
racemosa
  Actaea r.
  Aralia r.
  Cimicifuga r.
  Sambucus r.
rachial
rachidial
rachidian
rachilysis
rachiopagus
rachis
rachischisis
rachitic
  r. pelvis
  r. rosary
  r. scoliosis
rachitis
  r. fetalis
  r. fetalis annularis
  r. fetalis micromelica
  r. intrauterina
racket amputation
radiad
radial
  r. artery palpation
  r. border of forearm
  r. bursa
  r. clubhand
  r. collateral ligament
  r. collateral ligament of elbow
    joint
  r. collateral ligament of wrist
    joint
  r. deviation
  r. eminence of wrist
  r. flexor muscle of wrist
  r. fossa of humerus
  r. head
  r. head anterior
  r. head functional technique
  r. head posterior
  r. motion testing
  r. nerve
  r. nerve entrapment
  r. notch

  r. pulse
  r. styloid tendovaginitis
  r. tuberosity
  r. tunnel syndrome
radialis
  eminentia carpi r.
  flexor carpi r.
  incisura r.
  musculus flexor carpi r.
  sulcus nervi r.
  vagina tendinis musculi flexoris
    carpi r.
radialium
  vagina tendinum musculorum
    extensorum carpi r.
radial-ulnar deviation
radiance breathwork
radiate
  r. ligament
  r. ligament of head of rib
  r. ligament of wrist
  r. sternocostal ligament
radiating pain
radiation
  direct infrared r.
  electromagnetic r. (EMR)
  r. fibrosis
  indirect infrared r.
  infrared r.
  microwave r.
  r. myelitis
  r. myelopathy
  r. of pain
  segmental pain r.
  r. treatment
  UVB r.
radiation-induced interstitial cystitis
radical
  free r.
radicans
  Toxicodendron r.
radicle
radicula
radicularia
  fila r.
radicular pain
radiculitis
  acute brachial r.
radiculopathy
  discogenic r.

345

radiculopathy *(continued)*
    lumbar r.
    spinal nerve r.
radii *(pl. of* radius)
radioactivity
radiobicipital
radiocarpal
    r. articulation
    r. joint
radiocarpalis
    articulatio r.
radiodigital
radiograph
    plain r.
radiographic mensuration
radiohumeral joint
radioimmunoassay
radiology
    chiropractic r.
radiomuscular
radiopalmar
radiotherapy
radioulnar
    r. disk
    r. joint
    r. joint motion
    r. syndesmosis
radioulnaris
    syndesmosis r.
radish
    black r.
radius, pl. **radii**
    anular ligament of r.
    articular circumference of head
      of r.
    articular pit of head of r.
    caput radii
    carpal articular surface of r.
    circumferentia articularis capitis
      radii
    collum radii
    corpus radii
    dorsal tubercle of r., pl. dorsal
      vertebra
    r. dysfunction
    r. fixus
    fovea articularis capitis radii
    head of r.
    interosseous border of r.
    margo anterior radii
    margo interosseus radii
    margo posterior radii
    neck of r.

orbicular ligament of r.
posterior border of r.
posterior surface of r.
reciprocal motion or r.
shaft of r.
styloid process of r.
tuber radii
tuberculum dorsale radii
tuberositas radii
tuberosity of r.
radix
    bupleuri r.
    r. cardopatiae
    r. ginseng
    glycyrrhizae r.
    r. glycyrrhizae uralensis
    pareira r.
    polygalae r.
    rhei r.
    scutellariae r.
    r. valerianae
rage
    inadequate r.
Raggedy Ann syndrome
ragweed
ragwort
    golden r.
raising
    crossed straight leg r.
    rib r.
    straight leg r.
rajas
Raja yota
rakta
    r. moksha
ram-goat rose
ramosum
    Clostridium r.
ramus, pl. **ramus**
    auricular rami
    ischial r.
    ischiopubic r.
    r. of mandible
    mandibular r.
    peroneal anastomotic r.
    posterior border of r.
    primary dorsal r.
    primary ventral r.
    pubic rami
    superior pubic r.
randomized
    r. controlled trial (RCT)
    r. trial

R

range
    r. of active movement
    r. of ease
    r. of freedom
    lateral bucket-handle r.
    r. of motion (ROM)
    r. of motion abnormality
    r. of motion treatment
    r. of passive movement
    reduced r.
    red visible r.
    therapeutic r.
Ranunculus
    R. ficaria
rao
    dan yu tan r.
    tan zhou shang r.
RAPD
    rapid amplification of polymorphic
    DNA
rape
    California r.
raphanistrum
    Raphanus r.
Raphanus
    R. raphanistrum
    R. sativus
raphe
    r. descending system
    r. magnus
    r. nucleus
    r. serotonin effect
raphe-DLT-serotonin system
raphespinal fibers
rapid amplification of polymorphic
DNA (RAPD)
rapidly ascending end feel
Rapi-Snooze
rapport
Rapuntium inflatum
rasa
rasayana
rasceta
Ras El Hanout
raspatory
raspberry
    black r.

ground r.
    r. leaf tea
    red r.
raspbis
ratanhiawurzel
rate
    cranial rhythmic impulse r.
    CRI r.
    flow r.
    glomerular filtration r.
    metabolic r.
    relapse r.
    sedimentation r.
rating
    impairment r.
    RISCC r.
ratio
    body-weight r.
    cardiothoracic r.
    hand r.
    international normalized r.
    (INR)
    LDL/HDL r.
    risk-benefit r.
    r. of saturated fat and
      cholesterol to calories
    therapeutic r.
rational chiropractic
rat root
rattle
    medicine r.
rattlebush
rattleroot
rattlesnake
    r. meat
    r. root
    r. weed
rattleweed
RAU
    recurrent aphthous ulcer
Raudixin
Rauwiloid
Rauwolfia
    R. root
    R. serpentina
raw
    r. bile

NOTES

raw *(continued)*
    r. garlic
    r. lemon rub
    r. pituitary glandular
    r. potato juice
    r. potato poultice
    r. spleen glandular
raw-food vegetarian
ray
    sonar r.
Raynaud disease
RCT
    randomized controlled trial
RDA
    recommended daily allowance
    recommended dietary allowance
re
    r. disturbance
    gan dan shi r.
    pi yun shi r.
reaction
    adverse r.
    anaphylactoid r.
    antigen-antibody r.
    articular r.
    immune rejection r.
    irreversible r.
    local anesthetic r.
    Mantoux test skin r.
    neurobehavioral r.
    periarticular tissue r.
    periosteal r.
    positive transference r.
    telesomatic r.
    type A r.
    type B r.
    type C r.
    type D r.
reactive catecholamine
reactivity
    autonomic r.
reading
    diagnostic r.
read the tissue
realignment
    structural r.
reamer
    intramedullary r.
rebalance
rebellious qi
rebirthing
rebound
    r. scurvy

    r. of skin
    r. thrust
rebounding
rebreathing
recalcitrant osteomyelitis
receiver operating characteristic curve
receptaculum
receptivity
    mental r.
receptor
    articular r.
    conical r.
    fusiform r.
    globular r.
    skin r.
recess
    subpopliteal r.
recessus subpopliteus
recidivism
    alcoholic r.
reciprocal
    r. inhibition
    r. innervation
    r. motion or radius
    r. nervous system
    r. tension membrane (RTM)
    r. tension membrane function
recoil
    pulmonary elastic r.
    r. thrust
recombinant hirudin
recommended
    r. daily allowance (RDA)
    r. dietary allowance (RDA)
reconstructive therapy
record
    problem-oriented medical r. (POMR)
rectal
    r. balloon
    r. distention
    r. lymphatic drainage
    r. venous plexus
rectangular amputation
rectococcygeal
rectus
    r. abdominis muscle
    r. capitis anterior muscle
    r. capitis lateralis muscle
    r. capitis posterior major
    r. capitis posterior major muscle

r. capitis posterior minor
r. capitis posterior minor
muscle
r. femoris
r. femoris muscle
r. femoris muscle exercise
r. muscle of thigh
recumbent
lateral r.
self-stretch position lateral r.
recurrent
r. ankle sprain
r. aphthous ulcer (RAU)
r. inhibition
recurvatum
genu r.
pectus r.
r. test
recutita
Chamomilla r.
Matricaria r.
red
r. aura
r. beet crystal
r. blood cell
r. blood cell thiamine
r. bush tea
r. cinchona
r. clover
r. clover blossoms
R. Clover Cleanser
r. clover combo
R. Clover Plus
R. Clover Tops
r. color
R. Cross Toothache Medication
r. elderberry
r. elm
r. eyebright
r. ink plant
r. lapacho
r. muscle
r. pepper
r. periwinkle
r. poppy
r. puccoon
r. raspberry

r. raspberry leaf
r. raspberry tea
r. reflex
r. rhatany
r. root
r. squill
r. sunflower
r. valerian
r. visible range
r. yeast
r. yeast rice
red-beam
r.-b. laser
r.-b. laser pen
red-fruited elder
redressement forcé
redressment
redroot
reduce
reduced range
reducible
reducing
r. agent
r. method
reduction
5-alpha r.
r. deformity
hip r.
r. mammoplasty
seizure r.
weight r.
redwood
reeducation
muscular r.
neuromuscular r.
r. position
reef shark
reestablish
reference
point of r.
r. point
r. value
reflex
Achilles r.
Achilles deep tendon r.
Achilles tendon r.
r. activity

NOTES

349

reflex *(continued)*
  adductor r.
  r. arc
  asymmetric tonic r.
  Babinski r.
  baroreceptor r.
  biceps r.
  bowman's r.
  brachioradialis r.
  breathing r.
  celiac plexus r.
  r. change
  Chapman r.
  clasp-knife r.
  conditioned r.
  cremasteric r.
  crossed extensor r.
  cry r.
  deep tendon r.
  fencer's r.
  flexor r.
  Golgi tendon r.
  Hering-Breuer inflation r.
  r. inhibition
  inverse stretch r.
  ipsilateral flexor r.
  load r.
  modify r.
  Moro r.
  muscle spindle r.
  muscle stretch r.
  neck r.'s
  neurolymphatic r.
  neuromuscular r.
  nociceptive r.
  oculocephalogyric r.
  patellar deep tendon r.
  patellar tendon r.
  r. pathway
  r. pattern
  r. point
  polysynaptic r.
  r. procedure
  propriospinal pathway r.
  red r.
  righting r.
  somatosomatic r.
  somatovisceral r.
  somatoviscerosomatic r.
  static stretch r.
  stretch r.
  supporting r.'s
  r. sympathetic dystrophy (RSD)

  sympathetic nervous system r.
  tendo Achillis r.
  tendon r.
  triceps r.
  upper extremity r.
  vagovagal r.
  vibration-induced flexion r.
  visceral traction r.
  viscerosomatic r.
  viscerosomatovisceral r.
  viscerovisceral r.
  wind-up r.
  withdrawal r.
reflexologist
reflexology
  foot r.
  r. socks
reflexotherapy
reflux
  gastroesophageal r.
refractor
refractory period
refracture
refusion
regalis
  Consolida r.
regelii
  Smilax r.
regenerate
regeneration
  nerve r.
  psychophysical r.
regia
  Juglans r.
regimen
  Livingston-Wheeler r.
regio, pl. **regiones**
  r. antebrachialis anterior
  r. antebrachialis posterior
  r. axillaris
  r. brachialis anterior
  r. brachialis posterior
  r. calcanea
  r. carpalis anterior
  r. carpalis posterior
  regiones cervicales
  r. cervicalis anterior
  r. cervicalis lateralis
  r. cervicalis posterior
  regiones corporis
  r. cruralis posterior
  r. cruris anterior
  r. cubitalis anterior

r. cubitalis posterior
r. deltoidea
regiones dorsales
r. femoralis posterior
r. femoris
r. femoris anterior
r. genus anterior
r. genus posterior
r. hypochondriaca
r. infraclavicularis
r. infrascapularis
r. lumbalis
regiones membri inferioris
regiones membri superioris
r. nuchalis
r. pectoralis
r. plantaris
r. presternalis
r. sacralis
r. scapularis
r. sternocleidomastoidea
r. suralis
r. talocruralis
r. vertebralis
region
   ankle r.
   axillary r.
   r.'s of back
   r.'s of body
   calcaneal r.
   chakra r.
   r.'s of chest
   costochondral r.
   deltoid r.
   diseased r.
   elbow r.
   femoral r.
   gluteal r.
   hypochondriac r.
   iliac r.
   r.'s of inferior limb
   infrascapular r.
   junctional r.
   lateral abdominal r.
   r.'s of lower limb
   lumbar r.
   r.'s of neck

nuchal r.
pectoral r.
popliteal r.
posterior antebrachial r.
posterior brachial r.
posterior carpal r.
posterior crural r.
posterior cubital r.
posterior knee r.
posterior neck r.
presternal r.
proximal r.
pubic r.
sacral r.
scapular r.
shoulder r.
sternocleidomastoid r.
suboccipital r.
r.'s of superior limb
sural r.
transitional r.
translational r.
r.'s of upper limb
urogenital r.
vertebral r.
wrist and hand r.
regional
   r. anatomy
   r. anesthesia
   r. extension
   r. flexion
   r. hypothermia
   r. lymphatics
   r. motion testing
   r. stretch
regiones (*pl. of* regio)
Reglan
regression
   age r.
regulate
Regulate the Middle Decoction
regulation
   psychophysiologic self r.
regulator
   female r.
regulatory adaptation

NOTES

regurgitation
    tricuspid valve r.
rehabilitation
    biomechanical r.
    neuromuscular r.
    physical medicine and r.
    (PM&R)
    stroke r.
    work r.
Rehmannia glutinosa
Reichert cartilage
Reichian and Lowenian Bioenergetic Analysis technique
Reiki
reinforcement
    positive r.
reishi
rejection
    acute cellular r.
    chronic allograft r.
    hyperacute r.
rejuvenate
rejuvenation therapy
relapse
    r. prevention program
    r. rate
relationship
    acausal r.
    spatial r.
relative
    r. humidity
    r. sensitivity
    r. specificity
Relax-a-Cizor
relaxant
    muscle r.
    neuromuscular r.
    nondepolarizing r.
    smooth muscle r.
relaxation
    biofeedback-assisted r.
    deep r.
    isometric r.
    muscle r.
    passive r.
    positometric r.
    postisometric r.
    progressive r.
    progressive muscle r.
    r. response
    r. technique
    r. therapy
    r. training

relaxing
    r. effect
    r. exercise
relaxin level
release
    articular ligamentous r.
    balanced ligamentous r.
    r. of diaphragm
    diaphragmatic r.
    endorphin r.
    facilitated positional r. (FPR)
    integrated neuromusculoskeletal r.
    mesenteric r.
    myofascial r. (MFR)
    pectoral r.
    r. phenomenon
    r. by positioning functional technique
    r. by positioning technique
    prone mesenteric r.
    somatoemotional r.
    supine mesenteric r.
    thyroid hormone r.
    urogenital diaphragm r.
released ulnar intrinsic muscle
ReleaseWork
    Quantum R.
Relief
    Cran R.
religion
relocation test
remedial therapist
remediation
remedy
    allovedic r.
    Bach flower r.
    flower r.
    folk r.
    homeopathic r.
    magnetically influenced homeopathic r. (MIHR)
    naturopathic r.
    No. 2040 Headache R.
    No. 2090 Indigestion R.
    r. potion
    Rheumatic Pain R.
Remifemin
remind
    Ginexin R.
remineralization

remission

    character, onset, location,
    duration, exacerbation, r.
    (COLDER)
    condition, onset, location,
    duration, exacerbation, r.
    (COLDER)

remodeling

remote

    r. diagnosis
    r. healing

remove, replace, reinoculate, repair (four Rs)

ren

    ren mai channel (ren)
    r. channel
    r. 4 guanyuan
    huo ma r.
    hu tao r.
    r. 15 jiuwei
    r. 14 juque
    r. 23 lianquan
    r. mai
    r. 6 qihai
    r. 2 qugu
    rou cong r.
    r. 17 shanzhong
    r. shen
    r. 8 shenque
    r. 5 shimen
    tao r.
    r. 22 tiantu
    yi zhi r.
    r. 3 zhongji
    r. 12 zhongwan

renal

    r. artery
    r. calcinosis
    r. colic
    r. dialysis
    r. function
    r. interstitial fibrosis
    r. nanism
    r. osteodystrophy
    r. oxalate stone
    r. tubular necrosis
    r. tubular toxicity

renn

    r. mai
    r. mo

Renshaw inhibitory system

Rentone

renzhong

    du 26 r.

repair

    remove, replace, reinoculate, r.
    (four Rs)

repatterning

    biosonic r.
    neurocellular r.

repens

    Amomum r.
    lipidosterolic extract of
      Serosa r. (LSESR)
    Mitchella r.
    Serenoa r.

reperfusion injury

repetitive

    r. motion
    r. strain disorder
    r. strain injury (RSI)
    r. stress disorder
    r. stress injury (RSI)

Repha-OS

repigmentation

replacement

    r. bone
    fatty r.
    selective fatty r.

replenish

replication

    viral r.

repositioning

    muscle r.

repress

repressed memory

repression

research

    Foundation for Chiropractic
      Education and R. (FCER)
    National Institute for
      Healthcare R. (NIHR)

resect

resectable

R

NOTES

resection
reserpine
reserve force
reservoir
    chi r.
    Dantian r.
    energy r.
    qi r.
residual
    r. abscess
    postvoid r. (PVR)
residue
    postmicturition r.
resilience
    tissue r.
resiliency
resilient
resin
    jalap r.
    melamine r.
    podophyllum r.
    propolis r.
resina tolutana
resistance (R)
    electrode r.
    electrodermal skin r.
    host r.
    isokinetic r.
    isometric r.
    low immune r.
    mutual r.
    needle r.
    skin-electrode r.
    R. Support Formula
    vascular r.
resistant
    r. barrier
    r. hypertension
resistive
    r. duction
    r. movement
resolution
resolve
resolvent
resorption
    bone r.
respirable
Respiraprime
respiration
    artificial r.
    Cheyne-Stokes r.
    episodic inhibition of r.
    r. feedback

    mouth-to-mouth r.
    qigong r.
respirator
    cuirass r.
respiratory
    r. assist
    r. assistance
    r. axis
    r. axis of sacrum
    r. circulatory model
    r. cooperation
    r. diaphragm
    r. disorder
    r. effort technique
    r. force
    r. gas exchange
    r. mechanism
    r. movement
    r. rib dysfunction
    r. rib restriction
    r. syncytial virus
    r. tract
respirometer
    Wright r.
Respirtone
responder
    vascular r.
response
    adaptive r.
    cellular immune r.
    deep parasympathetic r.
    electrodermal r. (EDR)
    fight-or-flight r.
    galvanic skin r.
    general adaptation r.
    hypersensitivity r.
    immune r.
    lymphocyte stimulation r.
    maladaptive r.
    muscular r.
    neuroreflexive r.
    nocebo r.
    nonadaptive lumbar r.
    nonvolitional r.
    patient r.
    placebo r.
    psychophysiological r.
    quieting r. (QR)
    relaxation r.
    stress r.
    T-cell r.
    therapeutic r.
    tissue r.

responsiveness
  hypnotic r.
REST
  restriction of environmental
  stimulation therapy
rest
  bed r.
  r., ice, compression, elevation
  (RICE)
  r., ice, heat, elevation
restful alertness
resting length
restlessness
restoration
  noiseless r.
  painless r.
  r. of symmetrical movement
  pattern
restorative
restore coordinated activity
restraining orthopedic device
restricted
  r. abduction
  r. abduction and adduction
  r. abduction test
  r. adduction
  r. barrier
  r. coupled movement
  r. dorsiflexion
  r. elbow
  r. elbow muscle energy
  technique
  r. environmental stimulation
  r. environmental stimulation
  therapy
  r. external rotation
  r. horizontal flexion
  r. internal rotation
  r. motion barrier
  r. movement
  r. sacral base
restriction
  r. barrier
  bilateral extension r.
  dural r.
  r. of environmental stimulation
  therapy (REST)

exhalation r.
extension r.
fascial r.
flexion r.
inhalation r.
r. of internal-external rotation
r. of intervertebral motion
membranous tension r.
r. of motion
motion r.
neural r.
respiratory rib r.
rotation r.
rotational r.
sagittal plane r.
self-correction position for
  extension r.
sensory r.
talar r.
type I r.
restrictive
  r. barrier
  r. barrier to motion
restrictor
  short r.
restructuring
  body r.
  cognitive r.
resultant current (I)
resuscitate
resuscitation
  cardiopulmonary r.
  mouth-to-mouth r.
resveratrol
retaining position standing
retard
  Venostasin r.
rete
  r. acromiale arteriae
  thoracoacromialis
  r. articulare cubiti
  r. articulare genus
  r. calcaneum
  r. carpale dorsale
  r. carpi posterius
  r. malleolare laterale
  r. malleolare mediale

R

NOTES

rete *(continued)*
  r. patellare
  r. vasculosum articulare
  r. venosum dorsale manus
  r. venosum dorsale pedis
  r. venosum plantare
retention
  r. enema
  sodium r.
  water r.
reticular fiber
reticularis paragigantocellularis
reticulata
  Citrus r.
reticulated bone
reticulospinal tract
Retin-A
retinacula
  r. of extensor muscles
  r. of nail
  r. of peroneal muscles
  r. unguis
retinaculum
  antebrachial flexor r.
  r. of articular capsule of hip
  r. capsulae articularis coxae
  caudal r.
  r. caudale
  deep part of flexor r.
  flexor r.
  r. of flexor muscles
  inferior extensor r.
  lateral patellar r.
  medial patellar r.
  r. musculorum extensorum
  r. musculorum extensorum
    inferius
  r. musculorum extensorum
    superius
  r. musculorum fibularium
  r. musculorum flexorum
  r. musculorum flexorum
    membri inferioris
  r. musculorum peroneorum
  r. patellae laterale
  r. patellae mediale
  patellar r.
  peroneal r.
  r. of skin
  superior extensor r.
  r. tendinum
  wrist r.
retinoic acid

retinoid
retinol
retract
retractile
retraction stretch
retractor
retraining
  r. exercise
  gluteus maximus muscle r.
  gluteus medius muscle r.
  muscle r.
  r. position hands and knees
  r. position prone
  r. position supine
  r. in sitting position
  r. with curl-up
  r. with sit back
retreat
retroadductor space
retroauricular lymph node
retrobulbar anesthesia
retrocalcaneobursitis
retrocervical
retrograde degeneration
retrolisthesis
retroorbital area
retroperitoneal
retroperitoneum
retrospective study
retrospondylolisthesis
retrosternal
retrotarsal
retroversion
  angle of r.
retrovirus
return phase
Retzius ligament
reversal
  narcotic r.
  pressure r.
reverse
  r. pinocytosis
  r. torso curl
  r. torso curl exercise
reversible alopecia
Revici
  R. guided chemotherapy
  R. treatment
revivification
rewarming
Rexed layers of spinal cord
R-Gel

Rhamnus
 R. *cathartica*
 R. *purshiana*
rhaponticum
 Rheum r.
rhatanhia
rhatany
 Peruvian r.
 red r.
rhatany root
rhei
 r. radix
 r. rhizoma
rheostosis
Rheum
 R. *palmatum*
 R. *rhaponticum*
Rheumaid
Rheuma-Tee
rheumatic
 r. pain
 R. Pain Remedy
rheumatism
 chronic r.
 nodose r.
 r. root
 soft tissue r.
 tuberculous r.
rheumatoid
 r. arthritis (RA)
 r. disease
 r. nodule
 r. spondylitis
rheumatological
 r. condition
 r. test
Rheumex
rhinitis
 allergic r.
rhinovirus
rhizoma
 r. galangae
 rhei r.
rhizome
 ginger r.
 jessamine r.

 kava kava r.
 temu lawak r.
rhizomelia
Rhododendron
 R. *ferrugineum*
rhoeas
 Papaver r.
rhombic
rhomboatloideus
 musculus r.
rhombocele
rhomboid
 r. impression
 r. ligament
 r. major
 r. major muscle
 r. minor
 r. minor muscle
 r. muscle
 nerve to r.
rhomboidal sinus
rhomboideus major musculus
rhubarb
 Chinese r.
 Himalayan r.
 Turkish r.
Rhuli Gel
Rhus
 R. *venenata*
rhus
 R. tox
 R. *toxicodendron*
 R. *toxicodendron*
 rhythm
 biological r.
 circadian r.
 cranial rhythmic impulse r.
 CRI r.
 free-running circadian r.
 inherent body r.
 lumbar-pelvic r.
 melatonin r.
 scapulohumeral r.
 ultradian r.
rhythmic change
rib
 r. anatomy

NOTES

rib *(continued)*
    r. angle
    articular facet of head of r.
    articular facet of tubercle of r.
    r. articulation
    atypical r.
    beading of the r.'s
    bifid r.
    body of r.
    bucket-handle motion of r.
    r. cage dysfunction
    r. cage somatic dysfunction
    caliper motion of r.
    cervical r.
    r. compression
    costosternal joint of first r.
    crest of head of r.
    crest of neck of r.
    r. dysfunction
    elevator muscle of r.
    exhalation r.
    false r.
    first r.
    floating r.'s [XI–XII]
    group of r.'s
    r.'s of head of r.
    head of r.
    r. head motion
    inhalation r.
    r. [I–XII]
    key r.
    r. landmark
    lateral flexed r.
    laterally flexed superior r.
    r. lesion
    lumbar r.
    r. motion
    r. motion testing
    muscle energy technique
        for r.'s
    neck of r.
    pump-handle motion of r.
    radiate ligament of head of r.
    r. raising
    single r.
    r. tender point
    r. torsion
    r. torsional dysfunction
    true r.'s [I–VII]
    tubercle of r.
    typical r.
    vertebral r.'s

    vertebrochondral r.'s
    vertebrosternal r.'s
Ribes nigrum
riboflavin
ribonucleic acid (RNA)
rib-raising technique
ribwort
RICE
    rest, ice, compression, elevation
rice
    r. body
    r. bran
    brown r.
    R. Dream
    red yeast r.
richleaf
Richter-Monro line
rich weed
Ricinus communis
rickets
    acute r.
    adult r.
    celiac r.
    hemorrhagic r.
    nutritional r.
    vitamin D-resistant r.
rider's
    r. bone
    r. bursa
    r. leg
    r. muscles
ridge
    bicipital r.
    epidermal r.
    lateral epicondylar r.
    lateral supracondylar r.
    medial epicondylar r.
    medial supracondylar r.
    pectoral r.
    petrous r.
    pronator r.
    supraorbital r.
    trapezoid r.
RidgeCrest Herbals
Rife machine
right
    r. anterior ilium
    r. anterior innominate
    atlas rotated r.
    easy normal r. (ENR)
    extended, rotated, sidebent r.
        (ERSR)
    r. extended sacrum

flexed, rotated, sidebent r.
(FRSR)
r. inferior innominate shear
dysfunction
r. inferior pubes
injury left to r.
r. innominate inflare
r. innominate internally rotated
lower thoracic scoliosis convex
to r.
r. lumbar lymph node
r. oblique lumbar spine film
r. orthogonal coordinate system
r. posterior nutated sacrum
rotation r.
rotation vertebral motion r.
sacroiliac torsioned anteriorly
right on r.
sacroiliac torsioned posteriorly
left on r.
r. sacrum extended functional
technique
sidebending r.
sidebending vertebral motion r.
r. superior innominate shear
r. symphysis inferior
r. track
right-eye dominant
right-handed
righting reflex
right-on-left
r.-o.-l. sacral torsion
r.-o.-l. torsion
r.-o.-l. torsion functional
technique
right-on-right torsion
rigida
Phytolacca r.
rigid skull
rigidus
hallux r.
ring
crural r.
femoral r.
r. finger
intercrural fibers of
superficial r.

r. ligament
Waldeyer r.
Zinn r.
ringworm
rinse
propolis mouth r.
Riolan bouquet
Ripped Fuel
ripple grass
RISCC rating
riser
stress r.
rising
fire r.
r. heart fire
liver fire r.
r. liver fire
r. liver yang
liver yang r.
r. stomach fire
stomach fire r.
risk-benefit ' ratio
Ritter-Rollet phenomenon
ritual
hypnotic induction r.
purging r.
purification r.
symbolic healing r.
river
R. of Life
r. of qi
riyue
gb 24 r.
r. point
Rizin
Bio R.
RNA
ribonucleic acid
robbia
robe
kimono r.
Robert
herb R.
robertianum
Geranium r.
robotic
robusta coffee

NOTES

R

robustum
> *Caulophyllum* r.

rock
> R. on Tai Mountain Decoction
> r. parsley
> r. poppy

rockberry
rocket
> golden r.

rocking
> temporal r.
> to-and-fro r.

rod
> Aaron's r.

Röhrer index
rokan
Roland Disability Scale
Roland-Morris scale
role
> r. playing
> r. strain

Rolfer
Rolfing movement integration
roll
> cervical r.
> lumbar r.
> moxa r.
> neck r.
> silver mylar r.

roller bandage
rolling
> skin r.

ROM
> range of motion

romaine lettuce
Roman
> R. chamomile
> R. myrtle
> R. plant

Romberg sign
rong
> lu r.

roof
rooibos tea
root
> ague r.
> aloe r.
> althaea r.
> alum r.
> angelica r.
> arnica r.
> astragalus r.
> r. bark

bitter r.
black r.
blue cohosh r.
bowman's r.
brinton r.
bryony r.
burdock r.
butcher's broom r.
cancer r.
r. cause
celandine tops and r.
cervical r.
China r.
clove r.
colic r.
columbo r.
comfrey r.
costus r.
cough r.
Culver's r.
damiana r.
dandelion r.
devil's claw secondary r.
dorsal r.
East Indian r.
elfdock r.
eye r.
false unicorn r.
r. of foot
gentian r.
ginger r.
ginseng r.
goldenseal r.
gravel r.
r. of the Holy Ghost
horseradish r.
jaundice r.
kava r.
knob r.
knot r.
krameria r.
licorice r.
life r.
madder r.
mahuuanggen r.
mandrake r.
marshmallow r.
mortification r.
r. of nail
nerve r.
Nu Veg goldenseal r.
Oregon grape r.
papoose r.

parsley-leaved yellow r.
physic r.
pleurisy r.
poke r.
pokeweed r.
polygala r.
primrose r.
queen's r.
rat r.
rattlesnake r.
Rauwolfia r.
red r.
rhatany r.
rheumatism r.
scurvy r.
Seneca r.
senega r.
shrub yellow r.
slippery r.
soap r.
Solaray licorice r.
Solomon's seal r.
squaw r.
sweet r.
tartar r.
true unicorn r.
tuber r.
unicorn r.
wild alum r.
yellow r.
rooting
ropiness
Rosa
  R. *acicularis*
  R. *canina*
  R. *cinnamomea*
  R. *rugosa*
rosa
  r. francesa
  r. laurel
rosamonte
rosary
  r. pea
  rachitic r.
rose
  r. bay
  Christmas r.

corn r.
Easter r.
r. geranium
r. hips
laurier r.
r. oil
ram-goat r.
rosin r.
stinking r.
rosea
  Althaea r.
  Vinca r.
rosemary
  marsh r.
  r. oil
  oil of r.
  wild r.
Rosenbach law
Rosenberg Self-Esteem Scale (RSES)
Rosen method
Rosenmüller node
rose-noble
Roser-Nélaton line
roseus
  Catharanthus r.
rosin
  r. rose
  r. weed
Rosmarinus officinalis
rostrate pelvis
rotary
  r. instability testing of knee
  r. joint
  r. torque trauma
rotated
  r. dysfunction of sacrum
  r. innominate
  left innominate externally r.
  navicular bone internally r.
  right innominate internally r.
  tibia externally r.
  tibia internally r.
rotation
  active trunk r.
  anterior iliac r.
  anterior innominate iliac r.
  r. around axis

NOTES

rotation (*continued*)
   axial r.
   center of r.
   cervical r.
   r. diet
   r. dysfunction of sacrum
   external r.
   Fayette principles of r.
   horizontal external r.
   horizontal internal r.
   instantaneous axis of r.
   r. left
   medial and lateral r.
   neutral external r.
   neutral internal r.
   neutral internal r. stage 1
   neutral internal r. stage 2
   r. on a point
   pelvic r.
   posterior innominate iliac r.
   restricted external r.
   restricted internal r.
   r. restriction
   restriction of internal-
     external r.
   r. right
   r. of sacrum
   trunk r.
   r. of vertebra
   r. vertebral motion
   r. vertebral motion left
   r. vertebral motion right
rotational
   r. restriction
   r. technique
   r. thrust
rotator
   r. cuff of shoulder
   medial r.
   r. muscle
   r. muscle of hip
rotatores
   r. breves musculi
   r. cervicis muscles
   r. longi musculi
   r. lumborum muscles
   r. muscle
   musculi r.
   r. thoracis muscles
   r. thoracis musculi
rotoscoliosis
   lumbar r.
   r. testing

rototome
rotundus
   Cyperus r.
rou
   r. cong ren
   r. gui wan
   r. gui yin
rough
   r. line
   r. voice
rough-smooth
round
   r. cell idiopathic syndrome
   r. ligament of elbow joint
   r. ligament of femur
   r. pronator muscle
round-leaved sundew
roxo
   ipe r.
royal jelly
Rs
   four Rs
     remove, replace, reinoculate,
     repair
RSD
   reflex sympathetic dystrophy
RSD
   reflex sympathetic dystrophy
RSES
   Rosenberg Self-Esteem Scale
RSI
   repetitive strain injury
   repetitive stress injury
RTM
   reciprocal tension membrane
rua
   hsiang r.
rub
   Act-On R.
   raw lemon r.
rubarbo
rubbed thyme
rubber
   r. pelvis
   r. spa bowl
Rubenfield Synergy Method
ruber
   Centranthus r.
Rubia
   R. Teep
   R. tinctorum
Rubicin
rubifacient

rubra
>Actaea r.
>Ulmus r.

rubric
rubriflora
>Schisandra r.

rubrospinal tract
Rubus
>R. frondosus
>R. fruticosus
>R. idaeus
>R. occidentalis

Rudolf Weiss Formula
rue
>common r.
>garden r.
>German r.
>goat's r.
>oil of r.
>r. oil
>r. point
>r. tea

Ruffini corpuscle
rugen
>st 18 r.

rugger jersey vertebra
rugosa
>Agastache r.
>Rosa r.

rugosum
>Eupatorium r.

ruibarbo caribe
ruin
>maiden's r.

rule
>r. of the artery
>Mennell r.'s
>r. of the nerve

Rumalaya
Rumanian ginseng
rum cherry
Rumex
>R. acetosella

>R. crispus
>R. hymenosepalus

rumex
rumination
runner's knee
running
>r. box Ruscus
>r. start

ruo gui yin
rupestris
>Umbilicus r.

rupture
ruptured disk
Ruscorectal
Ruscus
>R. aculeatus
>running box R.

rush
>Dutch r.
>guarana r.
>scouring r.

Russian licorice
rusticana
>Armoracia r.

rustic treacle
rutaecarpa
>Evodia r.

Ruta graveolens
rutamarin
rutin
ru xiang
ruzhong
>st 17 r.

RV process down thrust technique
RX, Rx
>prescription
>>Diabetic Nutrition RX

rye
>wild r.

Ryodoraku method

NOTES

S-2000
    BTA S.
3s
    thoracic rule of 3s
sabal
Sabbatia, Sabatia
    S. angularis
sabdariffa
    Hibiscus s.
saber
    s. shin
    s. tibia
sac
    endolymphatic s.
saccharin
sacciform recess of distal
    radioulnar joint
saccular aneurysm
sachet
    woodruff s.
sacrad
sacral
    s. anesthesia
    s. base
    s. base declination
    s. base dysfunction
    s. base unleveling
    s. canal
    s. cornu
    s. counternutation
    s. crest
    s. extension
    s. flexion
    s. foramina
    s. ganglion
    s. hiatus
    s. horn
    s. involuntary mobility
    s. motion testing
    s. muscle energy technique
    s. nerves [S1–S5]
    s. part of spinal cord
    s. plexus
    s. postural motion
    s. pounding
    s. promontory
    s. region
    s. shear
    s. somatic dysfunction
    s. sulcus

    s. torsion
    s. triangle
    s. tuberosity
    s. urinary bladder point
    s. vertebrae [S1–S5]
sacrale
    cornu s.
    foramen s.
sacrales
    vertebrae s. [S1–S5]
sacralgia
sacralia
    ganglion s.
sacralis
    ala s.
    ansa s.
    canalis s.
    crista s.
    hiatus s.
    hiatus totalis s.
    regio s.
    tuberositas s.
sacralization
sacred
    s. bark
    s. bone
    s. hoop
    s. source
sacree
    herbe s.
sacri
    apex ossis s.
    basis ossis s.
    lineae transversae ossis s.
    pars lateralis ossis s.
    promontorium ossis s.
sacrococcygea
    articulatio s.
    junctura s.
sacrococcygeal
    s. disk
    s. joint
    s. joint mobilization
    s. junction
sacrococcygeus
sacrodural ligament
sacrodynia
sacroiliac
    s. articulation
    s. articulation dysfunction

S

sacroiliac *(continued)*
　　bilaterally nutated s.
　　s. bilaterally nutated anteriorly
　　s. bilaterally nutated posteriorly
　　s. cinch belt
　　s. dysfunction
　　s. functional technique
　　s. injection
　　s. joint
　　s. joint block
　　s. joint dysfunction
　　s. joint dysfunction muscle
　　　energy technique
　　s. joint four-point motion
　　s. joint injury
　　s. joint left-on-left torsion
　　s. joint ligamentous structure
　　s. joint motion
　　s. joint pain
　　s. joint right-on-left torsion
　　s. joint syndrome
　　s. ligament
　　s. motion by gapping test
　　s. motion spring test
　　s. rocking test
　　s. somatic dysfunction
　　s. syndrome
　　s. torsioned anteriorly left on
　　　left
　　s. torsioned anteriorly right on
　　　right
　　s. torsioned posteriorly left on
　　　right
　　s. torsioned posteriorly right
　　　on left
　　unilaterally nutated s.
sacroiliaca
　　articulatio s.
sacroiliitis
sacrolumbalis
　　musculus s.
sacrolumbar
sacrooccipital technique
sacropelvic surface of ilium
sacrosciatic notch
sacrospinal
sacrospinalis
　　musculus s.
　　s. musculus
sacrospinous ligament
sacrotuberous
　　s. ligament
　　s. ligament tension test

sacrovertebral
sacrum
　　anterior s.
　　anterior translated s.
　　apex of s.
　　assimilation s.
　　base of s.
　　dorsal surface of s.
　　s. extended
　　extension dysfunction of s.
　　extension lesion of the s.
　　s. flexed
　　flexion dysfunction of s.
　　flexion somatic dysfunction of
　　　the s.
　　inferior lateral angle of s.
　　lateral part of s.
　　left unilateral anterior
　　　nutated s.
　　oblique axis of the s.
　　os s.
　　pelvic surface of s.
　　posterior s.
　　posterior translated s.
　　promontory of the s.
　　respiratory axis of s.
　　s. restriction dysfunction
　　right extended s.
　　right posterior nutated s.
　　rotated dysfunction of s.
　　rotation of s.
　　rotation dysfunction of s.
　　somatic dysfunction of s.
　　superior articular process of s.
　　translated s.
　　transverse axis of s.
　　transverse ridges of s.
　　unleveling of s.
　　wing of s.
SAD
　　seasonal affective disorder
　　serial-agitated dilution
saddle
　　s. back
　　s. block anesthesia
　　s. joint
safe
　　generally recognized as s.
　　　(GRAS)
safety
　　margin of s.
　　triangle of s.

safflower
  s. oil
  s. tea
saffron
  American s.
  bastard s.
  dyer's s.
  false s.
  Indian s.
  meadow s.
  s. stigma
  true s.
safira
safrole
sage
  clary s.
  garden s.
  garlic s.
  Indian s.
  Jerusalem s.
  s. leaf
  meadow s.
  muscatel s.
  s. poultice
  scarlet s.
  s. tea
  tree s.
  true s.
sagitta
sagittal
  s. curve
  s. line
  s. plane
  s. plane extension
  s. plane flexion
  s. plane postural
    decompensation
  s. plane posture
  s. plane restriction
  s. plate
  s. section
  s. suture
  s. territory
sagittalis
sagittata
  Lactuca s.

sagrada
  cascara s.
Sahaja yoga
Sahasrara
SAHEM
  self-applied health enhancement
    method
Saigon
  S. cassia
  S. cinnamon
sailor
  blue s.'s
Sakau
salad
  s. burnet
  s. chervil
  poke s.
salakya
salet
  poke s.
salicylate
  methyl s.
salicylism
saline
  s. cathartic
  physiologic s.
  s. solution
  s. treatment
Salix alba
S-allyl cystein
Salmonella
  S. enterica
  S. typhimurium
salmon oil
saloop
salpingooophoritis
salpingopharyngeal muscle
salpingopharyngeus
  s. muscle
  musculus s.
salsalate
salsaparilha (*var. of* sarsaparilla)
salsepareille (*var. of* sarsaparilla)
salt
  berberine s.
  earth s.'s
  Epsom s.'s

NOTES

367

salt *(continued)*
    sea s.
    s. sensitive
    s. solution
saltwater fish
Salus Haus
Salve
    Golden S.
Salvia
    S. lavandulaefolia
    S. miltiorrhiza
    S. officinalis
Samadhi cushion
Sambaar Podi
sambac
    Jasminum s.
Sambucus
    S. canadensis
    S. cerulea
    S. ebulus
    S. niger
    S. pubens
    S. racemosa
samento
samhita
    susruta s.
sampling
    biological s.
    chemical s.
sampson
    black s.
san
    bai zhen s.
    ba zhen s.
    ba zheng s.
    chong xian s.
    da chi s.
    s. jiao
    ji ming s.
    s. lin
    ping wei s.
    sang piao xie s.
    san miao s.
    shen ling bai zhu s.
    shi xiao s.
    xiang su s.
    xiao yao s.
    yin qiao s.
    zhong s.
sanctum
    semen s.
sandalwood
sand painting

Sandström bodies
sang
    s. pian xiao
    s. piao xie san
    seng and s.
    s. shen
    s. zhi
sangrel
sanguinaria
Sanguinaria canadensis
sanguinary
sanguinea
    Datura s.
Sanguisorba
    S. minor
    S. officinalis
sanguisorba
    pimpinella s.
Sanhelio's Circu Caps
sanicle
sanjiao
    s. channel (sj)
    s. meridian
    s. meridian of hand
sanjiao-gallbladder axis
sanjiaoshu
    ub 22 s.
santa
    S. Maria
    yerba s.
santal oil
Santalum
    S. album
    S. album wood
Santane
santo
    cardo s.
santonica
Santorini muscle
Santos coffee
Sanvita Maen
sanyangluo
    sj 8 s.
sanyinjiao
    sp 6 s.
sap
Sapec
sapheni
    margo falciformis hiatus s.
saphenus
    hiatus s.
sapida
    Blighia s.

saponaria
>Quillaja s.

Saponaria officinalis

saponin

sarcodes

sarcoidosis
>pulmonary s.

sarcoma
>Ewing s.
>juxtacortical osteogenic s.
>Kaposi s.
>osteogenic s.
>periosteal s.
>synovial s.
>telangiectatic osteogenic s.

sardine

sargassam seaweed

Sargassum pallidum

sarothamni herb

Sarothamnus scoparius

sarsa

sarsaparilla, salsaparilha, salsepareille
>Ecuadorian s.
>English s.
>German s.
>Honduran s.
>Jamaican s.
>Mexican s.
>s. root extract

sartorius
>s. muscle
>musculus s.

saso
>wild s.

Sassafras
>S. albidum
>S. officinalis
>S. varifolium

sassafras
>bois de s.
>lignum s.
>s. tea
>s. wood

sassafrasholz

SAT
>spinal attunement technique

sat
>ad s.

satellite
>s. abscess
>s. cell of skeletal muscle

satinflower

sativa
>Allium s.
>Avena s.
>Cannabis s.
>Lactuca s.
>Medicago s.
>Oryza s.

sativum
>Allium s.
>Coriander s.
>Petroselinum s.

sativus
>Crocus s.
>Raphanus s.

sattva

sattvic

saturated fat

Satureja
>S. hortensis
>S. montana

saturnina
>arthralgia s.

sauce
>sour s.

saucerization

sauerkraut

sauna
>Aromist Personal Steam S.
>facial s.

Sauropus androgynus

savin
>horse s.

savory
>summer s.
>s. tea
>winter s.

saw
>s. palmetto
>s. palmetto berry
>s. palmetto formula
>s. palmetto fruit

S

NOTES

saw *(continued)*
    s. palmetto liposterolic extract
    S. Palmetto Pygeum Plus
sawi
saxifrage
saxifras
scabies
scabra
    Gentiana s.
scabwort
scale
    ASQ Internal S.
    ASQ Stability S.
    Attributional Style
      Questionnaire Global S.
    Brief Social Phobia S. (BSPS)
    Carleton University
      Responsiveness to
      Suggestion S.
    CGI s.
    Clinical Global Improvement s.
    Daily Hassles S.
    Harvard Group S. of Hypnotic
      Susceptibility, Form A
      (HGSHS:A)
    Impact of Events S.
    Marlow-Crown Social
      Desirability s.
    McGill s.
    nine-point s.
    Oswestry s.
    pentatonic s.
    Physical Activity Recall S.
    Roland Disability S.
    Roland-Morris s.
    Rosenberg Self-Esteem S.
      (RSES)
    Self-Rating Depression S.
    Social Readjustment Rating S.
    Stanford Hypnotic
      Susceptibility S., Form C
    Stanford Sleepiness S.
    State-Trait Anxiety S.
    Taylor Manifest Anxiety s.
    visual analog s. (VAS)
scalene
    s. hiatus
    s. muscle
    s. tubercle
  · s. tubercle of Lisfranc
scalenus
    s. anterior muscle
    s. anticus muscle

    s. medius muscle
    s. minimus muscle
    s. posterior muscle
scalloping of the tongue
scalp
    s. acupuncture
    s. muscle
scalprum
scammonia
    Convolvulus s.
scammony
    Mexican s.
scan
    bone s.
    three-phase bone s.
scanning
    s. examination
    functional brain s.
scanty and watery stool
scapha
    eminence of s.
scaphae
    eminentia s.
scaphohydrocephalus
scaphoid
    s. bone
    s. tuberosity
scaphoidei
    tuberculum ossis s.
scaphoideum
    os s.
scapula
    s. alata
    costal surface of s.
    dorsal surface of s.
    s. elevata
    elevator muscle of s.
    glenoid labrum of s.
    infraglenoid tubercle of s.
    lateral angle of s.
    lateral border of s.
    medial border of s.
    neck of s.
    spine of s.
    superior angle of s.
    superior border of s.
    vertebral border of s.
    winged s.
scapulae
    angulus inferior s.
    angulus lateralis s.
    angulus superior s.
    collum s.

dorsum s.
incisura s.
labrum glenoidale s.
levator s.
margo lateralis s.
margo medialis s.
margo superior s.
musculus levator s.
musculus levator anguli s.
spina s.
scapulalgia
scapular
s. line
s. notch
s. region
s. spine
s. stabilization
s. winging
scapularis
linea s.
regio s.
scapulary
scapuloclavicular
scapulocostal
s. junction
s. syndrome
scapulodynia
scapulohumeral
s. atrophy
s. joint motion
s. muscle
s. rhythm
scapulothoracic
s. joint
s. muscle
scar
scarf bandage
scarlet
s. berry
s. sage
Scarpa triangle
scarring
scattered energy
SCD
sudden cardiac death

scented
s. fern
s. geranium
sceptic (*var. of* skeptic)
Schatz-style yoga
schedule I drug
schema
schematic
schematograph
schidigera
Yucca s.
schindylesis
schindyletic joint
schinsent
schisandra
S. chinensis
s. extract
S. rubriflora
schistomelia
schistorrhachis
schizandra
schizoaffective disorder
schizophrenia
sciadopitysin
sciage
sciatic
s. foramen
s. nerve
s. nerve irritation
s. scoliosis
s. spine
sciatica
science
Christian S.
Heart S.
s. of life
Master of Ayurvedic S.
(MASc)
noetic s.
scientific-clinical theory of Janda
scilla
Scilla sibirica
scilliroside
scimitar sign
scintillation camera
scissor gait
scleroblastema

S

NOTES

scleroderma
scleromere
sclerosant injection
sclerose
sclerosing osteitis
sclerosis
    amyotrophic lateral s. (ALS)
    bone s.
    combined s.
    multiple s. (MS)
    posterior s.
    posterior spinal s.
sclerotherapy
Sclerotium Poriae cocos
sclerotomal
    s. pain
    s. pattern
scoke
scoliokyphosis
scoliometer
scoliosis
    cervical s.
    Cobb measurements in s.
    coxitic s.
    C-type compensated
      structural s.
    empyemic s.
    habit s.
    infantile idiopathic s.
    juvenile s.
    left cervical s.
    left lumbar s.
    lumbar s.
    myopathic s.
    ocular s.
    osteopathic s.
    paralytic s.
    rachitic s.
    sciatic s.
    static s.
    structural s.
    S-type compensated
      structural s.
scoliotic pelvis
scoparius
    Cytisus s.
    Sarothamnus s.
scopolamine
scordiifolia
    Scutellaria s.
score
    International Prostate
      Symptom S. (IPSS)

Lequesne index s.
Marlow-Crowne s.
pain s.
scorodonia
    Teucrium s.
Scotch
    S. broom
    S. broom top
    S. fir
    S. pine
Scot's pine
Scotty
    S. dog appearance
    S. dog's eye
scourge
    devil's s.
scouring rush
scout film
screen
    lower extremity s.
    total body lymphatic s.
    upper extremity s.
screening
    s. examination
    hypertrophy dysfunction s.
scrofula plant
scullcap, skullcap
    s. herb
sculpting
    deep tissue s.
scurvy
    s. grass
    rebound s.
    s. root
Scutellaria
    S. baicalensis
    S. galericulata
    S. laterifolia
    S. scordiifolia
scutellariae radix
scyphiform
scyphoid
sea
    s. cucumber
    s. girdle
    s. grape
    s. holly
    s. holme
    s. hulver
    s. mussel
    s. of qi
    s. onion
    s. parsley

s. salt
s. squill
s. of vital energy
s. wormwood
s. wrack
Seabands
sea-oak
Season
One-A-Day Cold S.
seasonal
s. affective disorder (SAD)
s. purification
seated
s. bending test
s. flexion test
s. thrust technique
s. trunk bending test
Seatone
seaweed
s. bath
sargassam s.
seawrack
sebaceous gland
Sebileau muscle
seborrhea
seborrheic dermatitis
sebum secretion
second
s. chakra
s. cuneiform bone
s. finger
s. tibial muscle
s. toe
secondary
s. amputation
s. anesthetic
s. center of ossification
s. deficiency
s. failure
s. hypermobility
s. inflammatory disease
s. joint motion
s. point of ossification
s. posttraumatic stress
s. somatic dysfunction
Secret
Nature's S.

secretion
acetylcholine s.
cortisol s.
gastric acid s.
growth hormone s.
prostate s.
sebum s.
secretolytic
secretomotor activity
secretory
s. diarrhea
s. IgA
sectio
section
axial s.
diagonal s.
frontal s.
longitudinal s.
median s.
midsagittal s.
oblique s.
parasagittal s.
sagittal s.
transverse s.
sectorial
secundarium
punctum ossificationis s.
secundus
digitus manus s. [II]
musculus tibialis s.
sedate
sedating method
sedation
sedative
s. effect
s. method
s. point
s. stimulation
sedge
sweet s.
sedimentation rate
see bright
seed
anise s.
blond plantago s.
borage s.
boxthorn s.

S

NOTES

seed *(continued)*
celery s.
cola s.
dill s.
ear s.
fenugreek s.
guarana s.
horse chestnut s.
Indian plantago s.
ispaghula s.
jequirity s.
s. of life
loco s.
nutmeg s.
Nux vomica s.
oil from s.
plantago s.
poppy s.
s. powder
psyllium s.
sunflower s.
tonka s.
tung s.
wild carrot s.
seed-shell
ispaghula s.-s.
Seem
Mark S. needling
seesaw
pelvic s.
seetang
segment
anterior s.
atypical s.
cervical s.'s of spinal cord
[C1–C8]
coccygeal s. of spinal cord
[Co]
dysfunctional s.
facilitated s.
hypermobility of s.
lateral s.
medial s.
posterior s.
spinal motion s.
transitional s.
transitional vertebral s.
vertebral motion s.
segmenta
s. cervicalia medullae spinalis
s. coccygea medullae spinalis
s. sacralia medullae spinalis
s. thoracica medullae spinalis

segmental
s. anesthesia
s. definition
s. diagnosis
s. distribution
s. dysfunction
s. effect
s. fracture
s. innervation
s. mechanism
s. motion
s. muscle function
s. pain radiation
segmentalization
nervous system s.
segmentum
s. anterius
s. mediale
s. posterius
s. renale anterius inferius
s. renale anterius superius
Seirin acupuncture needle
seismotherapy
seizure
s. reduction
s. state
vitamin B_6-dependent s.
selection
point s.
selective
s. amnesia
s. fatty replacement
s. nerve block
Selenicereus
S. grandiflorus
selenium toxicity
self-actualization
**self-applied health enhancement
method (SAHEM)**
self-attention
self-correction
s.-c. position
s.-c. position for extension
restriction
s.-c. position prone
s.-c. position standing
s.-c. position supine
self-defense
self-efficacy
self-heal
self-healing
self-massage acupressure for s.-
h. (SMASH)

s.-h. style of qigong (SHQ)
s.-h. technique
self-hypnosis
self-massage acupressure for self-healing (SMASH)
self-mobilizing
  s.-m. exercise
  s.-m. technique
Self-Rating
  S.-R. Depression Scale
  S.-R. of Insomnia
self-recovery
self-regulation
  s.-r. of blood flow
  parasympathetic s.-r.
  psychosomatic s.-r.
self-regulatory mechanism
self-statement
  adaptive s.-s.
self-stretch
  s.-s. position kneeling
  s.-s. position lateral recumbent
  s.-s. position prone
  s.-s. position supine
  s.-s. sitting
  s.-s. standing
  s.-s. thoracic spine elongation position
self-stretching
self-talk
self-touching
self-treatment
sellae
  diaphragm s.
  diaphragma s.
  dorsum s.
sellaris
  articulatio s.
semen
  s. cinae
  s. sanctum
semicanalis
semicartilaginous
semiconduction
  fascial s.
  perineural s.
semiflexion

semilunar
  s. bone
  s. cartilage
  s. fascia
  s. fasciculus
  s. fibrocartilage
semiluxation
semimembranosus
  s. muscle
  musculus s.
semimembranous muscle
seminal hillock
semispinal
  s. muscle
  s. muscle of head
  s. muscle of neck
  s. muscle of thorax
semispinalis
  s. cervicis muscle
  s. muscle
  musculus s.
semisulcus
semitendinosus
  s. muscle
  musculus s.
semitendinous muscle
sempervirens
  Gelsemium s.
Seneca
  S. root
  S. snakeroot
Senecio
  S. aureus
  S. cineraria
senecio
  golden s.
senega
  northern s.
  Polygala s.
  s. root
  s. snakeroot
senegal
  Acacia s.
Senexon
seng and sang
senile
  s. hip disease

NOTES

senile *(continued)*
   malum coxae s.
   s. osteomalacia
senna
   Aden s.
   Cassia s.
   s. concentrate
   s. leaf
   Mecca s.
   Nubian s.
   s. tea
   Tinnevelly s.
   wild s.
sennoside
Senokot Granules
Senokot-S
Senolax
sensation
   boggy s.
   cutaneous s.
   deep nerve s.
   de qi s.
   de qi needling s.
   end feel s.
   palpatory s.
   pinprick s.
   pressure s.
   s. testing
   unyielding s.
   vagrant pain s.
sense
   kinesthetic s.
   motion s.
   muscular s.
sensitive
   salt s.
sensitivity
   clinical s.
   diagnostic s.
   insulin s.
   relative s.
sensitization
sensory
   s. conduction time
   s. event
   s. loss
   s. motor balance
   s. motor balance training
   s. nerve
   s. neuropathy
   s. organ
   s. polyneuropathy

   s. restriction
   s. therapy
sensory-motor-rhythm feedback
SensualiTea
senticosa
   Hedera s.
senticosus
   Acanthopanax s.
   Eleutherococcus s.
separation
   acromioclavicular joint s.
   s. of muscle origin and
      insertion
   s. phase
   suture s.
separation-type movement
sepia
sepium
   Periploca s.
sepsis
septa *(pl. of* septum)
septal defect
septfoil
septi
   nucleus accumbens s.
septicemia
   Staphylococcus s.
septic phlebitis
Septilin
septum, pl. septa
   Bigelow s.
   s. canalis musculotubarii
   cartilaginous s.
   intermuscular s.
   s. intermusculare
   septa interradicularia
      mandibulae et maxillae
   s. transversum
sequela, pl. sequelae
sequence
   altered muscle firing pattern s.
   circadian s.
   Feldenkrais s.
   lift therapy s.
   muscle patterning s.
   stacking s.
   treatment s.
sequestra
sequestral
sequestration
   disk s.
sequestrum
   primary s.

Serene
  HR 129 S.
  PMS S.
Serenoa
  S. repens
  S. serrulata
serial-agitated dilution (SAD)
serofibrinous inflammation
serofibrous
serology
seromembranous
serosa
  peritendinitis s.
serosanguinous exudate
serotina
  Prunus s.
serotinum
  Phoradendron s.
serotonin
  s. reuptake inhibition
  s. uptake
serotype
serous
  s. inflammation
  s. ligament
  s. synovitis
serovar
Serpasil
serpentaria
  Aristolochia s.
serpentina
  Rauwolfia s.
serpentine aneurysm
serrated sutural contour
serratus
  s. anterior muscle
  s. anterior treatment
  Fucus s.
  s. muscle
  s. posterior inferior muscle
  s. posterior superior muscle
serriola
  Lactuca s.
serrulata
  Serenoa s.
serum
  s. accelerator globulin

  Born Again's DHEA
  Eyelift S.
  s. cholesterol
  s. cholesterol level
  s. fatty acid level
  s. globulin
  s. glutamic-pyruvic
    transaminase (SGPT)
  s. lipid
  s. magnesium level
  s. melatonin level
  s. potassium
  s. sickness
  s. triglycerides
sesame oil
sesamoid bone
sesamoideum
  os s.
sesquiterpene lactone
session
  acupuncture s.
  acupuncture treatment s.
  treatment s.
set
setewale capon's tail
S-ethyl cystein
setwell
seven
  s. barks
  s. emotions
  s. leaf
  s. star needle
seven-step Spencer technique
seventh chakra
sexdigitate
sexuality
  harmonious s.
sexually transmitted disease (STD)
SFE
  supercritical fluid extraction
SGPT
  serum glutamic-pyruvic
    transaminase
shabda
shadow work
shaft
  s. of femur

S

NOTES

shaft *(continued)*
  s. of fibula
  s. of humerus
  s. of radius
  s. of tibia
  s. of ulna
shagal el ketira
shallow breathing
sham
  s. acupuncture
  s. needle
shaman
shamanic
  s. healing
  s. therapy
shamanism
  Pima Indian s.
shameface
sham-point
  s.-p. needling
  s.-p. stimulation
shamrock
  Indian s.
  water s.
shan
  s. chi
  s. dzao
  s. sheng jiang
shank
Shankhapushpi herbal preparation
Shanti Bori
shanzhong
  ren 17 s.
shao
  bai s.
  s. shen mail men dong tang
  s. yang disease
  s. yang lateral cervical
    spondylitis
  s. yang type
  s. yin
  s. yin channel
  s. yin-tai yang principal
    meridian subcircuit
shaochong
  he 9 s.
shaofu
  he 8 s.
shaohai
  he 3 s.
shaolin
shaoshang
  lu 11 s.

shao-yang, shaoyang
  s.-y. axis
  s.-y. channel axis
  s.-y. type headache
shao-yin, shaoyin
  s.-y. axis
  s.-y. channel axis
shaoze
  si 1 s.
shark
  s. cartilage
  s. cartilage-induced hepatitis
  s. derivative
  hammerhead s.
  s. liver oil
  reef s.
  spiny dogfish s.
Sharpey fiber
shatavari
shavegrass, shave grass
shawl
  s. area
  s. muscle
shear
  s. force
  iliosacral caudad s.
  iliosacral cephalic s.
  iliosacral inferior s.
  iliosacral superior s.
  s. of innominate
  innominate s.
  pubic s.
  right superior innominate s.
  sacral s.
  superior innominate iliac s.
  symphysial s.
sheath
  anulus of fibrous s.
  axillary s.
  common peroneal tendon s.
  fibrous s.'s
  fibrous tendon s.
  intertubercular tendon s.
  s. ligament
  muscle s.
  s. of styloid process
  synovial s.
  synovial tendon s.
  s. of thyroid gland
she chuang zi
sheepberry
sheep sorrel

sheet
> wet s.

shelf
> s. fungi
> s. procedure

shell
> abalone s.

shellac

shen
> dan s.
> dang s.
> s. fu tang
> s. jing xu
> s. ling bai zhu san
> s. physioemotional release
>   therapy
> s. qi xu
> ren s.
> sang s.
> s. therapy
> s. yang xu
> s. yin xu

shendao
> du 11 s.

sheng
> s. di huang
> wei huo shang s.
> s. ye cheng qi tang

Sheng-mai-san

shenmai
> ub 62 s.

shenmen
> he 7 s.

shenque
> ren 8 s.

shenshu
> ub 23 s.

shensu point

shenting
> du 24 s.

shepherd's
> s. knapperty
> s. knot
> s. needle
> s. purse

Sheridan's Formula

Sherrington law

shesha

shi
> s. bai di huang wan
> s. chang pu
> s. condition
> s. disturbance
> s. excess
> qian s.
> s. symptom
> s. xiao san
> s. zi bai bu

shiatsu
> macrobiotic s.
> water s.

shield
> s. fern
> Pumpkin Seed S.
> qi s.

shielding
> stress s.

shift
> circadian s.
> hip s.

Shigella sonnei

shigoka

shiitake mushroom

shilajit

shim
> 1/2-inch s.
> 1/4-inch s.
> 1/8-inch s.
> 3/8-inch s.

shimen
> ren 5 s.

shin
> s. bone
> saber s.
> s. splint

shingles

shirsh zallouh

shi-type condition

shivering

shock
> anaphylactic s.
> anesthetic s.
> insulin s.
> surge s.

S

NOTES

shoe
>whippoorwill's s.
>yellow Indian s.

shonny

shoot
>bamboo s.

short
>s. abductor muscle of thumb
>s. adductor muscle
>s. bone
>s. extensor muscle of great
>toe
>s. extensor muscle of thumb
>s. extensor muscle of toe
>s. fibular muscle
>s. flexor muscle of great toe
>s. flexor muscle of little
>finger
>s. flexor muscle of little toe
>s. flexor muscle of thumb
>s. flexor muscle of toe
>s. foot
>s. head
>s. head of biceps brachii
>s. head of biceps femoris
>s. leg/pelvic tilt
>s. leg/pelvic tilt syndrome
>s. leg syndrome
>s. levatores costarum muscle
>s. lever
>s. lower extremity
>s. muscle barrier
>s. palmar muscle
>s. peroneal muscle
>s. radial extensor muscle of
>wrist
>s. relaxation technique
>s. restrictive barrier
>s. restrictor

shortened psoas muscle

shortening
>myofascial s.

short-lever manipulation

short-term memory

sho-saiko-to

shotgun
>s. prescription
>s. technique

shoulder
>s. apprehension sign
>s. blade
>bursitis of s.
>capsulitis of s.

>critical zone of s.
>s. dislocation
>frozen s.
>s. girdle
>s. girdle dysfunction
>s. girdle functional technique
>s. joint
>s. level
>s. region
>rotator cuff of s.
>s. somatic dysfunction
>s. tender point

shoulder-girdle syndrome

shoulder-hand syndrome

shou-wu-pian

shovelweed

shower
>Hydrokinetic Vichy s.
>Vichy s.

SHQ
>self-healing style of qigong
>SHQ breathing exercise

shrub
>devil's s.
>tallow s.
>s. yellow root

shrug
>thoracic spine s.

shu
>s. II
>s. III
>s. IV
>s. V
>s. I
>s. point
>s. points: jing, ying,
>shu/yuan, jing, and he

shuaigu
>gb 8 s.

shuffling gait

shui
>feng s.
>s. niu jiao

shuiquan
>ki 5 s.

shunt muscle

shu-stream point

si
>small intestine channel
>si 3 houxi
>si 9 jianzhen
>si jun zi tang
>si 10 naoshu

si 18 quanliao
si 1 shaoze
si 17 tianrong
si 11 tianzong
si 19 tinggong
si wu tang
si 8 xiaohai
si 6 yanglao
sialidase
Siam benzoin
sibai
st 2 s.
Siberian
S. ginseng
S. motherwort
sibirica
Scilla s.
Sibson
S. fascia
S. groove
S. muscle
sicca
s. syndrome
synovitis s.
sick
s. chi
s. energy
sickle cell disease
sicklewort
sickness
S. Impact Profile (SIP)
morning s.
motion s.
serum s.
staying s.
wandering s.
Siddha
side
s. bending
contralateral s.
s. effect
ulnar s.
yang s.
yin s.
sidebending
coupled s.
s. dynamic film

s. left
s. right
s. rotational curve
s. rotation test
s. vertebral motion
s. vertebral motion left
s. vertebral motion right
sidebent
extended, rotated, s. (ERS)
flexed, rotated, s. (FRS)
flexed, rotated, s. (FRS)
sideroblastic anemia
sideshift
pelvic s.
sign
blush s.
drawer s.
drop-off s.
eye roll s.
impingement s.
Lasègue s.
Lhermitte s.
Ludloff s.
Naffziger s.
painful arc s.
patellar apprehension s.
Phalen s.
Romberg s.
scimitar s.
shoulder apprehension s.
stress s.
Tinel s.
tootsie roll s.
trough s.
signal
electromagnetic s.
frontal EMG s.
signature
Silent Night
silica
silicea
silicon
silk
corn s.
Silvapin
silver
colloidal s.

S

NOTES

silver *(continued)*
    s. fir
    s. mylar roll
    s. needle
    s. pine
silver-fork
    s.-f. deformity
    s.-f. fracture
silverleaf
silverweed
silybin
Silybum marianum
silymarin
simethicone
similar
    doctrine of s.
    Law of S.'s
similia principle
Simmondsia chinensis
Simonton method
Simon and Travell spray and stretch
simple
    s. bone cyst
    s. dislocation
    s. disorder
    s. fracture
    Hemodren S.
    s. joint
simpler's joy
simples
simplex
    articulatio s.
    herpes s.
simplicissima
    Xanthorhiza s.
Simply Wet table
Sims position
sinapic acid
sinapine
sindbis virus
sinensis
    Angelica s.
    Camellia s.
    Cordyceps s.
sinew
sing
single
    s. finger grip
    s. rib
    s. vertebral motion segment dysfunction
single-blind study

single-plane thrust technique
sinica
    Ephedra s.
sinister
sinistrad
sinistral
sinistrous
sink
    diagonal hip s.
sinking
    s. qi
    qi s.
    spleen qi s.
    s. spleen qi
Sinomenium acutum
sinovertebral nerve
sinus
    basilar s.
    s. bradycardia
    S. and Catarrh Complex
    S. Check
    circular s.
    s. congestion
    dermal s.
    dural venous s.
    ethmoid s.
    inferior petrosal s.
    inferior sagittal s.
    maxillary s.
    milking of maxillary s.
    paranasal s.
    petrosal s.
    pilonidal s.
    rhomboidal s.
    straight s.
    superior petrosal s.
    superior sagittal s.
    tarsal s.
    s. tarsi
    transverse s.
    venous s.
    s. vertebrales longitudinales
sinusitis
    frontal s.
    s. headache
    maxillary s.
Sinustop Pro
SIP
    Sickness Impact Profile
sireniform
sirenomelia
sishencong
    Ex-HN 6 s.

sismotherapy
sit back
sitosterol
    beta s.
sitting
    s. flexion test
    isometric strengthening
      position s.
    s. to kneeling exercise
    s. lumbar spine functional
      technique
    s. position
    self-stretch s.
    s. sternoclavicular joint
      dysfunction muscle energy
      technique
    s. up
situational depression
sitz bath
Six Flavor Tea
sixth chakra
six-word method
size
    aerodynamic s.
    luminal s.
sj
    sanjiao channel (sj)
    s. 21 ermen
    s. 14 jianliao
    s. 8 sanyangluo
    s. 5 waiguan
    s. 17 yifeng
    s. 3 zhongzhu
    s. 6 zigou
Skeffington method
skeletal
    s. dysfunction
    s. dysplasia
    s. extension
    s. muscle
    s. muscle fibers
    s. structure
    s. survey
    s. system
    s. traction
skeletale
    systema s.

skeletalis
    pars cartilaginea systematis s.
    pars ossea systematis s.
skeletology
skeleton
    appendicular s.
    s. appendiculare
    articulated s.
    axial s.
    s. axiale
    s. of free inferior limb
    s. of free superior limb
    s. hand
    s. thoracicus
    visceral s.
skeptic, sceptic
skewerwood
skills
    mind-body s.
    psychomotor s.
skin
    s. barrier
    s. battery
    s. brushing
    s. burning
    s. capacitance
    s. disorder
    s. drag
    s. eruption
    S. Gel Aloe Life
    s. lesion
    s. motion
    rebound of s.
    s. receptor
    retinaculum of s.
    s. rolling
    s. rolling test
    s. temperature biofeedback
    s. tonic
    s. traction
    s. viscera
skin-electrode resistance
skull
    articulation of s.
    basilar axis of s.
    s. bone motion
    nonrigid s.

S

NOTES

skull *(continued)*
  posterior pole of s.
  rigid s.
  s. suture
  s. symmetry
  s. trauma
  vault of s.
skunk cabbage
skunkweed
slack
  joint s.
SLE
  systemic lupus erythematosus
sleep
  s. disturbance
  s. onset insomnia
  s. phase syndrome
sleeve
  nerve root s.
slide
  muscle s.
  pelvic tilt and heel s.
sliding filament hypothesis
slim
  Herbal S.
sling
slip angle
slipped capital femoral epiphysis
slipper
  lady's s.
  yellow lady's s.
slippery
  s. elm
  s. pulse
  s. root
slipping
  s. patella
  s. rib cartilage
sloe
slow
  s. breathing
  s. insertion
  s. method of insertion
  s. pulse
  s. twitch fiber
sluggish immune system
Slumber
small
  s. cranberry
  s. intestine-bladder channel
  s. intestine-bladder meridian
  s. intestine channel (si)
  s. intestine meridian

  s. intestine meridian of hand
  s. pudendal lip
  s. sciatic nerve
  s. trochanter
smallage
smaller
  s. pectoral muscle
  s. psoas muscle
smallest scalene muscle
Smart Longevity
SMASH
  self-massage acupressure for self-
  healing
smellage
Smilax
  S. aristolochiaefolia
  S. febrifuga
  S. medica
  S. officinalis
  S. ornata
  S. regelii
Smith drug treatment model
smoke
  earth s.
smokeless tobacco
smoking
  s. cessation
  Quit S.
smoldering mugwort
smooth
  s. cayenne pineapple
  s. cicely
  s. muscle relaxant
  s. strophanthus
SMT
  spinal manipulative therapy
smudging
snake
  s. bite
  s. butter
  s. lily
  s. weed
snakeberry
snakehead
snakeroot
  black s.
  Canada s.
  Indian s.
  Kansas s.
  Missouri s.
  Seneca s.
  senega s.
  Vermont s.

Virginia s.
white s.
snakeweed
snap finger
snapping
   s. hazel
   s. hip
sneezewort
snehana
SNMT
   systematic nutritional muscle testing
snowball tree
snow-drop tree
snow-flower
snuffbox
   anatomic s.
snuff dipping
Snuz Plus
SN-X Vegitabs
soap
   s. root
   tea tree oil s.
   s. tree
soapbark
soapwort
soaring crane qigong
Social Readjustment Rating Scale
Society for Clinical and
  Experimental Hypnosis
sock
   reflexology s.'s
socket
   dental s.
   dry s.
   s. joint
socotrine aloe
SOD
   superoxide dismutase
soda
   baking s.
sodium
   s. bicarbonate
   s. dichromate
   s. oxylate
   s. retention
soft
   s. feel

s. laser
s. muscle inhibition
s. parts
s. tissue
s. tissue inhibition
s. tissue injury
s. tissue looseness
s. tissue manipulation
s. tissue mobilization
s. tissue myofascial technique
s. tissue procedure
s. tissue procedure dosage
s. tissue rheumatism
s. tissue stimulation
s. tissue technique
s. tissue texture abnormality
s. tissue therapy
s. tissue treatment (ST)
softgel
soft-hard tissue texture abnormality
soft-tissue dysfunction
Solanaceae poisoning
solanine
Solanum
   S. capsicastrum
   S. dulcamara
   S. nigrum
   S. tuberosum
solar
   s. plexus
   s. plexus chakra
Solaray licorice root
soldier's
   s. cap
   s. woundwort
sole
   s. of foot
   quadrate muscle of s.
soleal line
solei
   arcus tendineus musculi s.
   linea musculi s.
soleus
   s. muscle
   musculus s.
Solgar
solidified energy

S

NOTES

solid organ
solitary bone cyst
Solomon's seal root
soluble
 s. fiber
 s. glass
solution
 Burow s.
 Dakin s.
 ethanolic s.
 liquid s.
 proliferant s.
 saline s.
 salt s.
 tannic s.
 topical s.
Solvefort
soma
 S. bodywork
 s. neuromuscular integration
Somali myrrh
somatic
 s. component
 s. dysfunction
 s. dysfunction of
  carpometacarpal joint
 s. dysfunction of cuboid bone
 s. dysfunction of fibula
 s. dysfunction of forearm
 s. dysfunction of ilium
 s. dysfunction of pubes
 s. dysfunction of pubic
  symphysis
 s. dysfunction of sacrum
 s. dysfunction of tarsal bone
 s. effect
 s. energy
 s. monitoring
 s. nervous system
 s. psychology
 s. reflex arc
 s. sympathetic
 s. symptom
 s. system
somaticosomatic reflex pathway
somatics
somatic-tropic correspondence
somatid
somatization
somatoemotional release
somatogenic
somatology
somatomammotroph

somatomedin
somatoprosthetics
somatoscope
somatosensory
 s. distribution tome
 s. feedback
somatosomatic reflex
somatostatin
somatotopic system
somatotypology
somatovisceral
 s. reflex
 s. reflex arc
somatoviscerosomatic reflex
somatropin
somnifera
 Withania s.
somniferum
 Papaver s.
somnotherapist
son
 s. element
 s. point
 s. sedating point
sonar ray
songuafen
sonnei
 Shigella s.
sonogram
sonopuncture
soother
 Tummy S.
SOPA
 Survey of Pain Attitudes
sophium
Sophora
sorbitol
sore
 canker s.
 cold s.
 pressure s.
sororia
 Arnica s.
sorrel
 garden s.
 green s.
 sheep s.
 wood s.
sorrow
 cuckoo s.
sotai therapy
sound
 cavitation pop s.

popping s.
s. therapy
white s.
soup
herbal s.
sour
s. dock
s. odor
s. sauce
wood s.
source
S. Naturals
s. point
Primary S.
s. qi
sacred s.
soured milk products
sourgrass
sour-spine
soursuds
southern
s. prickly ash
s. wax myrtle
southernwood
sovereign fire
sowberry
soy
s. lecithin
s. milk
soya
soybean lecithin
soyfood
sp
spleen channel (sp)
s. 21 dabao
s. 15 daheng
s. 4 gongsun
s. 6 sanyinjiao
s. 3 taiai
s. 10 xuehai
s. 1 yinbai
s. 9 yinlingquan
SP-23 Eyebright Blend
SP-6 Cornsilk Blend
SP-8 Hawthorn Motherwort Blend
space
antecubital s.

Burns s.
central palmar s.
Chassaignac s.
disk s.
haversian s.
intercostal s. (ICS)
interosseous metacarpal s.
interosseous metatarsal s.
interspinous s.
lateral central palmar s.
lateral midpalmar s.
medial midpalmar s.
middle palmar s.
midpalmar s.
Mohrenheim s.
paraphysiological s.
Parona s.
plantar s.
popliteal s.
potential s.
quadrangular s.
quadrilateral s.
retroadductor s.
subarachnoid s.
suprasternal s.
thenar s.
Traube semilunar s.
vertebral epidural s.
spade hand
Spanish
S. bayonet
S. flu
S. fly
S. influenza
S. lavender
S. licorice
S. psyllium
S. Tummy Mixture
spark
Elixir S.
sparsha
sparshanam
Spartium junceum
spasm
diffuse esophageal s.
muscle s.
vascular s.

S

NOTES

spasmodic torticollis
spasmolytic effect
spasm-pain-spasm
spastic
    s. anemia
    s. constipation
    s. flat foot
    s. hamstring muscle
    s. muscle
    s. paresis
    s. quadratus lumborum muscle
    s. torticollis
SpaTable
    Wet S.
spa therapy
spatia
    s. interossea metacarpi
    s. interossea metatarsi
spatial relationship
spatium intercostale
spearmint
special anatomy
species tolerance
specific
    s. action
    s. effect
    s. hypnotherapy
    s. tonification point
specificity
    diagnostic s.
    relative s.
specimen
    cytologic s.
spectrochrome therapy
spectrometry
    gas chromatographic-mass s.
    (GCMS, GC-MS)
spectroscopy
    magnetoresonance s.
spectrum
    motion s.
speech therapy
speedwell
    tall s.
Speman
Spencer technique
sperm antibody
spermatic plexus
spermatorrhea
sphagnum moss
sphenobasilar
    s. compression
    s. extension

    s. flexion
    s. junction
    s. junction dysfunction
    s. symphysis
    s. synchondrosis
sphenocephaly
sphenoid
    s. angle
    s. articulation
    s. body
    s. bone
    great wing of s.
sphenoidale
    jugum s.
    os s.
sphenoidalis
    ala major ossis s.
    ala minor ossis s.
sphenoiditis
sphenosquamous pivot
spheroidal joint
spheroid articulation
spheroidea
    articulatio s.
sphincter
    anal s.
    s. urethrae muscle
    urethral s.
sphinx
    s. position
    s. test
spica bandage
spicata
    Actaea s.
    Mentha s.
spice
    king of s.'s
    master s.
spicebush
spider
    wood s.
spierstaude
spigo
spike lavender
spikenard
spill
    cellular s.
spina
    s. bifida
    s. bifida aperta
    s. bifida cystica
    s. bifida manifesta
    s. bifida occulta

s. dorsalis
s. iliaca anterior inferior
s. iliaca anterior superior
s. iliaca posterior inferior
s. iliaca posterior superior
s. ischiadica
s. peronealis
s. pubis
s. scapulae
s. ventosa
spinae
erector s.
musculus erector s.
musculus multifidus s.
spinal
s. accessory nerve
s. adjustment
s. analgesia
s. anesthesia
s. anesthetic
s. arteries
s. attunement technique (SAT)
s. balancing
s. block
s. canal
s. column
s. concussion
s. cord
s. cord concussion
s. cord stimulation
s. cord transmission neuron
s. curvature
s. curve
s. decompression
s. dysraphism
s. fusion
s. ganglion
s. gate
s. headache
s. manipulation
s. manipulative therapy (SMT)
s. marrow
s. medulla
s. mobility
s. motion
s. motion segment
s. motion testing

s. muscle
s. muscle of neck
s. muscle of thorax
s. muscular atrophy, type I
s. muscular atrophy, type III
s. nerve
s. nerve radiculopathy
s. overlay
s. part of arachnoid
s. pathology
s. percussion
s. point
s. spondylarthrosis
s. spondylosis
s. stenosis
s. steroid
s. subluxation
s. surgery
s. tract
spinale
ganglion s.
spinalis
arachnoidea mater s.
canalis centralis medullae s.
s. capitis muscle
s. cervicis muscle
dura mater s.
filum durae matris s.
s. muscle
musculus s.
pars cervicalis medullae s.
pars coccygea medullae s.
pars lumbalis medullae s.
pars sacralis medullae s.
pars thoracica medullae s.
segmenta cervicalia medullae s.
segmenta coccygea medullae s.
segmenta sacralia medullae s.
segmenta thoracica medullae s.
sulcus nervi s.
s. thoracis muscle
spinalium
ansae nervorum s.
spinalized patient
spinate
spindle
muscle s.

NOTES

spindle *(continued)*
  tendon s.
  s. tree
spindle-shaped muscle
spindletree
spine
  anterior inferior iliac s.
  anterior nasal s.
  anterior superior iliac s.
    (ASIS)
  anteroposterior erect lumbar s.
  atlantoaxial cervical s.
  bamboo s.
  cervical s.
  cleft s.
  coupled motion of s.
  crest of scapular s.
  dorsal s.
  erector muscle of s.
  flattened lower cervical s.
  flattening of thoracic s.
  hemal s.
  iliac s.
  ischiadic s.
  ischial s.
  lateral lumbar s.
  lumbar s.
  lumbosacral s.
  middle to lower thoracic s.
  s. motion testing
  s. muscle hypertonicity
  neural s.
  neutral lumbar s.
  nonneutral lumbar s.
  occipitoatlantal cervical s.
  s. orientation
  s. patterning
  poker s.
  posterior inferior iliac s.
  posterior superior iliac s.
    (PSIS)
  pubic s.
  s. of scapula
  scapular s.
  sciatic s.
  thoracic s.
  thoracolumbar and lumbar s.
  upper thoracic s.
  weightbearing of s.
spinning disk nebulizer
spinocostalis
spinoglenoid ligament
spinomuscular

spinoneural
spinosa
  Capparis s.
spinosus
  sulcus s.
spinothalamic
  s. system
  s. tract (STT)
spinotransversarius
spinous
  s. process
  s. process of tibia
  s. process of vertebra
spiny dogfish shark
Spiraea ulmaria
spiral
  s. bandage
  s. fracture
  s. groove
  s. joint
  s. line
spiramycin
Spireadosa
spirit-calling ceremony
spirit guide
spiritism
spiritual
  s. care counselor
  s. emergence trauma
  s. healing
  s. imbalance
  s. mentoring
spiritualism
Spirulina maxima
Spiru-tein
splanchnapophysial
splanchnapophysis
splanchnic
  s. anesthesia
  s. nerve
splanchnologia
splanchnology
splanchnoskeletal
splanchnoskeleton
splanchnosomatic
spleen
  s. channel (sp)
  damp cold in the s.
  damp heat in the s.
  s. deficiency
  s. meridian
  s. meridian of foot
  s. qi sinking

s. system
s. yang xu
splenial
splenica
   extremitas anterior s.
   extremitas posterior s.
spleniserrate
splenium
splenius
   s. capitis muscle
   s. cervicis muscle
   s. muscle
   s. muscle of head
   s. muscle of neck
splint
   active s.
   air s.
   airplane s.
   backboard s.
   coaptation s.
   dynamic s.
   functional s.
   inflatable s.
   ladder s.
   plaster s.
   shin s.
splintered fracture
splinting
split hand
spondylalgia
spondylarthropthy
spondylarthrosis
   spinal s.
spondylitis
   ankylosing s.
   cervical s.
   s. deformans
   rheumatoid s.
   shao yang lateral cervical s.
   tai yang medial cervical s.
   tuberculous s.
spondyloarthropathy
spondyloepiphyseal dysplasia
spondylolisthesis
   dysplastic s.
   isthmic s.
spondylolisthetic pelvis

spondylolysis
spondylomalacia
spondylopathy
spondyloptosis
spondylopyosis
spondyloschisis
spondylosis
   cervical s.
   hyperostotic s.
   spinal s.
spondylosyndesis
spondylothoracic
spondylous
Spongia Tosta Homeopathic
spongiosum
   osteoma s.
spongy feel
spontaneous fracture
spontaneously sensitive point
sports
   s. injury
   s. therapy
spot
   s. film
   flat s.
   s. lateral projection
   tender s.
spotted
   s. alder
   s. comfrey
   s. cranesbill
   s. thistle
   s. wintergreen
spotting
sprain
   acute lumbar s.
   s. fracture
   recurrent ankle s.
spray
   All-Purpose Bactericide S.
   Aloe Herbal Horse S.
   Arnica s.
   s. and stretch technique
spring
   s. finger
   s. grass
   s. ligament

S

NOTES

spring *(continued)*
    s. test
    s. water
springing
    s. force
    s. technique
    s. treatment
springy feel
S-propyl cystein
sprout
sprue
    celiac s.
spur
    calcaneal heel s.
    heel s.
spurge
    s. family
    garden s.
    pill-bearing s.
spuriae
    costae s. [VII–XII]
    vertebrae s.
spurious
    s. ankylosis
    s. torticollis
Spurling maneuver
spurt
    s. muscle
    s. and shunt action of muscle
squalamine
squalene
Squalus acanthias
squama
    occipital s.
    parietal s.
    s. portion
    temporal s.
squamous cell carcinoma
square
    carpenter's s.
    s. dancing
    s. pulse
    s. stalk
    s. wave pulse
squat
    polarity s.
    s. test
squaw
    s. root
    s. tea
    s. vine
    s. weed
squawberry

squawmint
squawroot
squawvine
squill
    enteric-coated s.
    European s.
    Indian s.
    Mediterranean s.
    red s.
    sea s.
    white s.
squirting cucumber
srotas
Ssssting Stop Homeopathic Gel
ST
    soft tissue treatment
St.
    St. Bartholomew's tea
    St. Benedict's thistle
    St. James wort
    St. John method of
        neuromuscular therapy
    St. Johnswort
    St. John's wort
    St. Mary's thistle
    St. Mary's thistle fruit
st
    stomach channel
    st 31 biguan
    st 1 chengqi
    st 5 daying
    st 4 dicang
    st 35 dubi
    st 32 femur-futu
    st 40 fenglong
    st 29 guilai
    st 6 jiache
    st 41 jiexi
    st 3 juliao
    st 21 liangmen
    st 44 neiting
    st 12 quepen
    st 18 rugen
    st 17 ruzhong
    st 2 sibai
    st 25 tianshu
    st 38 tiaokou
    st 8 touwei
    st 7 xiaguan
    st 39 xiajuxu
    st 43 xiangu
    st 36 zusanli

stability
  ligamentous s.
stabilization
  scapular s.
stabilizing ligament
stable
  s. factor
  s. fracture
Stachys
  S. betonica
  S. officinalis
stacking
  joint s.
  s. sequence
staff
  Jacob's s.
stagbush
stage
  tumor s.
staggerwort
staging
  TNM s.
stagnant area
stagnated
  s. area
  s. energy
stagnation
  blood s.
  s. of blood
  chronic s.
  s. of heart blood
  liver s.
  s. of liver qi
  lung qi s.
  s. of qi
  qi s.
  xue s.
Stago
stalk
  pituitary s.
  square s.
stamen
stamina
stammerwort
stance
  biped s.
  s. phase of gait

stanchgrass
standard
  dog s.
standardized extract
stander
  one-legged s.
standing
  s. bending test
  s. flexion test
  s. position
  retaining position s.
  self-correction position s.
  self-stretch s.
  s. trunk bending test
Stanford
  S. Hypnotic Susceptibility
    Scale, Form C
  S. Sleepiness Scale
Stanley cervical ligament
stanol ester
stanols
  plant s.
stapes
  anular ligament of s.
  base of s.
  head of s.
  posterior crus of s.
  posterior limb of s.
Staphylococcus
  S. aureus
  S. epidermidis
  methicillin-resistant *S. aureus*
    (MRSA)
  S. septicemia
staphysagria
star
  Bio S.
  blazing s.
  s. chickweed
  goldy s.
  s. grass
starflower
stargrass
  whitetube s.
start
  running s.
Starter

S

NOTES

starting
s. friction
s. point
starweed
starwort
stasimorphia
stasis
s. of blood
s. of qi
state
aesthenic s.
s. of excess
harmonious energy s.
Profile of Mood S.'s (POMS)
qi s.
seizure s.
trance-like s.
s. of weakness
State-Trait
S.-T. Anxiety Inventory
S.-T. Anxiety Scale
static
s. analysis
s. arthropathy
s. contraction
s. electricity
s. friction
s. malposition
s. mechanoreceptor
s. muscle
s. muscle contraction
s. palpation
s. posture
s. scoliosis
s. stretch
s. stretch reflex
s. symmetric examination
s. symmetry
stature
status
endocrine s.
financial s.
nutritional s.
staying sickness
STD
sexually transmitted disease
steam
s. bath
s. box
S. Embrace
s. inhalation
s. inhalation therapy
Mr. S.

steam-distilled water
steatorrhea
stechapfel
steeple
church s.
stegnotic
stellaria
Stellaria media
stellate
s. block
s. fracture
s. ganglion
s. ligament
stellatum
ganglion s.
stem
s. cell
clove s.
stemless gentian
stenosing tenosynovitis
stenosis
central canal s.
central spinal s.
lateral recess s.
lateral spinal s.
spinal s.
stenothorax
Stephania tetrandra
steppage gait
sterculia
s. gum
S. tragacantha
S. urens
S. villosa
stereoarthrolysis
stereognosis
stereospecific effect
sterile abscess
sterilization
blood s.
sterilize
sterilizer
hot air s.
sterna
sternad
sternal
s. angle
s. articular surface of clavicle
s. cartilage
s. end of clavicle
s. extremity of clavicle
s. joint
s. line

s. muscle
s. notch
s. origin
s. part of diaphragm
s. plane
s. synchondroses
sternale
planum s.
sternales
synchondroses s.
sternalis
linea s.
s. muscle
musculus s.
sternal-xiphoid junction
sternebra
sternen
sterni
angulus s.
corpus s.
manubrium s.
mucro s.
musculus triangularis s.
sternochondral articulation
sternochondroscapularis
musculus s.
sternochondroscapular muscle
sternoclavicular
s. angle
s. articulation
s. disk
s. joint
s. joint dysfunction muscle
  energy technique
s. joint mobility
s. ligament
s. muscle
sternoclavicularis
articulatio s.
discus articularis s.
musculus s.
sternocleidal
sternocleidomastoid
s. muscle
s. region
sternocleidomastoidea
regio s.

sternocleidomastoideus
musculus s.
sternocostal
s. articulations
s. head of pectoralis major
  muscle
s. joint
s. part of pectoralis major
  muscle
s. surface of heart
s. triangle
sternocostales
articulationes s.
sternocostalis muscle
sternofascialis
musculus s.
sternoglossal
sternohyoid muscle
sternoid
sternomanubrial
s. joint
s. junction
sternomastoid
s. artery
s. muscle
sternopagia
sternopericardial ligament
sternoschisis
sternothyroideus
musculus s.
sternothyroid muscle
sternotracheal
sternovertebral
sternum
body of s.
clavicular notch of s.
s. functional technique
manubrium of s.
steroid
epidural s.
s. hormone
oral s.
s. secretory modulation
spinal s.
sterol
plant s.
sthenometer

S

NOTES

sthenometry
sticklewort
stickwort
sticky feel
Stieda process
stiff
    s. man syndrome
    s. toe
stigma, pl. **stigmata**
    stigmata maydis
    saffron s.
Stik
    Witch S.
stilbamidine
Stillingia sylvatica
still point
stimulant
    centrally acting s.
    diffusible s.
    general s.
    immune s.
    local s.
    uterine s.
stimulation
    aberrant s.
    aberrant afferent s.
    ah shi point s.
    appetite s.
    central s.
    cranioelectrical s.
    electrical s.
    electroencephalogram-driven s.
    epidural s.
    high-frequency s.
    high-frequency low-intensity s.
    high-frequency low-intensity
      electrical s.
    intravaginal electrical s.
    large-fiber s.
    low-frequency s.
    low-frequency, high-intensity s.
    low-frequency, high-intensity
      electrical s.
    manual s.
    needle s.
    nerve s.
    neuromagnetic s.
    nociceptive pathway s.
    percutaneous electrical nerve s.
      (PENS)
    peripheral s.
    restricted environmental s.
    sedative s.

    sham-point s.
    soft tissue s.
    spinal cord s.
    strong s.
    sympathetic s.
    tender point s.
    tonifying s.
    transcutaneous electrical
      nerve s. (TENS)
    ulnar s.
    vigorous s.
stimulator
    acupoint s.
    biphasic s.
stimulus, pl. **stimuli**
    afferent s.
    habituation to monotonous
      stimuli
    noxious s.
    train-of-four s.
sting
    bee s.
stinging nettle
stinking
    s. benjamin
    s. Christopher
    s. cranesbill
    s. nanny
    s. rose
    s. willie
stinkweed
stippled epiphysis
stitch abscess
stitchwort
stoechas
    Lavandula s.
Stokes law
stomach
    s. channel (st)
    s. excess
    s. fire
    s. fire rising
    s. meridian
    s. meridian of foot
Stomachiagil
stomachic
stomatitis
    angular s.
stomatologic infection
stone
    artificial s.
    calcium oxalate renal s.
    S. Free

kidney s.
s. oak
oxalate s.
renal oxalate s.
stoneroot
stool
dry s.
loose s.
scanty and watery s.
stor
storage organ
storax
stored chi
storksbill
straight
s. chiropractic
s. leg raising
s. leg raising test
s. sinus
strain
s. and counterstrain
cranial s.
foot s.
s. fracture
lateral s.
ligamentous s.
ligamentous articular s.
muscle s.
pattern of s.
role s.
s.'s of sphenobasilar
synchondrosis
torsional s.
traumatic lateral s.
traumatic vertical s.
vertical s.
strain-counterstrain
s.-c. therapy
stramoine
stramonium
Datura s.
strangury
compulsive s.
strap muscle
stratiform fibrocartilage
straw
oat s.

strawberry
s. bush
s. leaf
s. tree
streak
s. hyperostosis
linear s.
streblodactyly
strength
BioGinkgo 27/7 Extra S.
fatigue s.
grip s.
inner s.
isokinetic muscle s.
isometric muscle s.
One-A-Day Bone S.
s. testing
ultimate s.
yield s.
strengthen
strengthening
ego s.
s. exercise
s. method
Streptococcus
S. agalactiae
S. thermophilus
stress
S. Aid
s. attenuation
s. bands
compressive s.
s. disorder
s. fracture
S. Free
gravitational s.
s. hormone
HR 133 S.
s. incontinence
s. inoculation training
s. management
s. management technique
mental s.
oxidative s.
physical excessive s.
postural gravitational s.
s. profile

S

NOTES

stress *(continued)*
s. response
s. riser
secondary posttraumatic s.
s. shielding
s. sign
s. test
torsional s.
stress-induced
s.-i. analgesia
s.-i. anxiety
s.-i. depression
Stressmelt
stressor
emotional s.
gravity s.
intrapsychic s.
nonphysical s.
physical s.
stress-strain curve
stretch
adductor s.
bilateral lateral s.
bilateral linear cervical
spine s.
elevation s.
expiration abdominal s.
extensor neck muscle linear s.
full body s.
hamstring muscle s.
inspiration rib s.
lateral s.
lateral and longitudinal s.
linear s.
long axis longitudinal s.
longitudinal s.
occipitoatlantal region linear s.
parallel s.
perpendicular s.
posterior capsule s.
prayer s.
prone lateral s.
protraction s.
quadratus lumborum s.
s. reflex
regional s.
retraction s.
Simon and Travell spray
and s.
static s.
unilateral lateral s.
unilateral linear s.

stretching
manual s.
PNF s.
proprioceptor neuromuscular
facilitation s.
tissue s.
striata
osteopathia s.
striate
s. muscle tension
s. voluntary system
striated muscle
stricta
Euphrasia s.
stride
length of s.
symmetry of s.
strike
heel s.
stringiness
Strogen
stroke
s. rehabilitation
s. rehabilitation control patient
thrombotic s.
strong
s. and rapid pulse
s. stimulation
strong-scented lettuce
strontium
strophanthus
S. gratus
smooth s.
strophocephaly
structural
s. balance
s. compensation
s. diagnosis
s. examination
s. force
s. integration
s. integrity
s. realignment
s. rib dysfunction
s. scoliosis
structure
arthrodial s.
articular s.
myofascial s.
periarticular s.
sacroiliac joint ligamentous s.
skeletal s.
vascular s.

structure-function
    s.-f. interface
    s.-f. interrelationship
struthiopteris
    Matteuccia s.
Strychnos nux-vomica
STT
    spinothalamic tract
    STT cell
stuck finger
study
    bone densitometry s.
    case s.
    Doppler s.
    double-blind s.
    dynamic s.
    electrodiagnostic s.
    nerve conduction s.
    nerve conduction velocity s.
    prospective s.
    retrospective s.
    single-blind s.
    urodynamic s.
stump
    s. hallucination
    s. neuralgia
stupor
stylet
styliform
styloauricularis
styloid
    s. process
    s. process of fibula
    s. process of radius
    s. process of temporal bone
    s. process of third metacarpal
      bone
    s. process of ulna
    s. prominence
styloidea
    prominentia s.
stylopodium
S-type compensated structural
  scoliosis
styptic
    s. collodion

    s. colloid
    s. cotton
styraciflua
    Liquidambar s.
styramate
su
    chan s.
    s. ferasyunu
    s. ye
suan
    da s.
    s. zao ren tang
subacromial
    s. bursa
    s. bursitis
subacute
    s. bacterial endocarditis
    s. combined degeneration of
      the spinal cord
    s. degeneration of cerebellum
    s. dysfunction
    s. necrotizing myelitis
Sub-Adrene
subanconeus muscle
subarachnoid
    s. anesthesia
    s. space
subastragalar amputation
subaxial
subaxillary
subcapital fracture
subcartilaginous
subchondral
subcircuit
    meridian s.
    principal meridian s.
    shao yin-tai yang principal
      meridian s.
subclavia
    ansa s.
subclaviae
    sulcus costae arteriae s.
subclavian
    s. artery
    s. duct
    s. groove
    s. loop

S

NOTES

subclavian *(continued)*
  s. lymphatic trunk
  s. muscle
  s. plexus
  s. sulcus
  s. triangle
  s. vein
subclavianus
  sulcus s.
subclavicular fossa
subclavii
  sulcus musculi s.
subclavius
  s. muscle
  musculus s.
  sulcus s.
subcoracoid
subcostal
  s. groove
  s. line
  s. muscle
  s. plane
subcostale
  planum s.
subcostalis
  linea s.
  musculus s.
subcostosternal
subcruralis
subcrural muscle
subcrureus
subcutaneous
  s. band
  s. fascia
  s. fat necrosis
  s. hirudin
  s. needle
  s. needling
  s. nodule
  s. operation
  s. tenotomy
  s. tissue
  s. tissue palpation
subcuticular
subcutis
subdeltoid bursitis
subdiaphragmatic
subdorsal
subdural
  s. hematoma
  s. hematorrhachis
subfascial prepatellar bursa
subglenoid

subiliac
subilium
sublatum
  Amomum s.
sublimis
  musculus flexor s.
  musculus flexor digitorum s.
sublumbar
subluxation
  anterior s.
  chiropractic s.
  first rib superior s.
  posterior s.
  spinal s.
  superior s.
  superior first rib s.
  vertebral s.
subluxation-based chiropractic
submandibular lymph node
suboccipital
  s. compression
  s. region
suboccipitale
  malum vertebrale s.
subpatellar
subpectoral
subpelviperitoneal
subperiosteal
  s. amputation
  s. fracture
subplexal
subpopliteal recess
subpopliteus
  recessus s.
subquadricipital muscle
subsartorial
  s. canal
  s. fascia
subscapular
  s. fossa
  s. muscle
  s. muscle tender point
subscapularis
  fossa s.
  s. muscle
  musculus s.
subscription
subserosa
  fascia s.
subserous
  s. fascia
  s. layer
subsidence

subspinous
substance
  amorphous ground s.
  controlled s.
  ground s.
substance P
substance-transporting organ
substantia
substernal angle
substernomastoid
substitute
  blood s.
substrate
  biochemical s.
subtalar
  s. articulation
  s. joint
subtalaris
  articulatio s.
subtarsal
subthyroideus
subtibiale
  os s.
subtle energy
subtrapezial
subvertebral
succedaneum
succenturiate
success
  long-lasting s.
succinate
  L-lysine s.
succirubra
  Cinchona s.
succory
  wild s.
succuss
succussion
Sucquet canal
Sucquet-Hoyer canal
Sucrets
  Wintergreen S.
sucrose
sudden cardiac death (SCD)
sudiferous gland
sudorific
suehirotake

sufficient cause
suffocate
suffocation
sugar
  blood s.
  s. wrack
suggestibility
suggestion
  direct s.
  failed test s.
  hypnotic s.
  s. technique
sukra artava
sulbactam
sulcoplasty
sulcus, pl. sulci
  s. arteriae vertebralis
  s. bicipitalis lateralis
  s. bicipitalis medialis
  calcaneal s.
  s. calcanei
  s. carpi
  s. costae
  s. costae arteriae subclaviae
  intertubercular s.
  s. intertubercularis
  s. musculi subclavii
  s. nervi radialis
  s. nervi spinalis
  s. nervi ulnaris
  s. popliteus
  sacral s.
  s. spinosus
  subclavian s.
  s. subclavianus
  s. subclavius
  talar s.
  s. tali
  s. tendinis musculi fibularis longi
  s. tendinis musculi flexoris hallucis longi
  s. tendinis musculi peronei longi
  s. test
  s. venae subclaviae sulfatidosis
  s. for vertebral artery

S

NOTES

sulfate
- Cadmium s.
- chondroitin s.
- chondroitin s. A
- dehydroepiandrosterone s. (DHEA-S)
- Enhanced Glucosamine s.
- glucosamine s.
- hydrazine s.
- keratan s.
- liquid glucosamine s.
- magnesium s.
- purified chondroitin s.
- Ultra Maximum Strength Glucosamine s.
- vanadyl s.

sulfatidosis
- sulcus venae subclaviae s.

sulfide
- dimethyl s. (DMS)

sulfite
sulforaphane
sulfoxide
- dimethyl s. (DMSO)

sulfur, sulphur
sulfur-containing foods
sulfured fruit
sulfuricum
- Natrum s.

suliao
- du 25 s.

sumac
- s. family
- poison s.

suma tea
Sumatra benzoin
summation
summer savory
Sun
- S. Dance
- Health From the S.

sundew
- common s.
- great s.
- round-leaved s.

sunflower
- red s.
- s. seed
- wild s.

sunshine view
suo
- s. yang
- yen hu s.

supai
super
- s. blue-green alga
- S. Octacosanol
- S. Supplemental

superabduction
superacromial
supercritical fluid extraction (SFE)
Superdophilus
superextensa
- manus s.

superextension
superficial
- s. back muscle
- s. branch
- s. dorsal sacrococcygeal ligament
- s. fascia
- s. flexor muscle of fingers
- s. head of flexor pollicis brevis
- s. lamina
- s. layer
- s. layer of deep cervical fascia
- s. nerve
- s. parotid lymph node
- s. posterior sacrococcygeal ligament
- s. pulse
- s. tightness
- s. transverse metacarpal ligament
- s. transverse metatarsal ligament

superficial-deep
superficialis
- arcus palmaris s.
- arcus venosus palmaris s.
- arcus volaris s.
- fascia s.
- fibrae intercrurales anuli inguinalis s.
- lamina s.
- musculus flexor digitorum s.
- s. volae

superficies
superflexion
supergenual
Superguarana
superincumbent vertebral column
superior
- s. angle of scapula

superior · supine

apertura thoracis s.
arcus palpebralis s.
s. articular facet
s. articular facet of atlas
s. articular process of sacrum
s. articular surface of tibia
s. belly of omohyoid muscle
s. border
s. border of scapula
s. branch
s. branch of the pubic bone
s. cervical ganglion
s. costal facet
s. costal pit
s. costotransverse ligament
s. extensor retinaculum
s. extremity
s. first rib subluxation
fovea costalis s.
s. gemellus muscle
s. hypogastric plexus
s. innominate iliac shear
s. limb
s. mesenteric ganglion
musculus gemellus s.
musculus obliquus s.
musculus obliquus capitis s.
musculus serratus posterior s.
musculus tarsalis s.
s. petrosal sinus
s. pharyngeal constrictor
  muscle
s. pole
s. posterior serratus muscle
s. pubic dysfunction
s. pubic ramus
s. pubis
s. radioulnar joint
s. retinaculum of extensor
  muscle
s. sagittal sinus
spina iliaca anterior s.
spina iliaca posterior s.
s. subluxation
s. surface of talus
s. tarsal muscle
s. temporal line

s. thoracic aperture
s. thyroid tubercle
s. tibial articulation
s. tibiofibular joint
s. transverse axis
s. transverse scapular ligament
s. trapezius myofascial
  technique
s. zygapophysial joint
superioris
articulationes cinguli membri s.
caput zygomaticum quadrati
  labii s.
cingulum membri s.
juncturae membri s.
ossa membri s.
regiones membri s.
vagina tendinis musculi
  obliqui s.
superius
ganglion cervicale s.
membrum s.
retinaculum musculorum
  extensorum s.
segmentum renale anterius s.
tuberculum s.
superolateral
superoxide
s. anion
s. dismutase (SOD)
supinate
supination
s. of the foot
foot s.
forearm s.
s. of the forearm
supinator
s. crest of ulna
s. muscle
supine
assisted eccentric
  strengthening s.
s. cervical flexion test
s. condylar glide
s. hypotensive syndrome
s. iliac crest height test
s. mesenteric release

NOTES

403

supine *(continued)*
    s. position
    s. pubic symphysis height test
    retraining position s.
    self-correction position s.
    self-stretch position s.
    s. sternoclavicular joint
    dysfunction muscle energy
    technique
    s. thrust technique
    unassisted eccentric
    strengthening s.
supplement
    Attention! dietary s.
    botanical s.
    dietary s.
    fish oil s.
    multinutrient s.
    phytonutrient s.
supplemental
    Super S.
supplementary tonification
supply
    blood s.
    peripheral bloody s.
support
    base of s.
    Bone S.
    CTR S.
    Joint S.
    mitochondria energy s.
    Mood S.
supporter
supporting reflexes
supportive care
suppository
    Key-E s.
    tea tree s.
suppression
    bone marrow s.
suppressor cell
suppurant
suppurate
suppuration
suppurative
    s. arthritis
    s. inflammation
supraacetabular groove
supraacromial
supraarytenoid cartilage
supraaxillary
supraclavicular
    s. lymph node

    s. muscle
    s. triangle
supraclavicularis
    musculus s.
supracondylar
    s. fracture
    s. process of humerus
supracondyloid
supracostal
supracrestal
    s. line
    s. plane
supracristale
    planum s.
supracristalis
    linea s.
supracristal plane
supraepicondylar process
suprahumeral joint
suprahyoid node technique
supralumbar
supraoptic nucleus
supraorbital
    s. notch
    s. ridge
suprapatellar
supraphysiologic dose
suprapleuralis
    membrana s.
suprascapular ligament
supraspinal
supraspinalis
    s. muscle
    musculus s.
supraspinata
    fossa s.
supraspinatus
    s. muscle
    s. muscle tender point
    musculus s.
    s. syndrome
supraspinous
    s. fossa
    s. ligament
    s. muscle
suprasternal
    s. bone
    s. notch
    s. plane
    s. space
suprasternalia
    ossa s.
suprathoracic

supratragic tubercle
supratragicum
    tuberculum s.
supraventricular
    s. crest
    s. tachycardia (SVT)
supraventricularis
    crista s.
supreme
    Bloodroot/Celandine S.
    Fennel/Wild Yam S.
    Feverfew/Dogwood S.
    Ginkgo/Gotu Kola S.
    s. nuchal line
    Wild Cherry S.
surae
    musculus triceps s.
surale di bierdji
suralis
    regio s.
sural region
suramin
surface
    anterior s.
    costal s.
    dorsal s.
    s. EMG
    external s.
    glenoid s.
    lateral s.
    medial s.
    palmar s.
    posterior s.
    synovial s.
    volar s.
surgery
    anorectal s.
    Bachelor of Ayurvedic
      Medicine and S. (BAMS)
    bladder suspension s.
    closed s.
    minor s.
    psychic s.
    spinal s.
surge shock
surgical
    s. anesthesia

    s. hypnoanalgesia
    s. maggot
    s. neck of humerus
    s. pathology
    s. sympathetectomy
surging pulse
survey
    Life Experiences S.
    S. of Pain Attitudes (SOPA)
    skeletal s.
Susan
    black-eyed S.
susceptibility
    Harvard Group Scale of
      Hypnotic S. (HGSHS)
    s. testing
suspension
    breath s.
suspensory
    s. ligament of axilla
    s. ligaments of breast
    s. ligaments of Cooper
suspicion
    index of s.
susruta samhita
Sustain
    Ultra Clear S.
sustained-release
    s.-r. form
    s.-r. niacin
sustentacular
sustentaculum tali
suterberry
Sutherland
    S. fulcrum
    S. technique
sutra
sutural
    s. bone
    s. motion test
    s. obliteration
sutura notha
suture
    coronal s.
    cranial s.
    false s.
    intermaxillary s.

S

NOTES

suture *(continued)*
 internasal s.
 s. joint
 lambdoid s.
 lambdoidal s.
 maxillofrontal s.
 maxillonasal s.
 metopic s.
 occipital mastoid s.
 occipitomastoid s.
 s. palpation
 parietomastoid s.
 patent s.
 sagittal s.
 s. separation
 skull s.
 tendon s.
Svadhishthana
SVT
 supraventricular tachycardia
swainsinone
swallowing disorder
swallow wort
swamp
 s. dewberry
 s. hellebore
swan neck deformity
Swanson Ultra Tea Tree oil
swayback posture
sweat
 s. gland
 s. gland activity
 s. lodge
 night s.
 s. therapy
sweating
 big s.
 night s.
 s. plant
sweat-lodge ceremony
swedana
Swedish-Esalen massage
Swedish massage
sweet
 s. Annie
 s. basil
 s. bay
 s. Betty
 s. birch oil
 s. bracken
 s. brake
 s. broom
 s. chervil

 s. cicely
 s. coltsfoot
 s. cumin
 s. elder
 s. elm
 s. false chamomile
 s. fennel
 s. fern
 s. flag
 s. goldenrod
 s. haw
 s. hemlock
 s. marjoram
 s. marjoram essential oil
 s. myrtle
 s. oak
 s. root
 s. sedge
 s. vernal grass
 s. violet
 s. woodruff
 s. wormwood
sweet-scented cactus
sweetweed
swelling
 levator s.
swimming
swing
 s. of arm
 s. phase of gait
sylvatica
 Stillingia s.
sylvestris
 Malva s.
 Pinus s.
sylvii
 caro quadrata s.
symbiotic bacteria
symbolic healing ritual
symbrachydactyly
Symington anococcygeal body
symmetrical gait
symmetry
 facet s.
 posterior plane s.
 skull s.
 static s.
 s. of stride
sympathetectomy
 surgical s.
sympathetic
 s. activation
 s. activity

s. arousal
s. block
s. blockade
s. ganglion
s. innervation
s. lateral chain ganglion
s. nerve
s. nervous system
s. nervous system reflex
s. part of autonomic division
  of peripheral nervous system
s. reflex pathway
somatic s.
s. stimulation
s. trunk
sympathicolytic
sympathovagal balance
symphalangism
symphysial, symphyseal
s. shear
symphysic
symphysis
intervertebral s.
s. intervertebralis
left superior s.
s. mandibulae
manubriosternal s.
s. manubriosternalis
mental s.
s. mentalis
s. menti
pubic s.
s. pubis
s. pubis dysfunction
somatic dysfunction of
  pubic s.
sphenobasilar s.
Symphytum
S. *asperum*
S. *officinale*
S. *x uplandicum*
sympodia
symptom
s. chart
cold s.
coldness s.
deficiency s.

s. diary
diffuse s.
s. dynamic
exacerbated s.
excess-type s.
four big s.'s
inhibited muscle s.'s
lower urinary tract s. (LUTS)
organic s.
pronounced s.
psychogenic urological s.
shi s.
somatic s.
traditional classification of s.'s
s. trigger
uncomfortable s.
vegetative s.
vegetative physical s.
yang xu s.
yin xu s.
symptomatic nanism
symptomatology
symptothermal method
sympus
s. apus
s. dipus
s. monopus
synaca
Asclepias s.
synadelphus
synapse
postsynaptic endorphin s.
synarthrodia
synarthrodial joint
synarthrophysis
synarthrosis
syncephalus
synchondrodial joint
synchondroses
sternal s.
s. sternales
synchondrosis
s. intraoccipitalis anterior
s. intraoccipitalis posterior
s. manubriosternalis
neurocentral s.
posterior intraoccipital s.

S

NOTES

synchondrosis *(continued)*
    sphenobasilar s.
    strains of sphenobasilar s.
    s. xiphosternalis
synchronization
    heart-brain s.
synchronize
synchronous function
syncope
syndesmectopia
syndesmitis metatarsea
syndesmodial joint
syndesmophyte
syndesmosis
    radioulnar s.
    s. radioulnaris
    tibiofibular s.
    s. tibiofibularis
syndesmotic
syndrome
    acquired immunodeficiency s.
    (AIDS)
    acute cauda equina s.
    aglossia-adactylia s.
    anterior tibial compartment s.
    Arnold-Chiari s.
    autoimmune deficiency s.
    Barr-Lieou s.
    basal cell nevus s.
    bi s.
    blue toe s.
    camptomelic s.
    carpal tunnel s. (CTS)
    Carpenter s.
    cauda equina s.
    cerebral insufficiency s.
    cervical s.
    cervical cranial s.
    cervical fusion s.
    cervicobrachial s.
    cervicocephalic s.
    cervicocranial s.
    Chinese s.
    chronic fatigue s. (CFS)
    cloverleaf skull s.
    cocktail s.
    cocktail party s.
    compartment s.
    complex regional pain s.
    (CRPS)
    compression s.
    crush s.
    cubital tunnel s.

Cushing s.
dead arm s.
deficiency s.
depersonalization s.
Di Ferrante s.
discogenic pain s.
disk s.
Down s.
Eaton-Lambert s.
Ehlers-Danlos s.
eosinophilia-myalgia s. (EMS)
exhaustion s.
failed lower back s.
fibromyalgia s. (FMS)
fibrositis s.
ginseng abuse s.
gracilis s.
Guillain-Barré s.
Horner s.
hypersympathetic s.
hyperuricemic s.
iliotibial band s.
iliotibial band friction s.
impingement s.
irritable bowel s. (IBS)
Janda lower crossed s.
Janda upper crossed s.
jiggling hands s.
Kasabach-Merritt s.
Landry-Guillain-Barré s.
layer s.
loin pain/hematuria s.
lower crossed s.
lumbar diskogenic pain s.
lumbar spine layer s.
Maigne s.
mandibulofacial dysotosis s.
Marfan s.
marfanoid hypermobility s.
milk-alkali s.
Morquio s.
Morton s.
myasthenic s.
myofascial s.
myofascial pain s. (MPS)
nail-patella s.
nephrotic s.
nutrient-dependency s.
oculomandibulofacial s.
oculovertebral s.
orofaciodigital s.
outlet s.
pachydermoperiostosis s.

pain s.
painful arc s.
patellofemoral s.
patellofemoral stress s.
pelvic tilt s.
Pfaundler-Hurler s.
piriformis s.
popliteal entrapment s.
posterior facet joint s.
postmastectomy pain s.
postpartum carpal tunnel s.
posttraumatic stress s.
premenstrual s. (PMS)
pronator teres s.
s. of psoas muscle
qigong deviation s. (QDS)
radial tunnel s.
Raggedy Ann s.
round cell idiopathic s.
sacroiliac s.
sacroiliac joint s.
scapulocostal s.
short leg s.
short leg/pelvic tilt s.
shoulder-girdle s.
shoulder-hand s.
sicca s.
sleep phase s.
stiff man s.
supine hypotensive s.
supraspinatus s.
tai yang s.
tarsal tunnel s.
temporomandibular joint s.
thoracic outlet s.
traditional Chinese s.
trochanteric s.
Tzietze s.
upper crossed s.
Venus s.
withdrawal s.
xue level s.
yang ming fu s.
ying level s.
synergetic
synergia
synergic

synergism
synergist
synergistic
  s. effect
  s. muscle
  s. muscle
synergistism
synergy
  S. Plus
synesthesia
synosteology
synosteosis
synostosis
synostotic
synovia
synovial
  s. bursa
  s. chondromatosis
  s. crypt
  s. cyst
  s. extremity joint
  s. fluid
  s. fold
  s. frena
  s. frenula
  s. fringe
  s. hernia
  s. joint
  s. joints of free lower limb
  s. joints of free upper limb
  s. ligament
  s. material
  s. membrane
  s. meniscoid
  s. mesenchyme
  s. sarcoma
  s. sheath
  s. sheaths of digits of foot
  s. sheaths of digits of hand
  s. surface
  s. tendon sheath
  s. tufts
synovialis
  articulatio s.
  junctura s.
  plica s.
synoviocyte

S

NOTES

synoviparous
synovitis
    bursal s.
    chronic hemorrhagic villous s.
    dry s.
    filarial s.
    hip s.
    pigmented villonodular s.
    serous s.
    s. sicca
    tendinous s.
    traumatic s.
synovium
synthesis
    GAG s.
    leukotriene s.
syntonic optometry
syntropic
syntropy
syphilis
syphilitic osteochondritis
Syrian tragacanth
syringocele
syringomeningocele
syringomyelia
syringomyelocele
syrup
    black cohosh s.
    ipecac s.
syssarcosic
syssarcosis
syssarcotic
system
    adrenal s.
    antioxidant defense s.
    autonomic nervous s. (ANS)
    autonomic part of peripheral
      nervous s.
    Bates eye s.
    biliary s.
    bioinformation s.
    blood circulation s.
    body-mind s.
    bodywork s.
    BTA S-2000 biofeedback s.
    cartilaginous part of skeletal s.
    central nervous s. (CNS)
    cerebrospinal s.
    chakra s.
    Chinese kidney s.
    circulatory s.
    collateral s.
    connective tissue s.

    coordinate s.
    craniosacral s.
    crossed s.
    cutaneous nervous s.
    descending serotonin-DLT
      inhibitory s.
    dynamical energy s.
    electromagnetic s.
    electromagnetic
      bioinformation s.
    endocrine s.
    endorphin-dependent s.
    enteric nervous s.
    functional s.
    Gravity Lumbar Traction s.
    immune s.
    Indian chakra s.
    jing-luo s.
    kinetic s.
    limbic s.
    low-energy laser s.
    lymphatic s.
    macrocosmic energy s.
    Max Nutrition S.
    microcosmic energy s.
    monoamine-dependent s.
    Morter Health S.
    motor s.
    muscular s.
    musculoskeletal s.
    Natchez Mobil-Trac s.
    nervous s.
    neuroendocrine s.
    neuromuscular s.
    neuromusculoskeletal s.
    osseous part of skeletal s.
    painful disorder of the
      locomotor s.
    parasympathetic nervous s.
    parasynaptic s.
    peripheral nervous s.
    pituitary-portal venous s.
    prospective outcomes
      monitoring evaluation s.
    (POMES)
    raphe descending s.
    raphe-DLT-serotonin s.
    reciprocal nervous s.
    Renshaw inhibitory s.
    right orthogonal coordinate s.
    skeletal s.
    sluggish immune s.
    somatic s.

somatic nervous s.
somatotopic s.
spinothalamic s.
spleen s.
striate voluntary s.
sympathetic nervous s.
sympathetic part of autonomic
  division of peripheral
  nervous s.
T s.
thoracolumbar s.
uncrossed s.
upper respiratory s.
urogenital s.
uropoietic s.
Vacuflex Reflexology S.
vascular s.
vertebral-basilar s.
vertebral-basilar artery s.
vertebral venous s.
vestibular s.

visceral s.
yang s.
systema skeletale
systematic
  s. desensitization
  s. nutritional muscle testing
    (SNMT)
systemic
  s. circulation
  s. homeostasis
  s. hyperkalemia
  s. illness
  s. lupus erythematosus (SLE)
  s. myelitis
systolic blood pressure
systremma
Syzygium
  S. aromaticum
  S. jambolanum
  S. paniculatum

NOTES

S

T

T cell
T lymphocyte
T system
T tubule

"T"

Autussan "T"

T1-4 group dysfunction
T1-5

T1-5 mobilization with impulse technique
T1-5 muscle energy technique

T1-12 vertebrae
T3-6 group dysfunction
T3-12 mobilization with impulse technique
T5-10 mobilization with impulse technique
T5-12

T5-12 mobilization with impulse technique
T5-12 muscle energy technique

Tabasco pepper
tabatière anatomique
Tabebuia

T. avellanedae
T. heptaphylla
T. impetiginosa

tabetic arthropathy
table

body t.
EZ Lift t.
t. heating pad
HiLo t.
HiLo MultiPro t.
Lloyd flexion distraction t.
MultiPro t.
pedestal massage t.
Simply Wet t.
traction t.
treatment t.

tablet

Advance Defense System T.'s
Bantron T.'s
charcoal t.
GB T.'s
Huang Lian Su T.'s
Jin Bu Huan Anodyne t.
milk thistle t.
Odorless Garlic T.'s

papaya t.
Poison Ivy/Oak T.'s
Potter's Antigian t.
tanning t.
Teething t.
Traumeel t.
White Cohosh t.

taboo

breach of t.

Tabs

Kelp Combination T.

tachyarrhythmia
tachycardia

supraventricular t. (SVT)

tachypnea
tacrine
tactile anesthesia
taenia
Tagamet
Tagetes patula
taheebo tea
tahitensis

Vanilla t.

Tahitian noni juice
Tahiti vanilla
tai, t'ai

t. chi
t. chi chuan
t. chi form
t. ji quan
t. yang
t. yang channel
t. yang medial cervical spondylitis
t. yang syndrome
t. yang type

taiai

sp 3 t.

taibai
taichong

liv 3 t.

Taidecanone
tail

t. bone
setewale capon's t.

tailor's muscle
taixi

ki 3 t.

tai-yang, taiyang

t.-y. axis

tai-yang, taiyang *(continued)*
   t.-y. channel axis
   Ex-HN 2 t.-y.
   t.-y. point
   t.-y. type headache
tai-yin, taiyin
   t.-y. axis
   t.-y. channel axis
   t.-y. point
taiyuan
   lu 9 t.
tajibo
talalgia
talar
   t. restriction
   t. sulcus
talepetrako
tali
   collum t.
   corpus t.
   sulcus t.
   sustentaculum t.
   trochlea t.
   tuberculum laterale processus
     posterioris t.
   tuberculum mediale processus
     posterioris t.
talipedic
talipes
   t. calcaneovalgus
   t. calcaneovarus
   t. calcaneus
   t. cavus
   t. equinovalgus
   t. equinovarus
   t. equinus
   t. plantaris
   t. planus
   t. transversoplanus
   t. valgus
   t. varus
tallow
   t. shrub
   vegetable t.
tall speedwell
talocalcaneal
   t. articulation
   t. dysfunction
   t. joint
   t. ligament
talocalcaneonavicularis
   articulatio t.
talocalcaneonavicular joint

talocrucalis
   pars tibionavicularis ligamenti
     collateralis medialis
     articulationis t.
talocrural
   t. articulation
   t. joint
talocruralis
   articulatio t.
   pars tibiocalcanea ligamenti
     collateralis medialis
     articulationis t.
   pars tibiotalaris anterior
     ligamenti collateralis medialis
     articulationis t.
   pars tibiotalaris posterior
     ligamenti collateralis medialis
     articulationis t.
   regio t.
talofibular ligament
talonavicular
   t. articulation
   t. joint
   t. ligament
taloscaphoid
talotibial
   t. joint
   t. joint dysfunction
   t. mechanics
talotibiofibular mortise
talus
   body of t.
   calcaneal articular surface of t.
   t. dorsiflexed
   head of t.
   interosseous groove of t.
   inverted t.
   lateral malleolar surface of t.
   lateral process of t.
   lateral tubercle of posterior
     process of t.
   medial malleolar facet of t.
   medial tubercle of posterior
     process of t.
   navicular articular surface of t.
   neck of t.
   t. plantar flexed
   posterior process of t.
   pulley of t.
   superior surface of t.
   trochlea of the t.
Tamarindus indica
tamas

tamer
    Tension T.
tamoxifen citrate
tamponade
    cardiac t.
tan
    t. shi zu fei
    t. tien
    t. zhong point
    t. zhou shang rao
Tanacetum
    T. cinerariifolium
    T. parthenium
    T. vulgare
tanakan
tang
    bai he gu jin t.
    bai hu t.
    ban xia huo po t.
    ba wei di huang wan gui
      zhi t.
    ba zhen t.
    ba zheng t.
    black t.
    blasen t.
    bu yang huang wu t.
    bu zhong yi qi t.
    chai hu su gan t.
    ching qi t.
    chuang gui er chen t.
    da cheng qi t.
    da ching qi t.
    dang gui si ni t.
    dan gui xhao yao t.
    er chan t.
    er chen t.
    fu mai t.
    ge gen t.
    ge xian zhu yu t.
    gua luo xie bai bai jiu t.
    gui pi t.
    gui yang t.
    gui zhi t.
    huang lian jie tu t.
    huang qi gui zhi t.
    jin gui shen qi t.
    jing wei t.

    ling jiao gou teng t.
    ling yang ge gen t.
    li zhong t.
    long dan xie gan t.
    long dong xie gan t.
    ma huang xi xin fu zi t.
    ma xing shi gan t.
    pa ting fen zhu t.
    qing su yi qi t.
    qing wei t.
    qing zao jie fei t.
    shao shen mail men dong t.
    shen fu t.
    sheng ye cheng qi t.
    si jun zi t.
    si wu t.
    suan zao ren t.
    tao he cheng qi t.
    tao he si wu t.
    tao hong si wu t.
    tian wan bu xing t.
    tian wang bu xing t.
    wen dan t.
    wen jing t.
    wu zhu yu t.
    xiao chai hu t.
    xi jiao di huang t.
    xue fu zhu yu t.
    xu fu zhu yu t.
    zheng ren yang zhong t.
    zhi gan cao t.
tangantangan oil plant
tangchi
tangential
    t. insertion
    t. needling method
tang-kuei
tangleweed
tankard
    cool t.
tanner's bark
tannic
    t. acid
    t. solution
tannin
tanning tablet

NOTES

tansy
    common t.
    t. extract
    t. oil
    wild t.
tao
    t. he cheng qi tang
    t. he si wu tang
    t. hong si wu tang
    t. ren
    t. te king
taodao
    du 13 t.
taoism
    Chinese t.
taoist
tap
Tap N' Tones
tapotement
tapping
Taraxacum
    T. mongolicum
    T. officinale
tardive dyskinesia
target
    t. end organ viscera
    T. Endurance
    T. Immune
    T. P-14
    T. TS-II
tarragon
    French t.
tarsal
    t. arch
    t. bone
    t. canal
    t. cartilage
    t. joint
    t. ligament
    t. plates
    t. sinus
    t. tunnel syndrome
tarsale
tarsales
    glandulae t.
tarsalgia
tarsalis
tarsectopia
tarsen
tarseus
    arcus t.
tarsi
    musculus tensor t.

    os centrale t.
    ossa t.
    sinus t.
tarsitis
tarsoclasia
tarsoepiphyseal aclasis
tarsomegaly
tarsometatarsal
    t. joint
    t. ligament
tarsometatarsales
    articulationes t.
tarsophalangeal
tarsotarsal
tarsotibial amputation
tarsotomy
TART
    tissue texture changes, asymmetry, restriction of motion, tenderness
tartar root
tartrazine
tarweed
task
    mastery t.
    t. motivational instruction
Tasmanian blue gum
taurine
Taurine Plus
Tawara node
taxation
taxine
taxis
Taxol
taxonomy
taxotere
Taxus
    T. baccata
    T. brevifolia
    T. cuspidata
Taylor Manifest Anxiety scale
TBI
    traumatic brain injury
T-cell
    cytotoxic T.-c.
    T.-c. response
TCM
    traditional Chinese medicine
TCMM
    traditional Chinese materia medica
tea
    arthritis t.
    Avena Sativa Compound in Species Sedative T.

Bartholomew's t.
black t.
blue mountain t.
Bountiful Harvest t.
Brazilian Herbal T.
Brigham t.
Canada t.
catnip t.
chamomile t.
clean air t.
clove t.
cumin-coriander-fennel t.
desert t.
echinacea t.
Essiac t.
eyebright t.
fennel t.
First Color t.
Full Bloom t.
goldenseal t.
green t.
Hemorrhoid T.
horehound t.
hot ginger t.
Inner Voice t.
Insight t.
Jesuit's t.
Kaffree T.
kombucha t.
Labrador T.
lemongrass t.
licorice root t.
linden t.
linden flower t.
liver tonic t.
maitake t.
maté bulk loose t.
Mexican t.
mint t.
Mormon t.
mountain t.
oat-herb t.
oat straw t.
oil of t.
Paraguay t.
pau d'arco t.
pennyroyal herb t.

potato peel t.
raspberry leaf t.
red bush t.
red raspberry t.
rooibos t.
rue t.
safflower t.
sage t.
sassafras t.
savory t.
senna t.
Six Flavor T.
squaw t.
St. Bartholomew's t.
suma t.
taheebo t.
teamster's t.
T. Tonic
t. tree
t. tree oil (TTO)
t. tree oil cream
t. tree oil lotion
t. tree oil oap
t. tree suppository
t. with mint
yellow dock t.
Yew T.
teaberry
teamster's tea
tear
  annular t.
  bucket-handle t.
  intimal t.
  ligamentous t.
  meniscal t.
  Our Lady's t.'s
teasel
tebofortan
tebonin
  T. forte
TECA
  titrated extract of *Centella asiatica*
technique
  acetabular labrum and posterior capsule stretch t.
  acromioclavicular joint functional t.

NOTES

technique *(continued)*

activation force t.
activator t.
active direct t.
active indirect t.
active muscle relaxation t.
active myofascial t.
Acuball t.
adjustive t.
Alexander t.
ankle functional t.
anterior ilium functional t.
articulatory t.
assisted reproductive t. (ART)
autosuggestion t.
awareness release t.
balanced ligamentous tension t.
balance and hold t.
balance and hold functional t.
bilateral lateral stretch t.
bioenergetic synchronization t.
breathing t.
Callahan t.
cellular repatterning t.
cervical articulatory t.
cervical spine functional t.
cervical spine muscle energy t.
cervical spine myofascial t.
cervicothoracic articulatory t.
clavicle muscle energy t.
clean needle t. (CNT)
cognitive avoidance t.
combined t.
concept therapy t.
consolidation t.
continuum movement t.
costal articulatory t.
counterstrain t.
Cox flexion/extension t.
cranial t.
craniosacral t.
craniosacral V t.
craniosacral vault t.
crossed-hand thrust t.
CV t.
CV4 t.
Dalrymple t.
deep tissue massage t.
desensitization t.
dialogue t.
direct t.
direct action t.
direct cranial molding t.

direct method t.
direct motion t.
direct osteopathic
   manipulative t.
disengagement t.
diversified t.
dynamic functional t.
ease-bind functional t.
effleurage massage t.
elbow muscle energy t.
exaggeration t.
external rotation with flexed
   hip muscle energy t.
external rotation with neutral
   hip muscle energy t.
facilitated segmental release t.
fascial release t.
Feldenkrais t.
fibular head functional t.
flexed knee muscle energy t.
flexion-distraction t.
fluid fluctuation t.
foot functional t.
functional t.
functional indirect t.
functional ligamentous
   balance t.
glenohumeral joint functional t.
glenohumeral joint glenoid
   labrum t.
glenohumeral seven step
   Spencer t.
glenoid labrum t.
Gonstead t.
Green glenoid labrum t.
hand functional t.
hand myofascial release t.
hand region myofascial
   release t.
high-velocity low-amplitude t.
high velocity low amplitude
   thrust t.
high velocity thrust t.
hip functional t.
hip myofascial t.
HVLA t.
HVLA thrusting t.
iliac muscle energy t.
iliosacral functional t.
immobilization t.
impulse t.
indirect t.
indirect action t.

indirect ligamentous balance t.
indirect motion t.
infrahyoid node t.
inhibitory myofascial t.
injection t.
innominate shear t.
internal rotation with neutral
hip muscle energy t.
Jacobson relaxation t.
Josephing t.
knee functional t.
lateral meniscus t.
lateral recumbent thrust t.
left on right torsion
functional t.
left sacrum flexed functional t.
leg functional t.
leverage t.
lift t.
ligamentous articular strain t.
Logan basic t.
long-lever t.
lumbar articulatory t.
lumbar spine functional t.
lumbar spine muscle energy t.
lumbosacral spine myofascial
release t.
manipulative therapeutic t.
manual organ stimulation t.
(MOST)
medial and lateral meniscus t.
medial meniscus t.
Mennell diagnostic and
therapeutic joint play t.
metamorphic t.
mind-body t.
mobilization t.
mobilization with impulse t.
mobilization with impulse
direct action t.
mobilization with impulse and
muscle energy t.
mobilization without impulse t.
mobilizing t.
molding t.
movement integration t.
multiple-plane thrust t.

muscle energy t.
muscle mobilizing t.
myofascial t.
myofascial passive t.
myofascial release t.
nasal sinus drainage t.
neuroemotional t.
occipitoatlantal junction
functional t.
Ohashiatsu t.
operator guiding t.
osteopathic manipulative t.
(OMT)
partially flexed hip muscle
energy t.
passive t.
passive myofascial t.
pectoral traction t.
pelvic articulatory t.
pelvis compression functional t.
percussion hammer t.
pétrissage massage t.
Pfrimmer t.
posterior diaphragm myofascial
release t.
posterior ilium functional t.
pressure-point massage t.
projective t.
prone myofascial release t.
prone thrust t.
proximal tibiofibular joint
muscle energy t.
psychosomatic t.
pubes functional t.
pubic muscle energy t.
radial head functional t.
Reichian and Lowenian
Bioenergetic Analysis t.
relaxation t.
release by positioning t.
release by positioning
functional t.
respiratory effort t.
restricted elbow muscle
energy t.
rib-raising t.

T

NOTES

419

technique *(continued)*
right-on-left torsion
functional t.
right sacrum extended
functional t.
rotational t.
RV process down thrust t.
sacral muscle energy t.
sacroiliac functional t.
sacroiliac joint dysfunction
muscle energy t.
sacrooccipital t.
seated thrust t.
self-healing t.
self-mobilizing t.
seven-step Spencer t.
short relaxation t.
shotgun t.
shoulder girdle functional t.
single-plane thrust t.
sitting lumbar spine
functional t.
sitting sternoclavicular joint
dysfunction muscle energy t.
soft tissue t.
soft tissue myofascial t.
Spencer t.
spinal attunement t. (SAT)
spray and stretch t.
springing t.
sternoclavicular joint
dysfunction muscle energy t.
sternum functional t.
stress management t.
suggestion t.
superior trapezius myofascial t.
supine sternoclavicular joint
dysfunction muscle energy t.
supine thrust t.
suprahyoid node t.
Sutherland t.
temporomandibular joint muscle
energy t.
Thompson terminal point t.
thoracic articulatory t.
thoracic spine functional t.
thoracic spine mobilization
with impulse t.
thoracic spine myofascial t.
thoracic spine and ribs
functional t.
thoracolumbar spine
functional t.

thrusting t.
T1-5 mobilization with
impulse t.
T3-12 mobilization with
impulse t.
T5-10 mobilization with
impulse t.
T5-12 mobilization with
impulse t.
T1-5 muscle energy t.
T5-12 muscle energy t.
tonifying t.
touch and relaxation t.
traction t.
transverse process up thrust t.
ulnohumeral joint dysfunction
muscle energy t.
upper cervical t.
venous sinus t.
ventral t.
visceral t.
visualization t.
V-spread t.
warming needle t.
wet towel t.
wrist functional t.
wrist muscle energy t.
tectology
**tectorial membrane of median
atlantoaxial joint**
tectospinal tract
tecuitlatl
Teep
Rubia T.
teeth (*pl. of* tooth)
Teething tablet
Tegafur
Tegam microprocessor thermometer
Tegreen 97
tei fu massage lotion
tejas
telangiectasia
telangiectatic osteogenic sarcoma
telesomatic reaction
temper
choleric t.
temperature
basal body t. (BBT)
core body t.
t. feedback
finger t.
peripheral and core t.

peripheral skin t.
t. variation
temporal
t. arteritis
t. articulation
t. articulation of mandible
t. bone
t. bone articulation
t. fossa
t. lift
t. line
mastoid portion of t.
petrous portion of t.
t. rocking
t. squama
t. tone
temporalis
ala t.
lamina superficialis fasciae t.
t. muscle
temporary
t. callus
t. cartilage
temporomandibular
t. joint (TMJ)
t. joint dysfunction
t. joint muscle energy
technique
t. joint pain
t. joint syndrome
t. joint tomography
t. ligament
t. ligament innervation
temu lawak rhizome
tenacula tendinum
tenaculum, pl. tenacula
tenalgia crepitans
tender
t. nodule
t. point
t. point stimulation
t. spot
tenderness
point t.
tissue texture changes,
asymmetry, restriction of
motion, t. (TART)

tenderpoint
Jones t.
tendinea
chordae t.'s
inscriptio t.
intersectio t.
tendineus
arcus t.
hiatus t.
tendinis
vagina fibrosa t.
vagina synovialis t.
tendinitis, tendonitis
bicipital t.
patellar t.
tendinomuscular meridian
tendinoplasty
tendinosuture
tendinous
t. arch
t. arch of soleus muscle
t. chiasm of the digital
tendons
t. cords
t. hiatus
t. inscription
t. intersection
t. opening
t. sheath of extensor carpi
radialis muscle
t. sheath of extensor carpi
ulnaris muscle
t. sheath of extensor digiti
minimi muscle
t. sheath of extensor hallucis
longus muscle
t. sheath of extensor pollicis
longus muscle
t. sheath of flexor carpi
radialis muscle
t. sheath of flexor hallucis
longus muscle
t. sheath of flexor pollicis
longus muscle
t. sheath of superior oblique
muscle

NOTES

T

tendinous *(continued)*
    t. sheath of tibialis anterior muscle
    t. sheath of tibialis posterior muscle
    t. synovitis
tendinum
    chiasma t.
    juncturae t.
    retinaculum t.
    tenacula t.
tendo
    t. Achillis
    t. Achillis reflex
    t. calcaneus
    t. conjunctivus
tendolysis
tendon
    Achilles t.
    calcaneal t.
    t. cell
    central t.
    t. changing qigong
    conjoined t.
    conjoint t.
    flexor t.
    t. graft
    hamstring t.
    heel t.
    influential point of t.
    t. insertion
    mucous sheath of t.
    t. palpation
    patellar t.
    pectoralis minor t.
    psoas minor t.
    t. reflex
    t. spindle
    t. suture
    tendinous chiasm of the digital t.'s
    t. transplantation
    trifoliate central t.
    vincula of t.'s
tendonitis *(var. of* tendinitis)
tendosynovitis
tendovaginitis
    radial styloid t.
tenesemus
teng, t'eng
    ji xue t.
    lei gong t., lei-kung teng
    lei-kung t.

tenia
teniposide
tennis
    t. elbow
    t. leg
    t. thumb
tenodesis
tenodynia
tenolysis
tenonitis
tenontitis
tenontodynia
tenontography
tenontology
tenontothecitis
tenophyte
tenostosis
tenosynovitis
    t. crepitans
    de Quervain t.
    localized nodular t.
    pigmented villonodular t.
    postpartum de Quervain t.
    stenosing t.
    villous t.
tenotomy
    subcutaneous t.
tenovaginitis
TENS
    transcutaneous electrical nerve stimulation
    acupuncture-like TENS
    conventional TENS
    TENS device
    TENS machine
    TENS pad
    TENS unit
tense pulse
tensiometer
tension
    t. back pain
    balanced t.
    balanced membranous t.
    chronic muscle t.
    t. curve
    dynamic t.
    dynamic reciprocal t.
    t. headache
    muscle t.
    myofascial t.
    t. neck
    striate muscle t.

T. Tamer
tissue t.
tensor
t. fasciae latae
t. fasciae latae muscle
t. of fascia lata
t. muscle of fascia lata
tent
Tentex Forte
tentorial notch
tentorium
t. cerebelli
t. cerebelli torsion
t. cerebri
Tenue
Extractum Filicis Maris T.
tenuifolia
Polygala t.
teratogenic
ter in die **(t.i.d.)**
teres
t. major muscle
t. minor muscle
t. muscle
musculus pronator t.
musculus pronator radii t.
teretis
caput humerale musculi
pronatoris t.
caput ulnare musculi
pronatoris t.
tergal
tergum
terminad
terminal
t. barrier
t. crest
excitatory t.
t. filum
inhibitory t.
t. line
t. objective
terminale
filum t.
Terminalia
T. bellerica
T. chebula

terminalis
crista t.
termini generales
terminus
terpene lactone
Terra Maxa
territory
sagittal t.
tertius
digitus manus t. [III]
musculus fibularis t.
musculus peroneus t.
peroneus t.
test
absorption t.
acromion drop t.
Adson t.
Allen t.
anterior apprehension t.
anterior superior iliac spine t.
anteroposterior translation t.
antinuclear antibody t.
Apley compression t.
Apley scratch t.
apprehension t.
arm drop t.
atlas motion t.
backward bending t.
backward bent t.
ballottement t.
Barlow t.
bending t.
bi-digital O-ring t.
blind t.
bulge t.
Bunnel-Littler t.
cervical flexion t.
compression t.
costoclavicular t.
crank t.
De Kleyn t.
discontinuation t.
dominant eye t.
drawer t.
drop arm t.
D-xylose t.
effusion knee joint t.

T

NOTES

test *(continued)*
Erichsen t.
erythema t.
extension compression t.
external compression t.
FABERE t.
Finkelstein t.
flexion t.
four-point sacral motion t.
Gillet t.
t. of hamstring muscle
hands-off t.
hip drop t.
Hoover t.
hyperabduction t.
iliac crest levelness t.
imbalance t.
impingement t.
inferior lateral angle t.
ischial tuberosity level t.
IV phentolamine t.
Jones t.
Kraus-Weber t.
Lachman t.
lateral translation t.
leg length t.
leg length at medial
malleolus t.
length t.
lumbar spring t.
Mantoux t.
McMurray t.
McMurray meniscal t.
motion t.
neural limb tension t.
neurophysiological t.
Ober t.
one-legged stork t.
palpatory t.
patellofemoral grinding t.
Patrick t.
Patrick FABERE t.
Phalen t.
pivot shift t.
posterior superior iliac spine,
sacral base, and L5 t.
t. profile
prone iliac crest height t.
provocative t.
psoas muscle tension t.
pubic symphysis levelness t.
recurvatum t.
relocation t.
restricted abduction t.
rheumatological t.
sacroiliac motion by gapping t.
sacroiliac motion spring t.
sacroiliac rocking t.
sacrotuberous ligament
tension t.
seated bending t.
seated flexion t.
seated trunk bending t.
sidebending rotation t.
sitting flexion t.
skin rolling t.
sphinx t.
spring t.
squat t.
standing bending t.
standing flexion t.
standing trunk bending t.
straight leg raising t.
stress t.
sulcus t.
supine cervical flexion t.
supine iliac crest height t.
supine pubic symphysis
height t.
sutural motion t.
Thomas t.
Trendelenburg t.
trunk bending t.
trunk sidebending t.
upper cervical complex
stress t.
upper extremity muscle
imbalance diagnostic t. 1
upper extremity muscle
imbalance diagnostic t. 2
upper extremity muscle
imbalance diagnostic t. 3
upper extremity muscle
imbalance diagnostic t. 4
varus-valgus stress t.
Yergason t.

testing
cervical spine motion t.
elbow motion t.
extensibility t.
gross motion t.
histocompatibility t.
indirect intersegmental
motion t.
individual vertebral motion t.
innominate motion t.

intersegmental motion t.
laboratory t.
leukocytotoxic t.
lumbar spine motion t.
mobility t.
motion t.
muscle t. (MT)
muscle strength t.
occiput motion t.
pelvic motion t.
posterior superior iliac spine
motion t.
radial motion t.
regional motion t.
rib motion t.
rotoscoliosis t.
sacral motion t.
sensation t.
spinal motion t.
spine motion t.
strength t.
susceptibility t.
systematic nutritional muscle t.
(SNMT)
thoracic spine motion t.
translatory motion t.
upper back strength t.
testosterone
tetanic
t. contraction
t. spastic contraction
tetanus
neonatal t.
tetany
tether
biomechanical t.
tethered cord
tethering
tetraamelia
tetrabrachius
tetrachirus
tetrachloride
carbon t.
tetracycline
tetradactyl
tetragon lumbale

tetragonoloba
Cyamopsis t.
tetragonus
musculus t.
tetrahydropalmatine
tetrandra
Stephania t.
tetraperomelia
tetrapus
tetrascelus
tetterwort, tetter wort
Teucrium
T. canadense
T. chamaedrys
T. scorodonia
teucrium
texture
asymmetry, range of motion, t.
TFT
Thought Field Therapy
Thai massage
thalictroides
Caulophyllum t.
thapsus
Verbascum t.
THC
delta-9-tetrahydrocannabinol
thebaine poppy
thecal
t. abscess
t. whitlow
thenad
thenal
thenar
t. eminence
t. muscle
t. prominence
t. space
thenaris
eminentia t.
thenen
Theobroma cacao
theophylline
theory
capsular compression t.
five element t.
gate-control t.

NOTES

theory *(continued)*
Integration of Natural
Systems T.
Jungian t.
meniscus entrapment t.
meniscus extrapment t.
meridian t.
Ollier t.
overproduction t.
wen bing t.
therapeutic
t. anesthesia
t. effect
t. enema
energy-field t.
t. environment
t. exercise
t. guidelines
t. imagery and dialogue
t. index
t. liquid
t. massage
t. measure
t. mode
t. monitoring
t. needling
t. nutrition
t. procedure
t. range
t. ratio
t. response
t. touch (TT)
t. use
t. vomiting
therapeutics
Aston t.
biofield t.
manipulative t.
physiologic t.
physiological t.
therapist
bioenergetic t.
chelation t.
colon t.
craniosacral t.
dance t.
neural t.
occupational t.
physical t.
remedial t.
therapy
alternative t.
Amma t.

anterior lift t.
antiaging drug t.
antineoplaston t.
art t.
attunement t.
autolymphocyte t.
behavior t.
behavioral t.
being t.
Benjamin system of
muscular t.
biofeedback t.
biomagnetic t.
bio-oxidative t.
body t.
Bristol diet t.
Callanetics t.
cell t.
cellular t.
chelation t.
chest physical t.
Chinese dietary t.
cleansing t.
cognitive t.
cognitive behavior t. (CBT)
cold t.
cold laser t.
colon t.
color t.
colored-light t.
complementary t.
conventional t.
cranial t.
craniosacral t.
cymatic t.
dance t.
detoxification t.
DHEA t.
diet t.
diurnal t.
doing t.
electrical stimulation t.
electromagnetic t.
energetic t.
energy t.
enzymatic t.
enzyme t.
exercise t.
fasting t.
fresh cell t.
glandular t.
growth hormone t.
heat t.

Heilig formula for lift t.
hematogenic oxidation t.
herbal t.
herbal bath t.
high-dose nutrient t.
high-dose vitamin t.
hormone replacement t.
humanistic t.
humor t.
humoral t.
hyperbaric oxygen t.
immunoaugmentative t. (IAT)
inhalation t.
intravenous nutrient t.
isometric t.
juice t.
ki-shiatsu bodywork t.
laughter t.
LeShan t.
lift t.
light t.
live cell t.
Livingston-Wheeler t.
LoowenWork t.
lymph drainage t.
maggot debridement t. (MDT)
magnet t.
magnetic t.
maintenance t.
manipulation t.
manual medicine t.
manual trigger point t.
marma t.
massage t.
meganutrient t.
megavitamin t.
meridian t.
metabolic t.
microwave resonance t.
mind-body t.
movement t.
muscle t.
music t.
myofascial release t.
neural t.
neural organization t.
occupational t.

oligo t.
oral t.
Oriental bodywork t.
orthomolecular t.
oxidative t.
oxygen t.
ozone t.
pain t.
past life t.
peripheral stimulation t.
pet t.
Pfrimmer deep muscle t.
Phoenix Rising yoga t.
photodynamic t.
physical t.
polarity t.
postural t.
prayer t.
pressure point t.
progressive relaxation t.
proliferant t.
proliferation t.
psychodynamic t.
psychophysiological t.
PUVA t.
reconstructive t.
rejuvenation t.
relaxation t.
restricted environmental
    stimulation t.
restriction of environmental
    stimulation t. (REST)
sensory t.
shamanic t.
shen t.
shen physioemotional release t.
soft tissue t.
sotai t.
sound t.
spa t.
spectrochrome t.
speech t.
spinal manipulative t. (SMT)
sports t.
steam inhalation t.
St. John method of
    neuromuscular t.

T

NOTES

therapy *(continued)*
 strain-counterstrain t.
 sweat t.
 thermal t.
 Thought Field T. (TFT)
 traditional t.
 Trager t.
 transfusion t.
 transpersonal t.
 trauma release t.
 trigger point t.
 trigger point injection t.
 (TPIT)
 Upledger craniosacral t.
 UV light t.
 virilization t.
 visual art t.
 water t.
 Zen t.
 zone t.
therapy-resistant case
theriacaria
thermal
 t. biofeedback
 t. feedback
 t. plastic wrap
 t. space blanket
 t. therapy
thermistor
thermodilution
thermography
thermology
thermomassage
thermometer
 Tegam microprocessor t.
thermophilus
 Streptococcus t.
theta
 t. EEG
 t. EEG wave
 t. wave
 t. wave production
thiamine
 t. deficiency
 red blood cell t.
thick tongue
thigh
 biceps muscle of t.
 t. bone
 deep fascia of t.
 t. joint
 t. pain
 posterior region of t.

 posterior surface of t.
 quadrate muscle of t.
 quadriceps muscle of t.
 rectus muscle of t.
Thim-J
thin
 t. acupuncture needle
 t. disposable cannula
 t. flow
 t. needle
 t. pulse
thin-layer chromatography (TLC)
thioctic acid
Thioproline
third
 t. chakra
 t. cranial nerve [CN III]
 t. cuneiform bone
 t. eye
 t. finger
 t. peroneal muscle
 t. toe
 t. trochanter
thirst
 big t.
Thisilyn Pro
thistle
 Beyond Milk T.
 bird-lime t.
 blessed t.
 carline t.
 holt t.
 holy t.
 lady's t.
 Marian t.
 milk t.
 spotted t.
 St. Benedict's t.
 St. Mary's t.
 tiger t.
thixotropic property
thixotropy
Thomas
 T. balsam
 T. test
Thompson terminal point technique
thoracal
thoraces (*pl. of* thorax)
thoracic
 t. aorta
 t. aperture
 t. articulatory technique
 t. axis

t. cage
t. cavity
t. connective tissue
t. cord tumor
t. dermatome
t. disk
t. duct
t. facet
t. ganglion
t. girdle
t. inlet
t. interspinales muscle
t. interspinal muscle
t. intertransversarii muscle
t. intertransverse muscle
t. lateral chain ganglion
t. limb
t. longissimus muscle
t. lymphatic pump
t. nerves [T1–T12]
t. outlet
t. outlet syndrome
t. pump
t. pumping
t. rotator muscle
t. rule of 3s
t. spine
t. spine extension
t. spine flattening
t. spine functional technique
t. spine mobilization with
  impulse technique
t. spine motion
t. spine motion testing
t. spine myofascial technique
t. spine osteology
t. spine and ribs functional
  technique
t. spine shrug
t. spine unwinding
t. tender point
t. tissue texture changes
t. vertebra
t. vertebrae [T1–T12]
t. wall
thoracica
  ganglion t.

thoracicae
  vertebrae t. [T1–T12]
thoracici
  pars abdominalis ductus t.
  pars cervicalis ductus t.
  pars thoracica ductus t.
thoracicoabdominal
thoracicoacromial
thoracicohumeral
thoracic-pelvic-phalangeal dystrophy
thoracicus
  ductus t.
  skeleton t.
thoracis
  cavitas t.
  cavum t.
  compages t.
  musculi t.
  musculi intertransversarii t.
  musculi rotatores t.
  musculus iliocostalis t.
  musculus interspinalis t.
  musculus longissimus t.
  musculus rectus t.
  musculus semispinalis t.
  musculus spinalis t.
  musculus transversus t.
thoracoabdominal diaphragm
thoracoacromialis
  rete acromiale arteriae t.
thoracoacromial trunk
thoracodorsal
thoracolumbalis
  fascia t.
thoracolumbar
  t. aponeurosis
  t. fascia
  t. ganglion
  t. and lumbar spine
  t. spine functional technique
  t. system
thoracolumbosacral orthosis
thoracopagus
thoracoplasty
thoracoschisis
thorax, pl. thoraces
  innervation of t.

T

NOTES

thorax *(continued)*
    muscles of t.
    semispinal muscle of t.
    spinal muscle of t.
    transverse muscle of t.
thormantle
thorn
    t. apple
    Egyptian t.
    goat's t.
thorny bur
thoroughwort
thought
    automatic t.
    danger t.
Thought Field Therapy (TFT)
thousand-leaf
thready pulse
threat perception
three
    balance testing level t.
    t. diaphragms
    Nature's T.
    t. times a day (t.i.d.)
three-cornered bone
three-dimensional assessment
three-phase bone scan
threonine
threshold
    cutaneous t.
    pain t.
thridace
throat chakra
throatwort
thrombin
    human t.
thrombocyte
thrombocytopenia
thrombosis, pl. **thromboses**
    cerebral t.
    coronary t.
    venous t.
thrombotic stroke
throwwort
thrust
    t. force
    high-velocity t.
    high-velocity short-amplitude t.
    quick t.
    rebound t.
    recoil t.
    rotational t.

thrusting
    t. force
    t. technique
    t. vessel
thryallis
thuja
Thuja orientalis
thumb
    adductor muscle of t.
    bifid t.
    carpometacarpal joint of t.
    gamekeeper's t.
    hitchhiker's t.
    long abductor muscle of t.
    long extensor muscle of t.
    long flexor muscle of t.
    opposer muscle of t.
    short abductor muscle of t.
    short extensor muscle of t.
    short flexor muscle of t.
    tennis t.
    t. walk
thunder god vine
Thursday Plantation Tea Tree oil
thus
    gum t.
thyme
    common t.
    garden t.
    rubbed t.
thymus
    t. gland
    T. vulgaris
thyroarytenoideus
    musculus t.
thyroarytenoid muscle
thyrocervical
thyroepiglottic muscle
thyroglossal
thyrohyal
thyrohyoid
thyroid
    t. axis
    t. body
    t. colloid
    t. disorder
    t. eminence
    t. gland
    t. hormone
    t. hormone level
    t. hormone release
    pyramid of t.
    underactive t.

thyroidea
t. accessoria
cartilago t.
glandula t.
thyroideae
cornu inferius cartilaginis t.
cornu superius cartilaginis t.
linea obliqua cartilaginis t.
musculus levator glandulae t.
thyroid-stimulating hormone (TSH)
thyropalatine
thyrotropin-releasing hormone
thyroxine
TIA
transient ischemic attack
tian
ba ji t.
t. kuei
middle dan t.
upper dan t.
t. wan bu xing tang
t. wang bu xing tang
tianchi
pe 1 t.
tianrong
si 17 t.
tianshu
t. point
st 25 t.
tiantu
ren 22 t.
tianzhu
ub 10 t.
tianzong
si 11 t.
tiaokou
st 38 t.
Tibetan
T. Buddhist meditation
T. medicine
tibia
body of t.
t. externally rotated
fibular articular surface of t.
t. internally rotated
interosseous border of t.
lateral condyle of t.

lateral surface of t.
malleolar articular surface of t.
medial border of t.
medial condyle of t.
medial surface of t.
posterior intercondylar area
of t.
posterior surface of t.
saber t.
shaft of t.
spinous process of t.
superior articular surface of t.
t. valga
t. vara
tibiad
tibiae
area intercondylaris anterior t.
area intercondylaris posterior t.
condylus lateralis t.
condylus medialis t.
corpus t.
margo anterior t.
margo interosseus t.
margo medialis t.
tuberositas t.
tibial
t. border of foot
t. collateral ligament
t. crest
t. lateral ligament
t. malleolus
t. muscle
t. nerve
t. torsion
t. tuberosity
tibiale posticum
tibialis
t. anterior
t. anterior muscle
apophysitis t.
t. posterior muscle
tibiocalcaneal
t. ligament
t. part of deltoid ligament
tibiocalcanean
tibiofascialis

T

NOTES

431

tibiofemoral
t. index
tibiofibular
t. articulation
t. joint
t. joint motion
t. ligament
t. syndesmosis
tibiofibularis
syndesmosis t.
tibionavicular
t. ligament
t. part of deltoid ligament
tibioperoneal
tibioscaphoid
tibiotarsal
t.i.d.
ter in die
three times a day
tidal fever
tien
tan t.
tiger
T. Balm
t. thistle
tightening end feel
tight-loose concept
tightness
superficial t.
tight pulse
tiglium
Croton t.
Tilia
T. cordata
T. platyphyllos
T. tomentosa
T. vulgaris
tilt
anterior pelvic t.
dorsal t.
metacarpal joint dorsal t.
pelvic t.
pelvis t.
short leg/pelvic t.
tilting of pelvis
time
bleeding t.
t. management
palliation, quality, radiation, severity, t. (PQRST)
partial prothrombin t. (PTT)
position, quality, radiation, severity, t. (PQRST)

prothrombin t. (PT)
sensory conduction t.
timo
tinctoria
Alkanna t.
Anchusa t.
Baptisia t.
Indigo t.
Podalyria t.
tinctorius
Carthamus t.
tinctorum
Rubia t.
tincture
aloe vesta perineal benzoin compound t.
t. of benzoin
T. Collinson
compound benzoin t.
croton t.
echinacea mother t.
homeopathic t.
lobelia t.
yerba maté t.
tinea pedis
Tinel sign
ting
t. point
t. zhi wan
tinggong
si 19 t.
tinghui
gb 2 t.
tingling
Tinnevelly senna
tinnitus
tip
bifid t.
t. of elbow
tiredness
Tirgon
tisane
tissue
adipose t.
areolar t.
cancellous t.
chondroid t.
connective t.
cutaneous soft t.
dense connective t.
fibrous t.
t. granulation
granulation t.

gut-associated lymphoid t.
  (GALT)
t. heating
t. level
t. loading
loose areolar t.
loose connective t.
muscle t.
muscular t.
necrotic t.
nervous t.
read the t.
t. resilience
t. response
soft t.
t. stretching
subcutaneous t.
t. tension
t. tension balance
t. texture abnormality (TTA)
t. texture changes
t. texture changes, asymmetry,
  restriction of motion,
  tenderness (TART)
thoracic connective t.
t. viability
violation of t.
wring out t.
titrated extract of *Centella asiatica*
  (TECA)
TLC
  thin-layer chromatography
TM
  transcendental meditation
TMJ
  temporomandibular joint
TM-Siddhi
  T.-S. meditation
  T.-S. program
TNF
  tumor necrosis factor
TNM staging
toad
  Chinese t.
  t. venom
to-and-fro
  t.-a.-f. anesthesia

t.-a.-f. oscillation
t.-a.-f. rocking
tobacco
  Indian t.
  t. leaf
  mountain t.
  smokeless t.
  t. wood
tocopherol
  alpha t.
  t. compound
  d-gamma t.
toe

  abductor muscle of great t.
  abductor muscle of little t.
  adductor muscle of great t.
  claw t.
  t. extensor muscle
  fifth t.
  t. flexor muscle
  fourth t.
  great t.
  hammer t., hammertoe
  lateral surface of t.
  long extensor muscle of t.
  long extensor muscle of
    great t.
  long flexor muscle of t.
  long flexor muscle of great t.
  medial surface of t.
  Morton t.
  muscle t.
  t. off
  painful t.
  plantar surface of t.
  second t.
  short extensor muscle of t.
  short extensor muscle of
    great t.
  short flexor muscle of t.
  short flexor muscle of great t.
  short flexor muscle of little t.
  stiff t.
  third t.
  web of t.'s
toe-drop

T

NOTES

toeing
    t. in
    t. out
toenail
    ingrowing t.
tofu
tolerance
    glucose t.
    species t.
tolerant
tolguacha
tolle causam
Tolu
    T. balsam
    balsam of T.
Toluifera balsamum
tolutana
    resina t.
tolutanum
    balsamum t.
tome
    somatosensory distribution t.
tomentosa
    Tilia t.
    Uncaria t.
tomentosum
    Phoradendron t.
tomography
    computed t. (CT)
    conventional t.
    temporomandibular joint t.
tonco (*var. of* tonga)
tone
    atonic muscle t.
    autonomic t.
    basal t.
    hypotonic muscle t.
    LC T.
    muscle t.
    pisiform t.
    Tap N' T.'s
    temporal t.
    vasomotor t.
tong
    mu t.
tonga, tonco, tonquin (*var. of*
    tonka)
tongli
    he 5 t.
tongue
    t. diagnosis
    furring of the t.
    furrowing of the t.

t. grass
green t.
t. moss
ox's t.
pale t.
purple t.
scalloping of the t.
thick t.
yellow t.
tongziliao
    gb 1 t.
tonic
    alfalfa t.
    cardiac t.
    t. contraction
    t. effect
    t. headache
    herbal t.
    Jade Screen Immune T.
    t. muscle
    skin t.
    Tea T.
tonification
    electrical t.
    t. point
    supplementary t.
tonify
tonifying
    t. effect
    t. method
    t. needling
    t. stimulation
    t. technique
toning exercise
tonka, tonga
    t. bean
    t. seed
tonquin (*var. of* tonga)
Tonquin musk
Tonsilgon-N
tonsillitis
tonus
    myogenic t.
tooth, pl. teeth
    t. grinding
    lion's t.
toothache tree
toothpick ammi
tootsie roll sign
top
    broom t.
    flowering t.
    Irish broom t.

Red Clover T.'s
Scotch broom t.
tophaceous gout
topical
- t. anesthesia
- t. anesthetic
- t. antiseptic
- t. boil
- t. capsaicin
- t. phototherapy
- t. podophyllotoxin
- t. solution
- t. vitamin C
topographic anatomy
topography
Toradol
tormentil
torque unwinding
torr
torsades de pointes
torsion
- angle of t.
- backward t.
- cranial t.
- t. dystonia
- external t.
- external rib t.
- forward t.
- forward sacral t.
- t. fracture
- left arm left sacral t.
- left on left forward sacral t.
- left-on-left sacral t.
- left-on-right sacral t.
- mandible t.
- t. neurosis
- occiput t.
- orbit t.
- rib t.
- right-on-left t.
- right-on-left sacral t.
- right-on-right t.
- sacral t.
- sacroiliac joint left-on-left t.
- sacroiliac joint right-on-left t.
- tentorium cerebelli t.
- tibial t.

torsional
- t. deformity
- t. dysfunction
- t. movement
- t. strain
- t. stress
torsionometer
torso
- t. curl
- t. curl exercise
- t. extension
- t. extension exercise
torticollis
- acute spastic t.
- congenital t.
- muscular t.
- spasmodic t.
- spastic t.
- spurious t.
tortipelvis
torula yeast
torus
- t. fracture
- t. manus
tosylate
- bretylium t.
total
- t. body hypothermia
- t. body lymphatic screen
- t. elasticity of muscle
- t. energy
- t. lesion osteopathy
- t. spinal anesthesia
t'ou
- niu she t.
touch
- deep t.
- healing t.
- T. for Health
- intentional t.
- Kofutu t.
- light t.
- noncontact therapeutic t.
- t. provider
- t. and relaxation technique
- therapeutic t. (TT)
TouchAmerica BodyTable

NOTES

435

touch-and-heal
    amber t.-a.-h.
touching
    pulse t.
touch-me-not
tough
tou mo
tourniquet
    Esmarch t.
toute-bonne
touwei
    st 8 t.
tox
    Rhus t.
toxemia
toxic
    t. congestion
    t. debris
toxicity
    aluminum t.
    dichromate t.
    endogenous t.
    exogenous t.
    nutmeg t.
    oleander t.
    oxygen t.
    podophyllin t.
    renal tubular t.
    selenium t.
toxicodendron
    t. dermatitis
    T. diversilobum
    T. quercifolium
    T. radicans
    Rhus t., Rhus tox
    Rhus t.
    T. vernix
toxicologic
toxicologist
toxicology
toxicopathic
toxigenic diarrhea
toxin
    cellular t.
    Coley t.
    emotional t.
    environmental t.
    t. load
toxin-induced cardiopathy
toxinosis
toxonosis
TPIT
    trigger point injection therapy

trabecula
trabecular network
trace
    t. element
    t. mineral
trachea
tracheal intubation
trachealis muscle
trachelalis
trachelian
tracheloclavicularis
    musculus t.
tracheloclavicular muscle
trachelomastoid
trachelos
tracheloschisis
track
    right t.
tracking
    joint t.
    lateral meniscal t.
    t. mechanism
    medial meniscal t.
    meniscal t.
    patellar t.
tract
    anterolateral t. (ALT)
    crossed t.
    dorsolateral t. (DLT)
    iliotibial t.
    lateral corticospinal t.
    lateral pyramidal t.
    lateral spinothalamic t.
    olivospinal t.
    t. plant
    respiratory t.
    reticulospinal t.
    rubrospinal t.
    spinal t.
    spinothalamic t. (STT)
    tectospinal t.
    uncrossed t.
    upper digestive t.
    urinary t.
    ventral cortical spinal t.
    vestibulospinal t.
traction
    t. epiphysis
    gravity lumbar t.
    halo t.
    t. headache
    head halter cervical t.
    isometric t.

436

isotonic t.
linear t.
lower neck linear t.
pelvic t.
perpendicular t.
perpendicular thoracic spine t.
skeletal t.
skin t.
t. table
t. technique
t. treatment
tractor
tractus iliotibialis
traditional
t. application
t. Chinese acupuncture
t. Chinese concept
t. Chinese diagnosis
t. Chinese materia medica
(TCMM)
t. Chinese medicine (TCM)
t. Chinese syndrome
t. classification of symptoms
t. diagnostic category
t. idea
t. medicine
t. method
t. pulse diagnosis
t. therapy
traditionally chosen point
traffic
neural t.
tragacanth
Bassora t.
gum t.
Indian t.
Syrian t.
t. tree
tragacantha
Sterculia t.
tragacanthae
gummi t.
Trager
T. bodywork
T. Mentastics
T. psychophysical integration
T. therapy

Tragering
Tragerwork
trailing mahonia
trail mix
training
alpha-theta brainwave t.
assertiveness t.
autogenic t.
biofeedback relaxation t.
gait t.
high-intensity progressive
resistance t.
home t.
movement t.
progressive relaxation t. (PRT)
relaxation t.
sensory motor balance t.
stress inoculation t.
train-of-four stimulus
train of pulse
trait anxiety
trajectory
trance
hypnotic t.
t. logic
trance-like state
tranquera
la t.
tranquilizer
transaminase
gamma aminobutyric acid t.
serum glutamic-pyruvic t.
(SGPT)
transcarpal ligament
transcendence
transcendental meditation (TM)
transcendent intuition
transcervical fracture
transcondylar fracture
**transcutaneous electrical nerve
stimulation (TENS)**
transfer
information t.
muscle t.
qi t.

T

NOTES

437

transferase
  catecholamine O-methyl t. (COMT)
transference
  positive t.
transferring
transfix
transformation
transfusion therapy
transient
  t. ischemic attack (TIA)
  t. synovitis of hip
transiliac
transischiac
transition
  cervicothoracic t.
  t. phase
transitional
  t. region
  t. segment
  t. vertebral segment
translated sacrum
translation
  t. along axis
  t. anterior
  t. caudad
  t. cephalic
  t. laterally
  t. posterior
translational region
translatory
  t. motion
  t. motion testing
  t. movement
transmission
  pain t.
  peripheral afferent t.
transmural
transosseous venography
transparent dressing
transpersonal
  t. imagery
  t. medicine
  t. therapy
transplant
  bone marrow t.
transplantar
transplantation
  t. genetics
  tendon t.
transport
  axoplasmic t.
  t. point

transpyloric plane
transpyloricum
  planum t.
transsegmental
transurethral resection of the
  prostate (TURP)
transversa
  articulatio tarsi t.
  diameter t.
transversalis
  arcus pedis t.
transversarium
  foramen t.
transverse
  t. arch
  t. arch of foot
  t. atlantal ligament
  t. atlas ligament
  t. axis
  t. axis of sacrum
  t. carpal ligament
  t. costal facet
  t. crural ligament
  t. diameter
  t. fasciculi
  t. foramen
  t. genicular ligament
  t. head
  t. humeral ligament
  t. ligament of acetabulum
  t. ligament of the atlas
  t. ligament of elbow
  t. ligament of knee
  t. ligament of leg
  t. metacarpal ligament
  t. metatarsal ligament
  t. muscle of abdomen
  t. muscle of nape
  t. muscle of thorax
  t. myelitis
  t. myelopathy
  t. plane
  t. process
  t. process up thrust technique
  t. process of vertebra
  t. ridges of sacrum
  t. section
  t. sinus
  t. tarsal articulation
  t. tarsal joint
  t. tibiofibular ligament

transversi
foramen processus t.
fovea costalis processus t.
transversocostal
transversoplanus
talipes t.
transversospinales muscle
transversospinal muscle
transversum
septum t.
transversus
t. abdominis muscle
t. nuchae muscle
t. thoracis muscle
Tranzone
trapezial
trapeziform
trapezii
tuberculum ossis t.
trapeziometacarpal
trapezium
t. bone
oblique ridge of t.
os t.
trapezius
t. muscle
t. muscle hypertonicity
musculus t.
trapezoid
t. bone
t. ligament
t. line
t. ridge
trapezoidea
linea t.
trapezoideum
os t.
Traube semilunar space
trauma
birth t.
Kundalini t.
physical t.
t. release therapy
rotary torque t.
skull t.
spiritual emergence t.
t. with hemorrhage

traumatic
t. alteration
t. amputation
t. anemia
t. anesthesia
t. aneurysm
t. bone cyst
t. brain injury (TBI)
t. cervical discopathy
t. compression
t. episode
t. lateral strain
t. synovitis
t. vertical strain
Traumeel
T. Homeopathic Formula
T. ointment
T. oral drops
T. oral liquid
T. tablet
Travel-Caps
Travell
T. myofascial trigger point
T. and Simons myofascial
trigger point
T. tender point
T. trigger point
Traxaton
treacle
rustic t.
treasure
Women's T.
treatment
acupuncture t.
antihypertensive t.
articulation t. (ART)
articulatory t.
balanced ligamentous tension t.
(BLT)
biobehavioral t.
blue light t.
cell t.
chakra acupuncture t.
contact, control, test,
evaluate, t. (CCTET)
craniosacral t. (CST)
Dalrymple t.

NOTES

T

treatment *(continued)*
    direct t. (D, DIR)
    electromagnetic energy t.
    emergency t.
    energetic t.
    equilibration t.
    exaggeration t.
    facilitated positional release t.
    fascial release t.
    FPR t.
    functional t.
    Galbraith t.
    herbal t.
    indirect t. (I, IND)
    kudzu t.
    laser t.
    learning-based t.
    Livingston t.
    long-term t.
    lymphatic pump t.
    manipulative t.
    manual t.
    ME t.
    MFR t.
    mobilization without impulse
      (articulatory) t.
    multimodal t.
    muscle energy t.
    myofascial release t.
    needle t.
    osteopathic manipulative t.
      (OMT)
    pain t.
    passive t.
    positional t.
    principle of t.
    radiation t.
    range of motion t.
    Revici t.
    saline t.
    t. sequence
    serratus anterior t.
    t. session
    soft tissue t. (ST)
    springing t.
    t. table
    traction t.
    UV light t.
    visceral manipulative t. (VIS)
treatment-emergent
tree
    African coffee t.
    African plum t.

    ague t.
    American dwarf palm t.
    angelica t.
    bay t.
    benjamin t.
    benzoin t.
    cacao t.
    camphor t.
    camptothecin t.
    chaste t.
    cola t.
    corkwood t.
    European spindle t.
    fever t.
    fish poison t.
    fringe t.
    God's t.
    gum t.
    hemp t.
    Jaborandi t.
    Joshua t.
    karaya t.
    kousso t.
    lime t.
    melon t.
    pipe t.
    t. sage
    snowball t.
    snow-drop t.
    soap t.
    spindle t.
    strawberry t.
    tea t.
    t. tea oil lozenges
    toothache t.
    tragacanth t.
    trumpet t.
    varnish t.
    wonder t.
tree-of-life
trefoil
    marsh t.
tremor
tremulor
Trendelenburg test
trepanation
tretinoin
Trevor disease
Trexam
triad
    diagnostic t.
    O'Donaghue t.

trial
  clinical t.
  controlled t.
  crossover t.
  Multiple Risk Factor
    Intervention T. (MRFIT)
  Phase I t.
  Phase II t.
  Phase III t.
  Phase IV t.
  placebo-controlled t.
  preclinical t.
  randomized t.
  randomized controlled t. (RCT)
triamelia
Triana
  Gonolobus condurango (T.)
  Nichols
triangle
  anal t.
  t. of auscultation
  axillary t.
  Béclard t.
  cervical t.
  Codman t.
  deltoideopectoral t.
  Elaut t.
  t. of elbow
  Farabeuf t.
  femoral t.
  Grynfeltt t.
  iliofemoral t.
  infraclavicular t.
  interscalene t.
  Labbé t.
  Langenbeck t.
  Lesshaft t.
  lumbar t.
  lumbocostoabdominal t.
  Marcille t.
  omoclavicular t.
  omotracheal t.
  Petit lumbar t.
  sacral t.
  t. of safety
  Scarpa t.
  sternocostal t.

  subclavian t.
  supraclavicular t.
  urogenital t.
  Ward t.
triangular
  t. bandage
  t. bone
  t. cartilage
  t. deltoid ligament
  t. disk of wrist
  t. muscle
triangulare
  os t.
triangularis
triangulum
tribe
  Muscle T.
tribrachia
tribrachius
triceps
  t. brachii muscle
  t. coxae muscle
  t. muscle of arm
  t. muscle of calf
  t. muscle of hip
  t. reflex
  t. surae muscle
  t. sura muscle
trichlorofluoromethane
trichloromethane
trichloromonofluoromethane
trichterbrust
tricipital
tricuspid valve regurgitation
tricyclic antidepressant
tridentata
  Artemisia t.
  Larrea t.
trident hand
tridigitate
tridosha
trifacial
Trifal
trifoliata
  Gillenia t.
trifoliate central tendon
Trifolium pratense

NOTES

trigeminal
   t. nerve
   t. nerve entrapment
   t. nerve neuralgia
   t. neuralgia
trigeminus
trigger
   t. finger
   t. point
   t. point infiltration
   t. point injection
   t. point injection therapy
      (TPIT)
   t. point therapy
   symptom t.
triglycerides
   plasma t.
   serum t.
trigona (*pl. of* trigonum)
trigonal
trigone
   deltoideopectoral t.
   lumbocostal t.
   t. muscle
trigonella
Trigonella foenum-graecum
trigonum, pl. **trigona**
   t. cervicale
   t. cervicale anterius
   t. cervicale posterius
   t. colli
   t. deltoideopectorale
   t. femorale
   t. lumbale inferius
   t. lumbocostale diaphragmatis
   t. musculare regionis cervicalis
      anterioris
   t. omoclaviculare
   os t.
Trikatu
trillium
   T. C
   T. erectum
   T. grandiflorum
   t. pendulum
   purple t.
Trim
   Herbal T.
   Power T.
trimalleolar fracture
trimethoprim
trip
   Ginger T.'s

tripartate
tripartita
   Bidens t.
triphala
triphalangia
triphosphate
   adenosine t.
triphylla
   Aloysia t.
triple
   t. arthrodesis
   t. burner
   t. burner channel
   t. heater channel
   t. warmer
   t. warmer channel
tripod
   t. fracture
   vital t.
tripodia
tripsis
triquetrous cartilage
triquetrum
   t. bone
   os t.
triradial
triradius
triticea
   cartilago t.
triticeal cartilage
Triticum aestivum
trochanter
   femoral t.
   greater t.
   lesser t.
   t. major
   t. minor
   small t.
   third t.
trochanterian
trochanteric
   t. bursitis
   t. crest
   t. fossa
   t. syndrome
trochanterica
   fossa t.
trochanterplasty
trochantin
trochantinian
trochlea
   t. femoris
   t. fibularis calcanei

t. humeri
t. of humerus
t. motion
t. muscularis
t. peronealis
t. phalangis manus et pedis
t. tali
t. of the talus
trochlear
t. nerve
t. process
trochleariform
trochlearis
incisura t.
trochleiform
trochoid
t. articulation
t. joint
Tropaeolum
tropane alkaloid
trophic
t. changes
t. function
trophicity
trophoneurosis
muscular t.
trophotropic
tropism
facet t.
zygapophysial t.
tropometer
trough sign
true
t. aneurysm
t. ankylosis
t. arthrodial joint
t. chamomile
t. jalap
t. lavender
t. muscles of back
t. ribs [I–VII]
t. saffron
t. sage
t. unicorn root
t. vertebra
true-point needling

trumpet
angel's t.
t. bush
devil's t.
t. tree
trumpet-weed
truncal
truncate
truncus
trunk
t. bending test
t. control exercise
costocervical arterial t.
extra point on the back of
the t. (Ex-B)
t. lift exercise
lumbar lymphatic t.
lumbosacral nerve t.
t. point
t. rotation
t. sidebending test
subclavian lymphatic t.
sympathetic t.
thoracoacromial t.
tryptophan
**tryptophan-associated eosinophilic
connective tissue disease**
tsang
chi nei t.
tsao
feng t.
gu jing t.
huang t.
tung t.
tsao-ho-hua
tschut
TSH
thyroid-stimulating hormone
TS-II
Target TS-II
Tso Tzu Otic Pills
tsri point
tsubos
TT
therapeutic touch
TTA
tissue texture abnormality

T

NOTES

TTO
tea tree oil
tub
ankle t.
hot t.
hydrotherapy t.
tuba
tube
Aromamist Steam T.
eustachian t.
intratracheal t.
neural t.
tuber
calcaneal t.
t. calcanei
t. calcis
t. ischiadicum
t. of ischium
Pinellia t.
t. radii
t. root
tubercle
t. of anterior scalene muscle
t. bacillus
calcaneal t.
crest of greater t.
crest of lesser t.
cuboid pronated medial t.
Gerdy t.
iliac t.
t. of iliac crest
inferior thyroid t.
intercondylar t.
Lisfranc t.
Lister t.
Lower t.
mental t.
obturator t.
postglenoid t.
pubic t.
t. of rib
scalene t.
t. of scaphoid bone
superior thyroid t.
supratragic t.
t. of trapezium bone
Wrisberg t.
tuberculosis
Mycobacterium t.
tuberculous
t. rheumatism
t. spondylitis

tuberculum
t. adductorium femoris
t. anterius vertebrarum
cervicalium
t. arthriticum
t. calcanei
t. costae
t. cuneiforme
t. dorsale radii
t. iliacum
t. intercondylare mediale et
laterale
t. intervenosum atrii dextri
t. laterale processus posterioris
tali
t. majus humeri
t. mediale processus posterioris
tali
t. minus humeri
t. musculi scaleni anterioris
t. obturatorium
t. ossis scaphoidei
t. ossis trapezii
t. posterius vertebrarum
cervicalium
t. pubicum
t. superius
t. supratragicum
tuberosa
Asclepias t.
tuberositas
t. coracoidea
t. costalis
t. deltoidea humeri
t. iliaca
t. musculi serrati anterioris
t. ossis cuboidei
t. ossis metatarsalis primi [I]
t. ossis metatarsalis quinti [V]
t. ossis navicularis
t. phalangis distalis manus et
pedis
t. radii
t. sacralis
t. tibiae
t. ulna
t. unguicularis
tuberosity
bicipital t.
calcaneal t.
coracoid t.
costal t.
t. of cuboid bone

t. of distal phalanx of hand
and foot
t. of fifth metatarsal bone [V]
t. of first metatarsal bone [I]
iliac t.
ischial t.
lateral femoral t.
lateral process of calcaneal t.
medial femoral t.
medial process of calcaneal t.
t. of navicular bone
radial t.
t. of radius
sacral t.
scaphoid t.
t. for serratus anterior muscle
tibial t.
t. of ulna
ungual t.
tuberosum
   Solanum t.
tuboligamentous
tuboovarian abscess
tubule
   T t.
tubus vertebralis
tuckahoe
tufted phalanx
tufts
   synovial t.
tug
tui-na, tuina, tui na
tulip
   angel t.
tumefacient
tumeric paste
Tummy Soother
tumor
   brown t.
   cord t.
   t. debulking
   endodermal sinus t.
   Ewing t.
   gynecological t.
   t. necrosis factor (TNF)
   t. stage

thoracic cord t.
vocal cord t.
Wilms t.
yolk sac t.
tumoral calcinosis
tung
   t. seed
   t. tsao
tunic
tunica
   t. fibrosa
   t. mucosa
   t. muscularis
tuning
tunnel
   carpal t.
   t. of Guyon
   palmar t.
turbinal
turbinate
   nasal t.
turbinated
turgor
Turkish rhubarb
Turlington's Balsam of Life
turmeric
   Indian t.
   jiang huang t.
TURP
   transurethral resection of the prostate
turpentine
   t. balsam
   t. bath
   gum t.
   t. oil
turtle-bloom
tu si zi
Tussilago farfara
twice a day (b.i.d.)
twig
twin berry
Twinlab
twirling
   manual t.
   manual needle t.
   needle t.

T

NOTES

twist
>point of entry, traction and t. (POET2, POETZ)

twisting
twitchgrass
two
>balance testing level t.
>Virility T.

two-column concept of backbone
two-eyed berry
two-eyed checkerberry
txiu kub nyug
Tylenol
Tylophora Plus
tympanic
>t. membrane
>t. part

type
>t. Ia fiber
>t. I immediate immunoreactivity
>t. I restriction
>t. I somatic dysfunction
>t. I vertebral motion
>t. II fiber
>t. II somatic dysfunction

>t. II vertebral motion
>t. III mechanics
>t. III vertebral motion
>t. IV delayed immunoreactivity
>t. A behavior
>acute t.
>t. A reaction
>blood t.
>t. B reaction
>chronic t.
>t. C reaction
>t. D reaction
>ectomorphic body t.
>muscle fiber t.
>t. O condition
>shao yang t.
>tai yang t.

typha pollen
typhimurium
>*Salmonella t.*

typical
>t. cervical vertebra
>t. rib

tyrosine
Tzietze syndrome

ub
　　urinary bladder channel
　　ub　53　baohuang
　　ub　36　chengfu
　　ub　25　dachangshu
　　ub　19　danshu
　　ub　11　dashu
　　ub　16　dushu
　　ub　13　feishu
　　ub　58　feiyang
　　ub　18　ganshu
　　ub　17　geshu
　　ub　26　guanyuanshu
　　ub　1　jingming
　　ub　14　jueyinshu
　　ub　60　kunlun
　　ub　3　meichong
　　ub　28　pangguangshu
　　ub　20　pishu
　　ub　24　qihaishu
　　ub　22　sanjiaoshu
　　ub　62　shenmai
　　ub　23　shenshu
　　ub　10　tianzhu
　　ub　21　weishu
　　ub　39　weiyang
　　ub　40　weizhong
　　ub　27　xiaochangshu
　　ub　15　xinshu
　　ub　2　zanzhu
　　ub　54　zhibian
　　ub　67　zhiyin
ubenimex
ubidecarenone
ubiquinone
UDCA
　　ursodeoxycholic acid
Udekinon
Ukrain
　　Venancapsan U.
ulcer
　　aphthous u.
　　decubitus u.
　　duodenal u.
　　gastric u.
　　Marjolin u.
　　Meleney u.
　　peptic u.
　　plantar foot u.
　　pressure u.

　　recurrent aphthous u. (RAU)
　　venous stasis u.
ulceration
ulcerative
　　u. colitis
　　u. gingivitis
uliginosum
　　Gnaphalium u.
Ullmann line
ulmaria
　　Spiraea u.
ulmariae
　　flores u.
ulmoides
　　Eucommia u.
Ulmus
　　U. fulva
　　U. rubra
ulna, pl. **ulnae**
　　articular circumference of head
　　　of u.
　　body of u.
　　circumferentia articularis
　　　capitis u.
　　corpus u.
　　crista musculi supinatoris u.
　　head of u.
　　incisura semilunaris u.
　　interosseous border of u.
　　margo anterior u.
　　margo interosseus u.
　　margo posterior u.
　　medial surface of u.
　　u. motion
　　posterior border of u.
　　posterior surface of u.
　　shaft of u.
　　styloid process of u.
　　supinator crest of u.
　　tuberositas u.
　　tuberosity of u.
ulnad
ulna-meniscal-triquetral articulation
ulnar
　　u. clubhand
　　u. collateral ligament
　　u. collateral ligament of elbow
　　　joint
　　u. collateral ligament of wrist
　　　joint

U

ulnar *(continued)*
  u. deviation
  u. eminence of wrist
  u. extensor muscle of wrist
  u. flexor muscle of wrist
  u. head
  u. margin of forearm
  u. nerve
  u. nerve entrapment
  u. notch
  u. side
  u. stimulation
ulnare
  caput u.
ulnaris
  capri u.
  caput humerale musculi
    flexoris carpi u.
  caput ulnare musculi flexoris
    carpi u.
  eminentia carpi u.
  extensor carpi u.
  incisura u.
  musculus extensor carpi u.
  musculus flexor carpi u.
  sulcus nervi u.
  vagina tendinis musculi
    extensoris carpi u.
ulnen
ulnocarpal
ulnohumeral
  u. joint
  u. joint dysfunction muscle
    energy technique
ulnomeniscotriquetral
  u. joint
  u. pseudojoint
ulnoradial
uloid
ultimate
  u. oil
  u. strength
  U. Zinc-C Lozenges
Ultra
  U. Clear Sustain
  U. Diet Pep
  U. Hair
  U. Maximum Strength
    Glucosamine sulfate
  U. Multiple vitamin
  U. Nails
  U. Nutrient

  U. Preventive III
  U. Scent Diffuser
ultradian rhythm
ultrasonic nebulizer
ultrasonography
ultrasound
ultraviolet (UV)
  u. light
  u. microscope
ultraviolet B (UVB, UV-B)
umbellata
  Chimaphilia u.
umbilicus
  U. rupestris
umbrella plant
umeboshi plum
una de gato
Unani medicine
unassisted eccentric strengthening
  supine
Uncaria tomentosa
unciform
  u. bone
  u. joint
uncinate Luschka joint
uncinatum
  Ptychopetalum u.
uncoiling
  u. motion
  u. process
uncomfortable symptom
uncompensated fascial patterning
uncontrolled
uncovertebral
  u. joint
  u. joint of Luschka
uncrossed
  u. system
  u. tract
underactive thyroid
underventilation
undisturbed function
undulata
  Mitchella u.
undulatum
  Xysmalobium u.
unequal
  u. length of hamstring muscle
  u. length of psoas muscle
uneven energy field
ungual
  u. phalanx
  u. tuberosity

ungues
unguicularis
  tuberositas u.
unguinal
unguis
  u. aduncus
  u. incarnatus
  retinacula u.
uniarticular
uniaxial joint
unicameral bone cyst
unicorn root
unifacet
unification
unifying force
unilateral
  u. disorder
  u. erector spinal muscle
  hypertonicity
  u. extension
  u. fallen arch
  u. lateral stretch
  u. linear stretch
  u. prone press-up
  u. sacral flexion
  u. thoracic lymphatic pump
  u. upper trapezius muscle
  hypertonicity
unilaterally nutated sacroiliac
union
  faulty u.
  fibrous u.
  vicious u.
unipennate muscle
unipennatus
  musculus u.
Unique E
unit
  biological standard u.
  functional u.
  integrated u.
  international u. (IU)
  Living Air XL-15 u.
  microamps TENS u.
  motor u.
  TENS u.
  vertebral u.

unitary person framework
UniTea Herbs
United
  U. States Food and Drug
  Administration (USFDA)
  U. States Pharmacopeia (USP)
uniting cartilage
unity
  body u.
  u. of body
Universal
  U. Nutrition
universal
  u. awareness
  u. pattern
unleveling
  u. of base
  u. of iliac crest
  pelvic u.
  sacral base u.
  u. of sacrum
unloaded position
unmyelinated C fiber
unpaired skull bone
unrefined
  u. canola oil
  u. food
  u. grain
unruffling
unstable
  u. angina
  u. fracture
  u. hypermobile joint
ununited fracture
unwind
unwinding
  fascial u.
  knee torque u.
  u. maneuver
  thoracic spine u.
  torque u.
  upper extremity u.
unyielding sensation
up
  course u.
  curl u.
  curling u.

U

NOTES

up (*continued*)
 hook and back u.
 sitting u.
upland cotton
uplandicum
 Symphytum x u.
Upledger craniosacral therapy
upper
 u. back strength testing
 u. burner
 u. cervical complex stress test
 u. cervical lordosis
 u. cervical technique
 u. chakra
 u. crossed syndrome
 u. dan tian
 u. digestive tract
 u. extremity
 u. extremity of fibula
 u. extremity lymphatic pump
 u. extremity muscle imbalance
  diagnostic test 1
 u. extremity muscle imbalance
  diagnostic test 2
 u. extremity muscle imbalance
  diagnostic test 3
 u. extremity muscle imbalance
  diagnostic test 4
 u. extremity reflex
 u. extremity screen
 u. extremity unwinding
 u. GI
 u. limb
 u. part
 u. quarter
 u. respiratory infection (URI)
 u. respiratory system
 u. respiratory tract infection
 u. rib cage dysfunction
 u. thoracic spine
 u. trapezius muscle
upright Bucky
Uprising
 Herbal U.
upset
 gastric u.
upslipped innominate
uptake
 oxygen u.
 serotonin u.
uptight muscle
upward
 injury below u.

Up Your Gas
uralensis
 Glycyrrhiza u.
 radix glycyrrhizae u.
Uralyt
urarthritis
Urban Air Defense
urea hydrochloride
uremia
uremic
 u. encephalopathy
 u. neuropathy
urens
 Sterculia u.
 Urtica u.
urethral sphincter
urethritis
Urginea
 U. indica
 U. maritima
URI
 upper respiratory infection
urinalysis
urinary
 u. acidification
 u. bladder channel (ub)
 u. bladder meridian
 u. bladder meridian of foot
 u. dribbling
 u. hesitancy
 u. incontinence
 u. infection
 u. oxalate
 u. tract
 u. tract infection (UTI)
 u. tract inflammation
urine
 acidic u.
 alkaline u.
 foul u.
urodynamic
 u. evaluation
 u. study
Uroflux
urogenital
 u. diaphragm
 u. diaphragm release
 u. organ
 u. region
 u. system
 u. triangle
urolithiasis
 calcium oxalate u.

urological disorder
uropoietic system
Uro-Pro
ursi
  uva u.
ursodeoxycholic acid (UDCA)
Urtica
  U. dioica
  U. urens
urticaria
  acute u.
  chronic u.
  contact u.
  idiopathic nocturnal u.
urticarial plaque
use
  therapeutic u.
USFDA
  Food and Drug Administration
  United States Food and Drug
    Administration
usnea
Usnea barbata
USP
  United States Pharmacopeia
uteri
  cervix u.
  glandulae cervicales u.
uterine
  u. bleeding

  u. contraction
  u. fibroid
  u. leiomyoma
  u. stimulant
uterocervical
uterosacral
Utero-Tone
uterotonic
uterus
  prolapsed u.
UTI
  urinary tract infection
utilization
  protein-energy u.
UV
  ultraviolet
  UV light therapy
  UV light treatment
uva
  u. ursi
  u. ursi capsule
Uvalyst
UVB, UV-B
  ultraviolet B
  UVB radiation
uvula
uvular
uvularis
uzara

U

NOTES

451

vaccination
homeopathic v.
vaccine
antituberculosis v.
Maruyama v.
vaccinia
Vaccinium
V. macrocarpon
V. myrtillus
V. oxycoccos
Vacuflex Reflexology System
vacuity
vacuum
v. disk phenomenon
v. phenomenon
vagal activity
vagi (*pl. of* vagus)
vagina
v. communis tendinum musculorum fibularium communis
v. communis tendinum musculorum flexorum manus
v. fibrosa tendinis
v. synovialis tendinis
v. tendinis musculi extensoris carpi ulnaris
v. tendinis musculi extensoris digiti minimi
v. tendinis musculi extensoris hallucis longi
v. tendinis musculi extensoris pollicis longi
v. tendinis musculi flexoris carpi radialis
v. tendinis musculi flexoris hallucis longi
v. tendinis musculi flexoris pollicis longi
v. tendinis musculi obliqui superioris
v. tendinis musculi peronei longi plantaris
v. tendinis musculi tibialis anterioris
v. tendinis musculi tibialis posterioris
v. tendinum musculi extensoris digitorum pedis longi

v. tendinum musculi flexoris digitorum pedis longi
v. tendinum musculorum extensorum carpi radialium
v. tendinum musculorum fibularium communis
vaginae
v. fibrosae digitorum manus
v. fibrosae digitorum pedis
v. synoviales digitorum manus
v. tendinum digitorum pedis
vaginal
v. delivery
v. opening
vaginitis
vaginosis
anaerobic v.
bacterial v.
vagovagal reflex
vagrant pain sensation
Vagtone
vagus, pl. **vagi**
v. nerve
vajikarana
valepotriate
valerian
American v.
v. extract
false v.
great wild v.
Indian v.
red v.
v. root extract
Valeriana
V. officinalis
valerianae
radix v.
valga
coxa v.
manus v.
tibia v.
valgoid
valgum
genu v.
valgus
cubitus v.
v. deformity
digitus v.
hallux v.
pes v.

V

453

valgus *(continued)*
    v. stress testing of knee
    talipes v.
validation
valine
valley
    lily of the v.
value
    core v.
    homing v.
    predictive v.
    prognostic v.
    reference v.
valve
valvula
vamana
vanadium
vanadyl sulfate
vandalroot
van Horne canal
Vanilla
    V. planifolia
    V. tahitensis
vanilla
    Bourbon v.
    v. cactus
    Mexican v.
    Tahiti v.
    Vera Cruz v.
vanillin
vapor
    anesthetic v.
    eucalyptus leaf v.
vaporization
vaporize
vaporizer
    eucalyptus oil in v.
    flow-over v.
VapoRub
    Vicks V.
vara
    coxa v.
    false coxa v.
    manus v.
    tibia v.
variation
    craniosacral vault technique,
      fourth v.
    frontal posture v.
    temperature v.
varicose vein
varifolium
    Sassafras v.

varnish tree
varum
    genu v.
varus
    cubitus v.
    v. deformity
    digitus v.
    hallux v.
    metatarsus v.
    pes v.
    v. stress testing of knee
    talipes v.
varus-valgus stress test
VAS
    visual analog scale
vas
    v. collaterale
    v. deferens
vasal
vasa vasorum
vascular
    v. complication
    v. element
    v. headache
    v. resistance
    v. responder
    v. spasm
    v. structure
    v. system
    v. toxic
    hyperhomocysteinanemia
    v. wall
vascularity
vascularization
    inflammatory v.
vasculature
vasculitis
    immune-complex v.
    pulmonary v.
vasculosus
    circulus articularis v.
vasculum
vasiform
vasoactive intestinal peptide
vasoconstriction
vasodilatation
    cutaneous v.
vasodilation
vasodilator
    peripheral v.
vasomotor
    v. dysfunction

v. instability
v. tone
vasorum
vasa v.
vasovagal
vastoadductor fascia
vastus
v. intermedius
v. intermedius muscle
v. lateralis
v. lateralis muscle
v. medialis
v. medialis muscle
v. medialis obliquus muscle
vata dosha
vata-pitta
vault
craniosacral v. (CV)
v. hold
v. of skull
vector
force v.
Vedic
V. astrology
V. medicine
vegan diet
Vegelax
vegetable
v. antimony
cruciferous v.
v. gelatin
green leafy v.
v. marrow
v. tallow
yin v.
vegetarian
ovolacteal v.
pure v.
raw-food v.
vegetative
v. physical symptom
v. symptom
Vegetex
Vegicap
Bilberry V.
Devil's Claw V.'s

Full Potency Licorice
Root V.'s
Vegitabs
SN-X V.
vein
accompanying v.
anonymous v.
axillary v.
brachiocephalic v.
Breschet v.
cerebral v.
companion v.
diploic v.
external jugular v.
innominate v.
internal jugular v.
jugular v.
v. palpation
perforating v.
subclavian v.
varicose v.
vertebral v.
veinlet
velocity
conduction v.
gait v.
muscle fiber conduction v.
nerve conduction v. (NCV)
velvet dock
vena diploica
Venancapsan Ukrain
venenata
Rhus v.
venenosum
Physostigma v.
veneris
herba v.
Venezuela aloe
venography
transosseous v.
vertebral v.
venom
dried v.
v. immunotherapy
toad v.
venorelbine
Venostasin retard

NOTES

V

Venostat
venous
    v. congestion
    v. drainage
    v. flow
    v. sinus
    v. sinus drainage
    v. sinus technique
    v. stasis ulcer
    v. thrombosis
venter
ventilation
    alveolar v.
    artificial v.
    high-frequency jet v.
ventosa
    spina v.
ventral
    v. border
    v. branch
    v. cortical spinal tract
    v. direction
    v. horn
    v. medial brainstem pathway
    v. medial pathway
    v. motor neuron
    v. sacrococcygeal ligament
    v. sacrococcygeal muscle
    v. sacrococcygeus muscle
    v. sacroiliac ligament
    v. surface of digit
    v. technique
ventralis
    musculus sacrococcygeus v.
ventricle
    cerebral v.
    compression of fourth v.
ventricular arrhythmia
venula
venular
venule
venulous
Venus syndrome
VePesid
vera
    aloe v.
    vertebra v.
Vera Cruz vanilla
verae
    costae v. [I–VII]
verapamil

Veratrum
    V. album
    V. viride
verbal conditioning
verbascum
    v. complex
    V. phlomoides
    V. thapsus
verbena
    lemon v.
Verbena officinalis
verde
    oropharynx v.
veris
    Primula v.
vermifuge
Vermont snakeroot
vernalis
    Adonis v.
vernix
    Toxicodendron v.
Veronica, Hebe
    V. virginica
veronica
    high v.
Veronicastrum virginicum
verruca vulgaris
versicolor
    Iris v.
vertebra, pl. **vertebrae**
    accessory process of lumbar v.
    arcus v.
    atlantoaxial v.
    atypical thoracic v.
    block v.
    body of v.
    butterfly v.
    C1–C7 vertebrae
    centrum of a v.
    cervical v.
    cervical vertebrae [C1–C7]
    v. cervicales [C1–C7]
    v. coccygeae [Co1–Co4]
    coccygeal vertebrae [Co1–Co4]
    codfish v.
    corpus v.
    false v.
    hourglass v.
    H-shape v.
    ivory v.
    L1–L5 vertebrae
    v. lumbales [L1–L5]
    lumbar vertebrae [L1–L5]

v. magna
occipitoatlantal v.
pedicle of arch of v.
pediculus arcus v.
picture-frame v.
v. plana
posterior tubercle of
    cervical v.
v. prominens
rotation of v.
rugger jersey v.
v. sacrales [S1–S5]
sacral vertebrae [S1–S5]
spinous process of v.
v. spuriae
thoracic v.
v. thoracicae [T1–T12]
thoracic vertebrae [T1–T12]
transverse process of v.
true v.
T1–T12 vertebrae
typical cervical v.
v. vera
vertebral
v. arch
v. artery
v. artery dissection
v. artery flow
v. axis
v. basilar artery
v. body
v. border of scapula
v. canal
v. column
v. column curve
v. column motion
v. column muscle
v. dysfunction
v. epidural space
ERS v.
extended, rotated and side
    bent v.
v. facet
flexed, rotated, and side
    bend v.
v. foramen
v. formula

FRS v.
v. fusion
v. ganglion
v. groove
v. gutter
v. motion
v. motion dysfunction
v. motion segment
v. nerve
v. notch
v. orientation
v. plexus
v. polyarthritis
v. region
v. ribs
v. somatic dysfunction
v. subluxation
v. unit
v. vein
v. venography
v. venous plexus
v. venous system
vertebral-basilar
v.-b. artery system
v.-b. system
vertebrale
foramen v.
ganglion v.
vertebralis
canalis v.
columna v.
incisura v.
pars intracranialis arteriae v.
regio v.
sulcus arteriae v.
tubus v.
vertebrarium
vertebroarteriale
foramen v.
vertebroarterial foramen
vertebrobasilar
v. accident
v. ischemia
vertebrochondral ribs
vertebrocostal
vertebrofemoral
vertebroiliac

NOTES

V

vertebropelvic ligament
vertebrosacral
vertebrosternal ribs
vertex
      flattened v.
vertical
      v. axis
      v. strain
verticalis
vertigo
      cervical v.
verum
      Cinnamomum v.
Vervain
      Blue V.
vervain
      American v.
      blue v.
      European v.
vesalianum
      os v.
Vesalius bone
vesical plexus
vesicant
vesicatoria
      Cantharis v.
      Lytta (Cantharis) v.
vesicobullous
vesicocervical
vesicospinal
vesiculosus
      Fucus v.
vessel
      afferent v.
      anastomosing v.
      blood v.
      collateral v.
      conception v.
      conceptional v. (cv)
      coronary v.
      efferent v.
      girdle v.
      governing v. (gv)
      governor v.
      influential point of the v.
      luo v.
      luo connecting v.
      qi v.
      thrusting v.
      yang heel v.
      yang linking v.
      yin heel v.
      yin linking v.

vestibula
vestibular
      v. system
vestibularis
vestibulate
vestibule
vestibulocerebellar ataxia
vestibulocochlear nerve
vestibulospinal tract
vestibulum
vestige
vestigial muscle
vestigium
vetch
      Missouri milk v.
vetivert
viability
      tissue v.
viable antiseptic
Viadent
vibesate
vibora
      carne de v.
      pulvo de v.
vibration
vibrational
      v. contact point
      v. medicine
vibration-induced flexion reflex
vibrative
vibrator
vibratory massage
vibromasseur
vibrotherapeutics
viburnum
      v. complex
      V. opulus
      V. prunifolium
vicarious hypertrophy
Vichy shower
vicious union
Vicks VapoRub
video fluoroscopy
Vieussens
      V. ansa
      V. loop
view
      v. box
      sunshine v.
Vigoran
vigorous stimulation
Vikonon Combination
villi (*pl. of* villus)

villosa
> *Dioscorea v.*
> polyarthritis chronica v.
> *Sterculia v.*

villosity

villosum
> *Amomum v.*

villous tenosynovitis

villus, pl. villi

vinblastine

Vinca rosea

vincristine

vincula

vincula of tendons

vinculum
> v. breve digitorum manus
> v. breve of fingers
> v. longum digitorum manus
> v. longum of fingers

vindesine

vine
> apricot v.
> bead v.
> squaw v.
> thunder god v.

vinegar
> apple cider v.

vingory

vinifera
> *Vitis v.*

Vinruta

Viocava

Viola odorata

violation of tissue

violet
> v. bloom
> blue v.
> English v.
> gentian v.
> sweet v.

violeta

viral
> v. hepatitis
> v. infection
> v. replication

Virchow cell

virechana

virginal membrane

Virginia
> V. poke
> V. snakeroot

virginiana
> *Hamamelis v.*
> *Prunus v.*

virginica
> *Leptandra v.*
> *Veronica v.*

virginicum
> *Veronicastrum v.*

virginicus
> *Chionanthus v.*

virgin oil

viride
> *Veratrum v.*

virile
> membrum v.

virilis
> *Acanthea v.*

Virility Two

virilization therapy

virosa
> *Lactuca v.*

virus
> Epstein-Barr v. (EBV)
> hepatitis C v.
> herpes simplex v. (HSV)
> herpes simplex type I v. (HSV-I)
> herpes simplex type II v. (HSV-II)
> human immunodeficiency v. (HIV)
> influenza v.
> respiratory syncytial v.
> sindbis v.

VIS
> visceral manipulative treatment

visagna
> *Ammi v.*

viscera (*pl. of* viscus)
> internal v.
> skin v.
> target end organ v.

V

NOTES

viscerad
visceral
   v. anesthesia
   v. condition
   v. dysfunction
   v. function
   v. layer
   v. manipulation
   v. manipulative treatment (VIS)
   v. organ
   v. pelvic fascia
   v. peritoneum
   v. reflex arc
   v. skeleton
   v. system
   v. technique
   v. traction reflex
visceralis
   fascia pelvis v.
   lamina v.
visceroskeletal
visceroskeleton
viscerosomatic
   v. reflex
   v. reflex dysfunction
   v. somatic dysfunction
viscerosomatovisceral reflex
viscerovisceral
   v. reflex
   v. reflex arc
viscosity
   blood v.
Viscum
   V. abietis
   V. album
   V. laxum
viscus, pl. viscera
Vishuddha
Vi-Siblin
vision
   v. deficiency
   v. quest
vis medicatrix naturae
visnagin
visual
   v. analog scale (VAS)
   v. art therapy
   v. deficiency
   v. feedback
visualization
   healing v.
   v. technique

Vita
   Gero V.
   V. Lemon
VitaCarte
vitae
   lignum v.
Vita-Flax
   Barlean's V.-F.
vital
   V. Balance
   v. energy
   v. energy exercise
   V. Eyes
   v. force
   v. tripod
VitaLife Sport Products
vitality
vitalization
   psychospiritual v.
vitalize
vitamin
   v. A
   activated B v.
   antioxidant v.
   antisterility v.
   v. B_2
   v. B_7
   v. B_{12}
   v. B_9
   v. B_3
   v. B_5
   v. B_1
   v. B_6
   v. B_{17}
   B-complex v.
   v. B_{12} deficiency
   v. B_6-dependent seizure
   v. C
   v. C with rose hips
   v. D
   v. D-resistant rickets
   v. E
   Freeda v.
   v. H
   v. K
   v. K_2
   megadose v.
   Ultra Multiple v.
   Wellness Formula v.
Vitapak
   Mega Men Men's V.
vitellin
Vitex agnus-castus

vitiligo
Vitis
  V. clignetiae
  V. vinifera
vitro
  in v.
vivation
vivo
  in v.
vocal
  v. cord tumor
  v. muscle
vocalis muscle
voice
  rough v.
vola
volae
  superficialis v.
volar
  v. carpal ligament
  v. forearm
  v. surface
volaris
  musculus interosseus v.
volatile anesthetic
volition
Voll
  electroacupuncture according
  to V. (EAV)
  V. machine
voltage
  applied v.
  v. current level
  v. intensity
voluntary
  v. component
  v. control
  v. exhalation
  v. inhalation
  v. motion
  v. movement

  v. muscle
  v. respiratory activity
vomer
  wing of v.
vomica
  Nux v.
vomiting
  anticipatory v.
  postoperative v.
  therapeutic v.
vomitoria
  Ilex v.
vomitwort
voodoo death
vortex, pl. vortices
VP-16
V-spread
  V.-s. procedure
  V.-s. technique
vulgare
  Chrysanthemum v.
  Foeniculum v.
  Hordeum v.
  Marrubium v.
  Tanacetum v.
vulgaris
  acne v.
  Alchemilla v.
  Aloe v.
  Artemisia v.
  Berberis v.
  Carlina v.
  Cydonia v.
  Proteus v.
  Prunus persica v.
  Thymus v.
  Tilia v.
  verruca v.
vulvar wart
VX-478

NOTES

V

waddling gait
wahoo bark
wai dan qigong
waiguan
    sj 5 w.
waiqiu
waist
wake-robin
waking hypnotic induction
Wakunaga of America
Waldeyer ring
waldmeister
walk
    w. cycle
    penguin w.
    thumb w.
walking
    cross-pattern pep w.
    w. cycle
wall
    chest w.
    w. germander
    pellitory of the w.
    w. pennywort
    w. press exercise
    thoracic w.
    vascular w.
walnut
    black w.
    w. fruit-shell
    otaheite w.
wan
    ba hui di huang w.
    ban he w.
    bao wei di huang w.
    bao yuan w.
    ba wei di huang w.
    da bu yin w.
    du huo ji sheng w.
    he che da zao w.
    hu jian w.
    kai kit w.
    liu wei di huang w.
    rou gui w.
    shi bai di huang w.
    ting zhi w.
    wu ren w.
    xiao yao w.
    you gui w.
    zhi bai di huang w.

    zhong w.
    zhou gui w.
    zuo gui w.
wand
    moxa w.
Wanderer
    Free & Easy W.
wandering
    w. abscess
    w. sickness
wang
    w. bu liu xin
    hua w.
wangu
    gb 12 w.
Ward's Balsam
Ward triangle
warfarin
Warix
Warmatowel
warm-cold
warmer
    triple w.
warming
    w. function
    w. needle technique
warm-up exercise
wart
    penile w.
    vulvar w.
    w. wort
    yellow w.
Wartec
wash
    eye w.
washbowl
    lady's w.
wasserkresse
wasting
    muscle w.
water
    w. agrimony
    w. birth
    w. bugle
    carbonaceous activated w.
    (CAW)
    catalyst altered w. (CAW)
    Concentrated Caraway W.
    deionized w.
    demineralized w.

W

water *(continued)*
 w. element
 five phase or five elements:
  wood, fire, earth, metal,
  and w.
 w. flag
 w. glass
 hamamelis w.
 w. hemlock
 w. horehound
 kidney w.
 w. lemon
 w. of life
 lime w.
 w. magnet
 w. path
 w. pipe
 w. principle
 w. qi
 w. qi circulation
 w. retention
 w. shamrock
 w. shiatsu
 spring w.
 steam-distilled w.
 w. therapy
 Willard w.
 Woodwards Gripe W.
watercress
watermelon
watsu
wave
 alpha w.
 brain w.
 cerebrospinal fluid pulse w.
 frontal and temporal theta w.
 pontine-geniculate-occipital w.
 theta w.
 theta EEG w.
wavelength
wax
 bone w.
 w. doll
 Horsley bone w.
 w. myrtle plant
 paraffin w.
 propolis w.
waxberry
way
 Nature's W.
way bennet
way-bread
waythorn

weak
 w. energy field
 w. pulse
weakness
 constitutional w.
 state of w.
 w. of willpower
web
 w. of fingers
 w. of toes
wedge
 w. bone
 knee w.
wedge-and-groove joint
weed
 asthma w.
 bear's w.
 bishop's w.
 butterfly w.
 consumptive's w.
 devil w.
 gall w.
 holy w.
 horse fly w.
 indigo w.
 Jamestown w.
 jimson w., jimsonweed
 Joe-pye w.
 klamath w.
 knob w.
 mad-dog w.
 Mexico w.
 moon w.
 rattlesnake w.
 rich w.
 rosin w.
 snake w.
 squaw w.
wei
 w. huo shang sheng
 w. qi
 w. yin xu
weichi
Weider
 Joe W.
weight
 w. distribution
 w. reduction
weightbearing
 w. of foot
 w. of ilium
 w. line of L3
 w. of spine

weiguan
weishu
    ub 21 w.
Weitbrecht
    W. cartilage
    W. cord
    W. fibers
    W. foramen
    W. ligament
weitbrechti
    apparatus ligamentosus w.
weiyang
    ub 39 w.
weizhong
    ub 40 w.
Welcker angle
wellness
    W. Formula vitamin
    Morning W.
    W. Multiple Max Daily
wen
    w. bing theory
    da bu yin w.
    w. dan tang
    w. jing tang
wenliu
wermut
Western
    W. acupuncture
    W. botanical medicine
    W. coltsfoot
    W. diagnosis
    W. ginseng
    W. medicine
    W. yew
West Indian dogwood
wet
    w. beriberi
    w. energy
    w. sheet
    W. SpaTable
    w. towel technique
we-wei-zu
WFC
    World Federation of Chiropractic
wheat
    w. flour

    w. germ
    w. germ oil
    w. grass
wheatgrass
    w. juice
Wheatstone bridge
wheel
    medicine w.
wheezing
whey
Whey to Go
whip
    Hiss plantar w.
whiplash
    w. injury
    w. injury mechanism
whipplei
    Yucca w.
whippoorwill's shoe
whirlpool
    w. bath
White
    W. Cohosh tablet
    W. Tiger Decoction
white
    w. aura
    w. birch
    w. bird's-eye
    w. blood cell magnesium
    w. cohosh
    w. cohosh liquid extract
    w. fringe
    w. hellebore
    w. horehound
    w. man's foot
    w. matter
    w. muscle
    w. mustard
    w. noise
    w. oak
    w. poplar
    w. potato
    w. rami communicantes
    w. sandalwood oil
    w. snakeroot
    w. sound
    w. sound machine

NOTES

W

white *(continued)*
  w. squill
  w. willow
  w. willow bark
whitethorn
whitetube stargrass
whitlow
  thecal w.
WHO
  World Health Organization
whole
  w. blood
  w. energy balance
  w. foods
  w. leaf aloe vera juice
  w. life health
  milk thistle seed w.
  w. oats
whole-blood serotonin measurement
whole-body immersion
whole-food diet
wholeness
whooping cough
whorl
  coccygeal w.
whortleberry
Wickram Experience Inventory
widening
width
  pulse w.
wild
  w. alum root
  w. angelica
  w. brier berry
  w. carrot
  w. carrot seed
  w. celery
  w. chamomile
  w. cherry
  w. cherry bark
  w. cherry bark compound
  W. Cherry Supreme
  w. chrysanthemum flower
  w. clover
  w. coleus
  w. cotton
  w. cranesbill
  w. cucumber
  w. endive
  w. fennel
  w. geranium
  w. ginger
  w. gobo

  w. goose
  w. hyssop
  w. indigo
  w. iris
  w. lemon
  w. lettuce
  w. marjoram
  w. mustard
  w. pansy
  w. passion flower
  w. pine
  w. plantain
  w. quinine
  w. rosemary
  w. rye
  w. saso
  w. senna
  w. succory
  w. sunflower
  w. sweet William
  w. tansy
  w. wormwood
  w. yam
  w. yarn
will
  divine w.
  personal w.
Willard water
William
  W. flexion exercise
  wild sweet W.
willie
  stinking w.
willow
  black w.
  white w.
willow-meadowsweet compound
Willowprin
willpower
  weakness of w.
Wilms tumor
wind
  liver w.
wind-cold
  w.-c. affects the lung
  w.-c. invasion
windflower
  meadow w.
wind-heat
  w.-h. affects the lung
  w.-h. invasion
window
  bone w.

wind-up
    w.-u. phenomenon
    w.-u. reflex
wing
    angel w.
    great w.
    w. of ilium
    w. of sacrum
    w. of vomer
winged scapula
winging
    scapular w.
wingxiang
    li 20 w.
Winslow ligament
winter
    w. bloom
    w. clover
    W. Formula
    w. savory
winterbloom
wintergreen
    W. Altoids
    w. leaf
    w. oil
    oil of w.
    spotted w.
    W. Sucrets
winterweed
wire
    measuring w.
    w. webbing handle
wiring
wispy pattern
wisteria
Witasu
witch
    w. doctor
    w. hazel
    W. Hazel Cream
    w. hazel gargle
    w. hazel liquid
    w. hazel pad
    W. Stik
witchcraft
witches' herb

Withania
    W. coagulans
    W. somnifera
withania
withdrawal
    w. from the environment
    quick w.
    w. reflex
    w. syndrome
Wobenzym N
Wolff law
Wölfler gland
wolf's
    w. bane
    w. foot
woman's sexuality herb
women's
    W. Comfort
    w. ginseng
    W. Precious Pills
    W. Treasure
wonder
    W. Gel
    w. tree
wood
    w. avens
    w. betony
    bitter w.
    cinnamon w.
    w. element
    master of the w.
    quassia w.
    Santalum album w.
    sassafras w.
    w. sorrel
    w. sour
    w. spider
    tobacco w.
    w. wool
woodruff
    w. sachet
    sweet w.
woodward
Woodwards Gripe Water
woody nightshade

NOTES

W

wool
 moxa w.
 wood w.
work
 energy w.
 percussion hammer w.
 w. rehabilitation
 shadow w.
 w. site modification
World
 W. Federation of Chiropractic
  (WFC)
 W. Health Organization
  (WHO)
wormian bone
wormseed
 levant w.
wormwood
 sea w.
 sweet w.
 wild w.
wort
 bee w.
 St. James w.
 St. John's w., St. Johnswort
 swallow w.
 tetter w.
 wart w.
 wound w.
wound
 w. debridement
 w. healing
 intrabuccal w.
 w. wort
woundwort
 hedge w.
 marsh w.
 soldier's w.
woven bone
wrack
 bladder w.
 sea w.
 sugar w.
wrap
 magnetic w.
 thermal plastic w.
Wright respirometer
wringing motion

wring out tissue
Wrisberg
 W. cartilage
 W. ligament
 W. nerve
 W. tubercle
wrist
 w. crease
 w. extension
 external collateral ligament
  of w.
 w. functional technique
 w. and hand region
 internal collateral ligament of
  the w.
 w. joint
 lateral ligament of w.
 long radial extensor muscle
  of w.
 medial ligament of w.
 w. muscle energy technique
 radial eminence of w.
 radial flexor muscle of w.
 radiate ligament of w.
 w. retinaculum
 short radial extensor muscle
  of w.
 w. somatic dysfunction
 triangular disk of w.
 ulnar eminence of w.
 ulnar extensor muscle of w.
 ulnar flexor muscle of w.
wrist-hand orthosis
writing hand
wry neck
wu
 he shou w.
 w. jia pi
 w. ren wan
 w. wei zi
 w. xing
 w. zhu yu
 w. zhu yu tang
wunderbaum
wurmfarn
wu-tieh-ni
wu-wei-zu

xanthine
xanthochlora
    Alchemilla x.
Xanthorhiza simplicissima
xanthorrhiza
    Curcuma x.
x axis
Xenical
xenobiotic
xenobiotics
xeronine
xerostomia
xi
    x. jiao
    x. jiao di huang tang
    x. point
    x. xin
xia
    x. ku cao
    pi x.
xiaguan
    st 7 x.
xiajuxu
    st 39 x.
xiang
    x. fu
    ru x.
    x. su san
xiangu
    st 43 x.
xian ma
xiao
    x. chai hu tang
    sang pian x.
    x. yao san
    x. yao wan
xiaochangshu
    ub 27 x.
xiaohai
    si 8 x.
xi-cleft point
xie method
ximen
    pe 4 x.
xin
    x. huo shang yang
    lian x.
    x. qi xu
    wang bu liu x.

    xi x.
    x. xue xu
    x. xue yu
    x. yang xu
    x. yin xu
xing
    wu x.
xingjian
    liv 2 x.
xinshu
    x. point
    ub 15 x.
xiphisternal
    x. joint
xiphisternum
xiphocostal
xiphoid
    x. cartilage
    x. process
xiphoiditis
xiphosternalis
    synchondrosis x.
xiyan
    Ex-LE 32 x.
x-radiation
x-ray
    plain x.-r.
X-Tablets
xu
    blood x.
    x. condition
    x. disturbance
    x. duan
    fei qi x.
    fei yin x.
    x. fu zhu yu tang
    gan xue x.
    gan yin x.
    heart yang x.
    kidney yang x.
    ming men x.
    pi qi x.
    pi yang x.
    qi x.
    qiu x.
    shen jing x.
    shen qi x.
    shen yang x.
    shen yin x.
    spleen yang x.

X

xu *(continued)*
    wei yin x.
    xin qi x.
    xin xue x.
    xin yang x.
    xin yin x.
    yang x.
    yin x.
    zhong qi x.
xuanzhong
    gb 39 x.
xue
    x. fu zhu yu tang

    x. level syndrome
    x. stagnation
xuehai
    sp 10 x.
xue-stage heat
xu-type disturbance
xu/weakness
Xylocaine
xyloidone
xylostyptic ether
xy plane
Xysmalobium undulatum
xz plane

y

y axis

ya

mo y.

yagona

yam

Mexican y.
Mexican wild y.
wild y.

yamen

du 15 y.

yan

gan shang y.

yang

y. activity
y. brightness
y. channel
y. channel axis
y. character
chuan y.
y. condition
y. deficiency
deficiency of heart y.
deficiency of kidney y.
deficiency of spleen y.
disharmony of yin and y.
y. energy
y. excess
y. function
greater y.
y. heel vessel
kidney y.
lesser y.
y. linking vessel
liver y.
y. ming fu
y. ming fu syndrome
y. ming heat
y. ming jing
y. organ
y. property
y. qi
y. quality
rising liver y.
y. side
suo y.
y. system
tai y.
xin huo shang y.
y. xu

y. xu symptom
yin and y.

yangbai

gb 14 y.

yangiiao

yanglao

si 6 y.

yanglingquan

gb 34 y.

yang-ming

y.-m. axis
y.-m. channel axis
y.-m. type headache

Yangqiao

yangqiao mai

yang-type condition

yangwei mai

yanhusuo

Corydalis y.

yao

yuen lian bai y.
zhong y.

yaoqi

Ex-B 20 y.

yaoshu

du 2 y.

yaoyangguan

du 3 y.

yarn

wild y.

yarrow

y. flower
y. grass extract

yaupon leaf

yawroot

Y cartilage

ye

ai y.
da qing y.
jin y.
su y.

yeast

brewer's y.
red y.
torula y.

Yeast-Gard

Yeast-X

yellow

y. astringent
y. button

Y

471

yellow *(continued)*
  y. cedar
  y. cinchona
  y. dock
  y. dock tea
  Y. Emperor's textbook of physical medicine
  y. gentian
  y. ginseng
  y. horse
  y. Indian shoe
  y. indigo
  jessamine y.
  y. lady's slipper
  y. ligament
  y. mustard
  y. paint
  y. puccoon
  y. root
  y. sandalwood oil
  y. tongue
  y. wart
yellowroot liquid extract
Yemen myrrh
yen hu suo
yerba
  y. maté
  y. maté tincture
  y. santa
yerba-de-mate
Yergason test
yew
  American y.
  California y.
  Oregon y.
  ornamental y.
  Pacific y.
  Y. Tea
  Western y.
yi
  y. guan jiang
  y. zhi ren
yield strength
yifeng
  sj 17 y.
yiming
  Ex-HN 7 y.
yin
  absolute y.
  y. channel
  y. channel axis
  y. condition

y. deficiency
deficiency of heart y.
deficiency of kidney y.
deficiency of liver y.
deficiency of lung y.
y. deficiency of the lung
deficiency of the stomach y.
y. deficient
y. evil
y. fluid
y. force
greater y.
y. heel vessel
kidney y.
lesser y.
y. linking vessel
liver y.
y. organ
pi xie feng qing y.
y. qi
qian wei qiang hua y.
y. qiao san
y. quality
rou gui y.
ruo gui y.
shao y.
y. side
y. vegetable
y. xu
y. xu symptom
y. and yang
y. and yang balance and exchange
y. yang huo
you gin gui y.
you gui y.
zuo gui y.
yinbai
  sp 1 y.
ying
  y. level syndrome
  y. point
  y. qi
yingu
  ki 10 y.
yinlingquan
  sp 9 y.
yinmen acupuncture point
yinqiao mai
yintang
  Ex-HN 1 y.
yin-type disturbance

yinwei
    confluent point of y.
      y. mai
yinxi
    he 6 y.
yin-yang energy
yin/yang pattern
yi-yi
ylang, ylang-ylang
    ylang y.
Y-ligament
    Bigelow Y.-l.
    Y.-l. of Bigelow
Yobinol
yoco
    y. bark
    Paullinia y.
Yocon
yoga
    Adhayatma y.
    Bhakti y.
    Buddhi y.
    Hatha y.
    holistic y.
    Integral y.
    Iyengar-style y.
    Japa y.
    Jnana y.
    Karma y.
    Kripalu y.
    Kriya y.
    Kundalini y.
    Laya y.
    mantra y.
    y. mat
    meditative y.
    Nada y.
    Nana y.
    Sahaja y.
    Schatz-style y.
yogic practitioner
yogurt douche
yohimbe
    Corynanthe y.
    Pausinystalia y.

yohimbehe
yohimbime
yohimbine
    y. HCl
    y. hydrochloride
Yohimex
yolk sac tumor
yong point
yongquan
    ki 1 y.
Yoshu-Nezu
yota
    Raja y.
you
    y. gin gui yin
    y. gui wan
    y. gui yin
Y-shaped ligament
yu
    y. niu jiao
    y. point
    wu zhu y.
    xin xue y.
yuan
    y. point
    y. qi
    y. zhi
yuan-source point
yuanzhi
Yucca
    Y. aloifolia
    Y. brevifolia
    Y. glauca
    Y. schidigera
    Y. whipplei
yucca
yuen lian bai yao
yuhao
    Ex-HN 3 y.
yunmen
    lu 2 y.
yunn point
Yuwipi
yz plane

NOTES

Y

Zac
Nutri Z.
zafran
Zaglas ligament
zallouh
shirsh z.
zang
z. fu
z. organ
zang-fu
Zanthoxylum americanum
zanzhu
ub 2 z.
Zanzibar aloe
zao
hai z.
z axis
Zea mays
Zen
Z. macrobiotic diet
Z. therapy
Zen-touch
zerboni
zero balancing
zeylanicum
Cinnamomum z.
ZGG
zinc gluconate glycine
zhangmen
liv 13 z.
zhaohai
ki 6 z.
zheng
bian z.
qi zhi z.
z. ren yang zhong tang
z. ti guan nian (ZTGN)
zhen jiu
zhi
z. bai di huang
z. bai di huang wan
z. bei di huang
bian zheng lun z. (BZLZ)
z. gan cao
z. gan cao tang
gui z.
z. mu
sang z.
yuan z.

zhibian
ub 54 z.
zhigancao
zhitai
zhiyin
ub 67 z.
zhizheng
zhong
z. deficiency
z. qi xu
z. san
z. wan
z. yao
zhongchong
pe 9 z.
zhongdu
liv 6 z.
zhongfu
lu 1 z.
z. point
zhongji
z. point
ren 3 z.
zhongwan
z. point
ren 12 z.
zhongzhu
sj 3 z.
zhou gui wan
zhu
bai z.
cang z.
da ding feng z.
e z.
zhubin
zi
bu gu z.
chi cuang z.
fu z.
fu pen z.
fu peng z.
z. he che
jing yin z.
jiu z.
she chuang z.
tu si z.
wu wei z.
zigbli
zigou
sj 6 z.

Z

475

zimbro
zinc
    ACES + Z.
    elemental z.
    z. gluconate glycine (ZGG)
    z. gluconate lozenge
    z. lozenge
    z. metabolism
Zinc-Loz
zingiber
    Z. officinale
Zink
    fascial patterning of Z.
Zinn ring
Ziziphus jujube
zombie's cucumber
zona
    z. dermatica
    z. epithelioserosa
    z. medullovasculosa
zonal
zonary
zone
    Looser z.'s
    z. therapy
zong qi
zonoskeleton

Zoom
zoster
    herpes z.
Zostrix
ZTGN
    zheng ti guan nian
zuo
    z. gui wan
    z. gui yin
zusanli
    st 36 z.
zygapophysial, zygapophyseal
    z. joint
    z. joint asymmetry
    z. joint block
    z. joint degenerative disease
    z. joint dysfunction
    z. tropism
zygapophysiales
    juncturae z.
zygoma
zygomatic
    z. arch
    z. margin of greater wing of
        sphenoid bone
zygomaticomaxillary
zygopodium

Appendix 1
Anatomical Illustrations

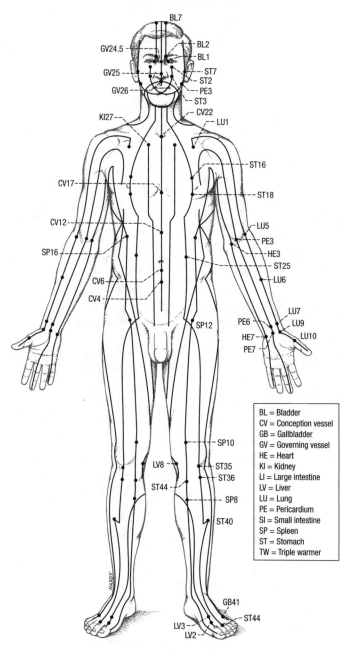

Figure 1. Acupressure/acupuncture points.

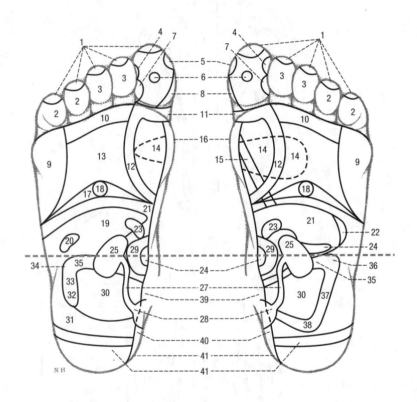

Figure 2. Reflexology points on the foot.

Reflexology Points on the Foot

Adrenal gland	23	Lung	13
Arm	9	Lymph drain for breast/chest	48
Ascending colon	33	Lymph drain for groin	52
Bladder	28	Mammary gland	49
Brain	1	Neck	10, 11, 45
Breast	49	Nose	53
Bronchial tube	12	Ovary	60
Cervical spine	8	Pancreas	24
Chest	13, 49	Parathyroid gland	11, 45
Colon	33–38	Penis	55
Diaphragm	17	Pituitary gland	6
Duodenum	29	Prostate	56
Ear	2, 3	Rectum	57
Esophagus	15	Sciatic nerve	42
Eye	3	Seminal vesicle	51
Fallopian tube	51	Shoulder	9
Gallbladder	20	Sigmoid colon	38
Head	1–8	Small intestine	30
Heart	14	Solar plexus	18
Helper to eye	10	Spine	8, 16, 39, 40, 41
Helper to inner ear	47	Spleen	22
Helper to thyroid	12	Stomach	21
Hip	58	Tailbone	41
Hip/sciatic nerve	59	Testicle	60
Hypothalamus	5	Thoracic spine	16
Ileocecal valve	32	Throat	11, 45
Intestine	29, 30, 32, 33, 35, 37, 38	Thymus	54
Kidney	25	Thyroid gland	11, 45
Knee	58	Tonsil	11, 45
Leg	58	Transverse colon	35
Liver	19	Ureter	27
Lower back	39, 40	Uterus	56
Lower spine	39, 40	Vagina	55
		Vas deferens	51

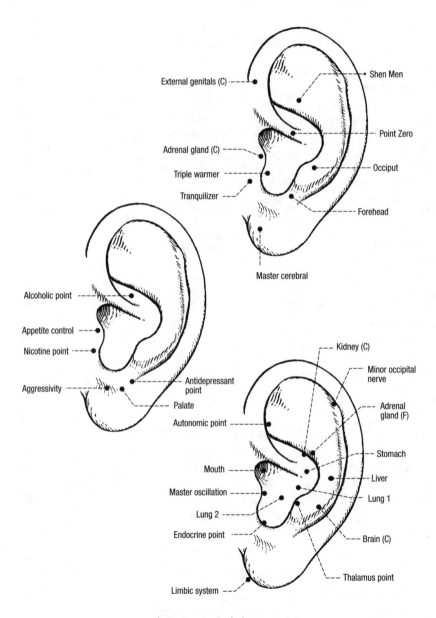

Figure 3. Auriculotherapy points.

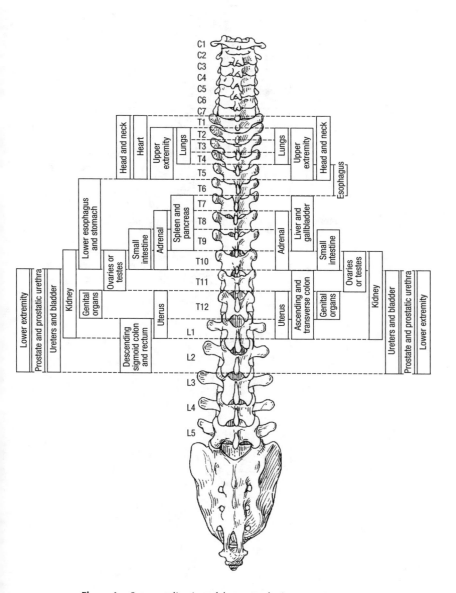

Figure 4. Segmentalization of the sympathetic nervous system.

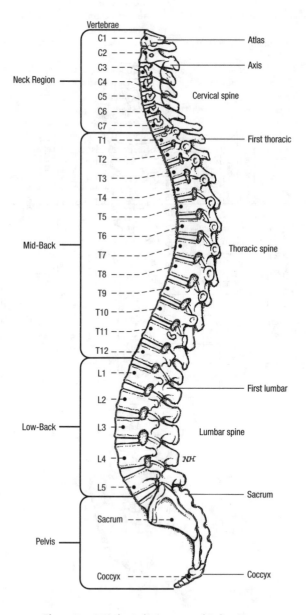

Figure 5. Spinal misalignments and indications.

Structures/Functions

C1	Blood supply to head, bones of the face, brain, inner ear, middle ear, pituitary gland, sympathetic nervous system	
C2	Auditory nerves, eyes, forehead, mastoid bones, optic nerves, sinuses, tongue	
C3	Cheeks, face bones, outer ear, teeth, trifacial nerves	
C4	Eustachian tube, lips, mouth, nose	
C5	Neck glands, pharynx, vocal cords	
C6	Neck muscles, shoulders, tonsils	
C7	Bursae in the shoulders and elbows, thyroid gland	
T1	Arms from elbows down, including hands, wrists, fingers; esophagus; trachea	
T2	Coronary arteries, heart including its valves and covering	
T3	Breast, bronchial tubes, chest, lungs	
T4	Common duct, gallbladder	
T5	Blood, liver, solar plexus	
T6	Stomach	
T7	Duodenum, pancreas	
T8	Diaphragm, spleen	
T9	Adrenal gland, suprarenal gland	
T10	Kidneys	
T11	Kidneys, ureters	
T12	Lymph circulation, small intestine	
L1	Inguinal ring, large intestine	
L2	Abdomen, appendix, upper leg	
L3	Bladder, knees, sex organs, uterus	
L4	Muscles of the lower back, prostate gland, sciatic nerve	
L5	Ankles, feet, lower legs	
SACRUM	Buttocks, hip bones	
COCCYX	Anus, rectum	

Indications

C1 — Amnesia, chronic tiredness, dizziness, headaches, head colds, high blood pressure, insomnia, migraine headaches, nervous breakdowns, nervousness

C2 — Allergies, certain cases of blindness, crossed eyes, deafness, earache, eye trouble, fainting, sinus trouble

C3 — Acne or pimples, eczema, neuralgia, neuritis

C4 — Adenoids, catarrh, hay fever, hearing loss

C5 — Hoarseness, laryngitis, throat conditions such as sore throat or peritonsillar abscess

C6 — Croup, pain in upper arm, stiff neck, whooping cough, tonsillitis

C7 — Bursitis, colds, thyroid conditions

T1 — Asthma, cough, difficulty breathing, pain in lower arms and hands, shortness of breath

T2 — Certain chest conditions, functional heart conditions

T3 — Bronchitis, congestion, influenza, pleurisy, pneumonia

T4 — Gallbladder conditions, jaundice, shingles

T5 — Anemia, arthritis, fevers, liver conditions, low blood pressure, poor circulation

T6 — Stomach troubles including dyspepsia, heartburn, indigestion, nervous stomach

T7 — Gastritis, ulcers

T8 — Hiccups, lowered resistance

T9 — Allergies, hives

T10 — Chronic tiredness, hardening of the arteries, kidney troubles, nephritis, pyelitis

T11 — Skin conditions such as acne, boils, eczema, or pimples

T12 — Certain types of sterility, gas pains, rheumatism

L1 — Colitis, constipation, diarrhea, dysentery, some ruptures or hernias

L2 — Acidosis, cramps, difficulty breathing, varicose veins

L3 — Bedwetting, bladder troubles, menopausal symptoms, impotency, many knee pains, menstrual troubles such as painful or irregular periods, miscarriage

L4 — Backache; difficult, painful, or frequent urination; lumbago; sciatica

L5 — Cold feet, leg cramps, poor circulation in legs, swollen ankles, weak ankles and arches, weakness in the legs

SACRUM — Sacroiliac conditions, spinal curvature

COCCYX — Hemorrhoids, pain at end of spine on sitting, pruritis

A7

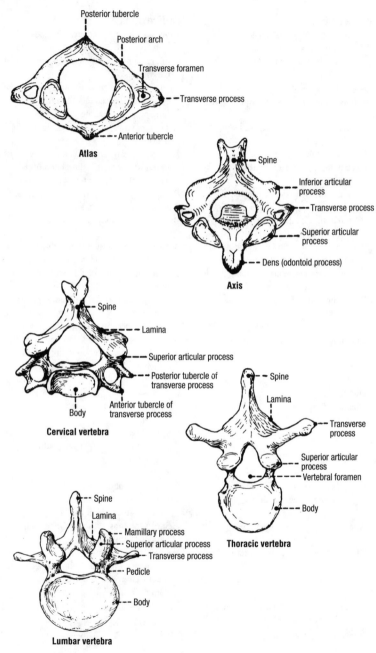

Figure 6. Typical cervical, thoracic, and lumbar vertebrae.

Acupuncture and Acupressure Meridians and Points (Chinese/English; English/Chinese)

Chinese Term/Phrase	English Meaning
ba gang	polar extremes
biao	exterior or external
bu	strengthening
dan yu tan rao	deficiency of the gallbladder and stagnation of phlegm
du mai or tou mo	governing vessel
fei	lung
fei qi xu	deficiency of lung qi
fei yin xu	deficiency of lung yin
feng han su fei	wind-cold affects the lung
feng re fan fei	wind-heat affects the lung
gan	liver
gan dan shi re	damp heat in the liver and gallbladder
gan feng nei dong	liver wind moving internally
gan qi yu jie	stagnation of liver qi
gan shang yan	rising liver fire
gan yang shang kang	rising liver yang
gan yin xu	deficiency of liver yin
gan xue xu	deficiency of liver blood
han	cold
han shi kun pi	damp cold in the spleen
han zhi gan mai	cold stagnation in the liver channel
hui xue point	influential point
jenn mo or ren mai	conceptional vessel
jiao	junction
jing or ting	channel
jing qi	vital energy that flows through the channels
li	interior or internal
luo	meridian
mu point	alarm point
neima	medial anesthesia
pi	spleen
pi qi xu	deficiency of spleen qi
pi yang xu	deficiency of spleen yang

pi yun shi re	damp heat in the spleen
qi	vital energy or life force
qi jingbamai or qi jingba mai	extraordinary channel
qi zhi zheng	state of excess
re	heat
ren mai or jenn mo	conceptional vessel
san	three
shen	spirit, consciousness, or kidney
shen jing xu	deficiency of kidney jing
shen qi xu	deficiency of kidney qi
shen yang xu	deficiency of kidney yang
shen yin xu	deficiency of kidney yin
shi	excess
tan shi zu fei	phlegm obstructs the lung
tan zhou shang rao	phlegm affecting the head
ting or jing	channel
tou mo or du mai	governing vessel
wei qi	protective gi or protecting qi
wei huo shang sheng	rising stomach fire
wei yin xu	deficiency of stomach yin
wu xing	five phases or five elements
xie	sedating, draining, dispersing, or reducing
xin	heart
xin huo shang yang	rising heart fire
xin qi xu	deficiency of heart qi
xin xue xu	deficiency of heart blood
xin xue yu	stagnation of heart blood
xin yang xu	deficiency of heart yang
xin yin xu	deficiency of heart yin
xu	weakness or deficiency
yang qi or zong qi	lung qi, chest qi, big qi, or gathering qi
yin	fluid
yin qi or ying qi	nutrient qi
ying qi or yin qi	nutrient qi
yuan qi	source qi or hereditary qi
zhen jiu	acupuncture
zong qi or yang qi	lung qi, chest qi, big qi, or gathering qi

English Term/Phrase	Chinese Term
acupuncture	zhen jiu
alarm point	mu point
big qi	zong qi or yang qi
channel	jing or ting
chest qi	zong qi or yang qi
cold	han
cold stagnation in the liver channel	han zhi gan mai
conceptional vessel	jenn mo or ren mai
consciousness	shen
damp cold in the spleen	han shi kun pi
damp heat in the liver and gallbladder	gan dan shi re
damp heat in the spleen	pi yun shi re
deficiency or weakness	xu
deficiency of the gallbladder and stagnation of phlegm	dan yu tan rao
deficiency of heart blood	xin xue xu
deficiency of heart qi	xin qi xu
deficiency of heart yang	xin yang xu
deficiency of heart yin	xin yin xu
deficiency of liver blood	gan xue xu
deficiency of liver yin	gan yin xu
deficiency of lung qi	fei qi xu
deficiency of lung yin	fei yin xu
deficiency of kidney jing	shen jing xu
deficiency of kidney qi	shen qi xu
deficiency of kidney yang	shen yang xu
deficiency of kidney yin	shen yin xu
deficiency of spleen qi	pi qi xu
deficiency of spleen yang	pi yang xu
deficiency of stomach yin	wei yin xu
dispersing	xie
draining	xie
excess	shi
exterior or external	biao
external or exterior	biao
extraordinary channel	qi jingbamai or qi jingba mai
five elements or five phases	wu xing
five phases or five elements	wu xing
fluid	yin
gathering qi	zong qi or yang qi

governing vessel	du mai or tou mo
heart	xin
heat	re
hereditary qi or source qi	yuan qi
influential point	hui xue point
interior or internal	li
internal or interior	li
junction	jiao
kidney	shen
life force or vital energy	qi
liver	gan
liver wind moving internally	gan feng nei dong
lung	fei
lung qi	zong qi or yang qi
medial anesthesia	neima
meridian	luo
nutrient qi	yin qi or ying qi
phlegm affecting the head	tan zhou shang rao
phlegm obstructs the lung	tan shi zu fei
polar extremes	ba gang
protecting qi or protective qi	wei qi
protective qi or protecting qi	wei qi
reducing	xie
rising heart fire	xin huo shang yang
rising liver fire	gan shang yan
rising liver yang	gan yang shang kang
rising stomach fire	wei huo shang sheng
sedating	xie
spirit	shen
spleen	pi
source qi or hereditary qi	yuan qi
stagnation of heart blood	xin xue yu
stagnation of liver qi	gan qi yu jie
state of excess	qi zhi zheng
strengthening	bu
three	san
vital energy or life force	qi
vital energy that flows through the channels	jing qi
weakness or deficiency	xu
wind-cold affects the lung	feng han su fei
wind-heat affects the lung	feng re fan fei

Appendix 3
Chakras

Chakra Number	Chakra English Name	Chakra Name
first chakra	base chakra	muladhara
second chakra	polarity chakra	svadhishthana
third chakra	solar plexus chakra	manipura
fourth chakra	heart chakra	anahata
fifth chakra	throat chakra	vishuddha
sixth chakra	third eye	ajna
seventh chakra	crown chakra	sahasrara

Appendix 4
Common Enzymes

acid protease
acylaminoacyl-peptidase
amylase
amyloglucosidase
arabinase
assemblin
astacin
autolysin
ß-glucanase
bromelain
calpain
carbohydrase
carboxypeptidase
caspase
catalase
cellobiohydrolase
cellulase
chymotrypsin
clostripain
coccidiodes endopeptidase
deuterolysin
dipeptidyl-peptidase
esterase
flavivirin
fragilysin
galactomannanase
gamma glutamyl hydrolase
glucanase
glucoamylase
glucosidase
glutamate carboxypeptidase
glutaminase
glutamyl aminopeptidase
glutamyl endopeptidase
GTG-ase
hemicellulase
hemoglobinase
kexin
lactase
leucine aminopeptidase
leucyl aminopeptidase
lipase
lysostaphin

lysozyme chloride
lysyl endopeptidase
papaya peptidase
maltose
mannanase
matrixin
methionyl aminopeptidase
mycolysin
mycozyme
neprilysin
omptin
pancrease
pancreatin
pancrelipase
papain
pectin esterase
pectin lyase
pectin esterase
pectinase
pentosanase
pepsin
peptidyl-dipeptidase A
picornain
pitrilysin
polygalacturonase
prolyl oligopeptidase
protease
pseudomonapepsin
pyroglutamyl-peptidase
reprolysin
retropepsin
scytalidopepsin
serralysin
streptopain
subtilisin
tentoxilysin
thermolysin
thermopsin
togavirin
tripeptidyl-peptidase
trypsin
urease
xylanase

Treatments by Indication

AMENORRHEA
herbal medicine
  blue cohosh
  chasteberry
  false unicorn root
  pennyroyal
  right upper extremity
  tansy

ANXIETY
acupressure
biofeedback training
bodywork
  Rolfing
diet therapy
  complex carbohydrates
environmental medicine
fasting
flower remedies
  aspen
  red chestnut
guided imagery
homeopathy
  Aconite
  Calcium carbonate
  Drosera
  Sulfur
hydrotherapy
  constitutional hydrotherapy
  immersion bath
  wet sheet pack
hypnotherapy
light therapy
magnetic field therapy
naturopathic medicine
nutritional therapy
  adrenal glandulars
  calcium

  kidney glandulars
  magnesium
  pantothenic acid
  vitamin B complex
orthomolecular medicine
qigong
yoga

ARTHRALGIA
acupuncture

ARTHRITIS
aromatherapy
Ayurveda
  medicated enema
bodywork
  prolotherapy
cell therapy
chiropractic
complementary alternative medicine
  (CAM)
diet therapy
  Gerson diet
herbal therapy
  alfalfa
  echinacea
  feverfew
  ginkgo biloba
  hawthorne
  kava root
  prickly ash bark
  St. John's wort
homeopathy
hydrotherapy
naturopathy
  glucosamine sulfate
pancreatic enzyme therapy
reflexology

ARTHRITIS, RHEUMATOID

applied kinesiology
aromatherapy
  benzoin
  camphor
  chamomile
  cypress
  fennel
  juniper
  lavender
  lemon
  rosemary
Ayurveda
biofeedback
chelation therapy
enzyme therapy
guided imagery
hydrotherapy
  constitutional hydrotherapy
  heating compress
  neutral bath
hypnotherapy
juice therapy
  cabbage
  carrot
  celery
  cherry
  cucumber
  garlic
  lemon
  parsley
  potato
  radish
magnetic field therapy
naturopathic medicine
orthomolecular medicine
  essential fatty acid
  zinc
  copper
  dietary modification

osteopathy
oxygen therapy
sound therapy
yoga

ATHEROSCLEROSIS

naturopathy

ATHLETIC INJURY

pancreatic enzyme therapy

BURSITIS

acupuncture
chiropractic

CARPAL TUNNEL SYNDROME

acupuncture
chiropractic
osteopathic
  manipulation

CENTRAL NERVOUS SYSTEM DISEASES

Ayurveda

CHILLS

acupuncture
applied kinesiology
colon therapy
environmental medicine
fasting
herbal therapy
  boneset
  chamomile
  pennyroyal
  yarrow
homeopathy
naturopathic medicine
nutritional therapy
  mixed amino acids
  niacin (B3)
  thyroid support

vitamin B complex
vitamin B12
vitamin C
oxygen therapy
  hydrogen peroxide IV
yoga

CIRRHOSIS

aromatherapy
Ayurveda
  aloe vera juice
  guduchi
  kutki
  shanka pushpi
cell therapy
colon therapy
detoxification therapy
diet therapy
  low-protein diet
  whole foods diet
fasting
flower remedies
herbal therapy
  licorice
  milk thistle
hydrotherapy
  cold friction
  constitutional hydrotherapy
  contrast application
juice therapy
  beet
  carrot
  raw flaxseed oil
  garlic
  wheat grass juice
magnetic field therapy
naturopathic medicine
nutritional therapy
  folic acid
  L-arginine
  L-carnitine
  L-cysteine

L-glutathione
L-methionine
lipotrophic factors
liver glandulars
multidigestive enzymes with HCl
    and ox bile extract
niacin (B3)
vitamin B complex
vitamin B12
vitamin C
qigong
reflexology
traditional Chinese medicine
  (TCM)
  bupleurum (chai-hu)

COLD SORES (HERPES SIMPLEX 1)

aromatherapy
biofeedback training
cell therapy
diet therapy
  whole foods diet
environmental medicine
fasting
guided imagery
herbal therapy
  calendula
  echinacea
  goldenseal
  myrrh
  nettle
  Siberian ginseng
homeopathy
hydrotherapy
  ice
magnetic field therapy
naturopathic medicine
nutritional therapy
  acidophilus
  thymus extract
  vitamin B complex

vitamin C with bioflavonoids
vitamin E
zinc gluconate lozenges
orthomolecular medicine
oxygen therapy
    hydrogen peroxide IV
ozone therapy
topical treatment
    butylated hydroxytoluene (BHT)
    vitamin E ointment
traditional Chinese medicine (TCM)

CONTUSION, SOFT-TISSUE
acupuncture

CONVULSIONS
acupressure
    nasal philtrum
aromatherapy
chiropractic
environmental medicine
fasting
guided imagery
herbal therapy
    asafetida
    mugwort
    skullcap
    valerian root
homeopathy
    Belladonna
    Cicuta
hydrotherapy
    constitutional hydrotherapy
light therapy
magnetic field therapy
naturopathic medicine
nutritional therapy
    dimethyl glycine
    DL-glutamic acid
    magnesium
    manganese
    taurine

vitamin B6
osteopathy
traditional Chinese medicine
    (TCM)

CORNS
aromatherapy
    lemon
    verucas
diet therapy
    whole foods diet
herbal therapy
    calendula
homeopathy
    Graphites
    Silicea
hydrotherapy
    hot Epsom salts foot bath
magnetic field therapy
naturopathic medicine
nutritional therapy
    essential fatty acids
    vitamin A
    vitamin E
reflexology
topical treatment
    aloe vera gel
    castor oil

COUGH
applied kinesiology
aromatherapy
    benzoin
    chamomile
    eucalyptus
    frankincense
    juniper
    myrrh
    peppermint
    sandalwood
    thyme
Ayurveda
    cinnamon powder

clove
ginger powder
ginger
honey
kant kari
lemon juice
Punarnava
raw sugar
salt
sesame seeds
shatavari
sitopaladi
turmeric powder
vasaka
yasti madhu
bodywork
chiropractic
colon therapy
diet therapy
  whole foods diet
  umeiboshi plum paste
    (dry cough)
environmental medicine
fasting
guided imagery
herbal therapy
  coltsfoot
  honey
  marshmallow leaves
  mullein
  onion juice
homeopathy
  Aconite
  Belladonna
  Bryonia
  Drosera
  Hyoscyamus
  Ipecac
  Phosphorus
  Pulsatilla
  Rumex
  Spongia

hydrotherapy
  benzoin steam inhalation
  hot pack
juice therapy
  cardamom
  cinnamon
  cumin
  fresh fruit/vegetable
  pear
magnetic field therapy
naturopathic medicine
neural therapy
nutritional therapy
  folic acid
  vitamin A
  vitamin C and
    bioflavonoids
  vitamin E
  zinc lozenges
osteopathy
oxygen therapy
  hydrogen peroxide therapy
traditional Chinese medicine
  (TCM)
yoga

CURVATURE OF THE SPINE
bodywork
  Rolfing

CUTS
acupuncture
Ayurveda
  aloe vera gel
  tikta ghee
  turmeric
fasting
guided imagery
herbal therapy
homeopathy
  Arnica
  Calendula

Hypericum
Ledum
hydrotherapy
  ice pack
naturopathic medicine
nutritional therapy
  aloe vera
  arginine
  pantothenic acid
  proteolytic enzymes
  vitamin A
  vitamin E oil
  vitamin C
  zinc oxide cream
  zinc
oxygen therapy
  hyperbaric oxygen
    therapy
topical treatment
  green clay

DANDRUFF
aromatherapy
  patchouli
  rosemary
  tea tree
detoxification therapy
diet therapy
  raw foods
  whole foods
environmental medicine
fasting
herbal therapy
  nettle
  oil of evening primrose
  rosemary
  sage
homeopathy
  Cantharis
  Graphites
  Lycopodium
  Sepia

Sulfur
Thuja
hydrotherapy
  contrast application
magnetic field therapy
naturopathic medicine
nutritional therapy
  beta carotene
  essential fatty acids (omega-6)
  kelp tablets
  vitamin B6
  vitamin E
  vitamin B complex
  vitamin A
  vitamin C
  zinc
topical treatment
  apple cider vinegar
  linseed oil
  selenium-based shampoo
  vitamin E oil
traditional Chinese medicine
  (TCM)

DECUBITUS ULCERS
massage therapy

DEGENERATIVE DISK DISEASE
acupuncture
chiropractic

DERMATITIS
acupuncture
aromatherapy
  benzoin
  bergamot
  chamomile
  geranium
  lavender
cell therapy
detoxification therapy

diet therapy
  gluten-free diet
environmental medicine
fasting
flower remedies
herbal therapy
  calendula flower
  chickweed
  cleavers
  nettle
  red clover
  St. John's wort
homeopathy
  Graphites
  Lycopodium
  petroleum
  Pulsatilla
  Sepia
  Sulfur
  Thuja
hydrotherapy
  cold compress
hypnotherapy
juice therapy
  apple
  beet
  cantaloupe
  carrot
  celery
  cucumber
magnetic field therapy
naturopathic medicine
nutritional therapy
  acidophilus
  evening primrose oil
  magnesium
  omega-6 fatty acids
  vitamin B complex
  vitamin B6
  zinc
osteopathy

oxygen therapy
  hydrogen peroxide IV
reflexology
relaxation
topical treatment
  aloe vera gel
  evening primrose oil
  honey
  pyridoxine ointment
  unflavored yogurt
vitamin A
vitamin E
zinc oxide
yoga

DISK HERNIATION
bodywork
  prolotherapy
chiropractic

DIZZINESS
acupressure
  GV26
biologic dentistry
bodywork
  acupressure
  Alexander technique
  massage
  shiatsu
cell therapy
chiropractic
craniosacral therapy
detoxification therapy
diet therapy
  whole foods diet
environmental medicine
fasting
guided imagery
herbal therapy
  ginger
  ginkgo leaf extract
homeopathy

Cocculus
Convallaria
Gelsemium
Granatum
Phosphorus
hydrotherapy
   hot foot bath
hypnotherapy
magnetic field therapy
naturopathic medicine
nutritional therapy
   calcium pantothenate
   iron
   niacin (B3)
   pantothenic acid
   vitamin B complex
   vitamin B5
   vitamin E
osteopathy
oxygen therapy
   hydrogen peroxide IV
reflexology
   cervicals
   ear reflex
   side of neck
traditional Chinese medicine (TCM)

DYSENTERY

applied kinesiology
aromatherapy
   black pepper
   chamomile
   cypress
   eucalyptus
   lemon
   melissa
colon therapy
fasting
herbal therapy
   chamomile
   electrolyte replacement
   garlic
   meadowsweet

   oak bark
hydrotherapy
   constitutional hydrotherapy
magnetic field therapy
naturopathic medicine
nutritional therapy
   acidophilus
   bifidobacteria
   citrus seed extract
   Lactobacillus bulgaricus
   vitamin A
osteopathy
traditional Chinese medicine (TCM)
yoga

DYSMENORRHEA

craniosacral therapy
herbal medicine
   black haw
   black cohosh
   chamomile
   chaste tree berry
   cramp bark
   dandelion leaf
   ginkgo biloba
   hospital
   red raspberry leaf
   skullcap
   white willow bark
homeopathy
   Chamomilla
   Lachesis
   Sepia
nutritional therapy
   calcium
   essential fatty acids
   magnesium
   potassium
   vitamin B3
   vitamin B6
   vitamin C
   zinc
traditional Chinese medicine (TCM)

ECZEMA

aromatherapy
  bergamot
  chamomile
  eucalyptus
  geranium
  juniper
  lavender
  melissa
  neroli
Ayurveda
  kutki
  manjista
  neem
  turmeric
bodywork
  acupressure
  reflexology
  shiatsu
diet therapy
fasting
flower remedies
herbal therapy
  burdock
  calendula flowers
  chamomile
  chickweed infusion
  cleavers
  figwort
  goldenseal
  linden flower
  nettle
  red clover
  skullcap
  St. John's wort
  yellowdock
homeopathy
  Dulcamara
  Graphites
  Petroleum
  Psorinum
  Rhus tox

Sulfur
hydrotherapy
  heating compress
juice therapy
  beet
  black currant
  carrot
  cucumber
  green juices
  parsley
  red grapes
  spinach
  wheat grass
mind/body therapy
naturopathic medicine
  zinc oxide
nutritional therapy
oxygen therapy
  hydrogen peroxide IV
reflexology
  adrenals
  diaphragm
  all glands
  intestines
  kidneys
  liver
  thyroid
topical treatment
yoga

EDEMA

aromatherapy
  fennel
  geranium
  juniper
  rosemary
Ayurveda
  Punarnava guggulu
bodywork
  acupressure
  massage
  reflexology
  shiatsu

chiropractic
craniosacral therapy
detoxification therapy
diet therapy
  whole foods diet
environmental medicine
fasting
herbal therapy
  dandelion leaf
hydrotherapy
  contrast application
  neutral bath
hydrotherapy
juice therapy
  carrot
  celery
  cranberry
  cucumber
  dandelion
  green juices
  parsley
  pear
  pineapple
  watermelon
magnetic field therapy
naturopathic medicine
nutritional therapy
  alfalfa tablets
  pantothenic acid
  potassium
  protein supplement (free-form
    amino acids)
  vitamin C
  vitamin B6
  vitamin B complex
osteopathy
oxygen therapy
  hyperbaric oxygen therapy
qigong
reflexology
traditional Chinese medicine (TCM)

EPILEPSY

acupressure
  see Convulsions
Ayurveda
  brahmi
  jatamansi
  Punarnava
  saraswati churna
bodywork
  abdominal massage
  acupressure
  Feldenkrais
  reflexology
  Rolfing
  shiatsu
diet therapy
  hypoglycemic diet
  low-carbohydrate diet
  low-fat diet
fasting
flower remedies
herbal therapy
  skullcap tincture
hydrotherapy
  constitutional therapy
  Epsom salts baths
juice therapy
meditation
mind/body therapy
  biofeedback
  hypnotherapy
  meditation
nutritional therapy
  amino acid blend formula
  B complex, IM
  calcium
  choline
  dimethyl glycine
  folic acid
  L-taurine
  L-tyrosine

magnesium
manganese
niacin (vitamin B3)
vitamin B complex
vitamin B5
vitamin B6
vitamin B12
zinc
reflexology
  colon
  diaphragm
  all glands
  ileocecal
  neck area
  whole spine
yoga

FAINTING
aromatherapy
  basil
  black pepper
  lavender
  neroli
  peppermint
  rosemary
bodywork
  acupressure
  reflexology
  shiatsu
diet therapy
  whole foods diet
environmental medicine
fasting
flower remedies
  Bach Flower Rescue Remedy
homeopathy
  Aconite
  Ignatia
hydrotherapy
  constitutional hydrotherapy
naturopathic medicine
nutritional therapy

oxygen therapy
reflexology
  pituitary
traditional Chinese medicine (TCM)

FIBROMYALGIA
massage therapy
  Trager method

FIBROSITIS
homeopathy
hydrotherapy

FLATULENCE
applied kinesiology
aromatherapy
  anise
  bergamot
  chamomile
  coriander
  fennel
  juniper
  lavender
  peppermint
  rosemary
biofeedback training
bodywork
  abdominal massage
cell therapy
chiropractic
colon therapy
detoxification therapy
  colon detoxification
  gastrointestinal detoxification
environmental medicine
fasting
herbal therapy
  anise water
homeopathy
  Lycopodium
  Chamomilla
  Cinchona
hydrotherapy

constitutional hydrotherapy
cold sitz baths
juice therapy
  beet
  carrot
  celery
  garlic
  papaya
  parsley
  yellow onion
light therapy
magnetic field therapy
naturopathic medicine
nutritional therapy
  acidophilus
  aloe vera
  charcoal tablets
  digestive enzymes
  hydrochloric acid
  lipotrophic factors
  niacin (vitamin B3)
  pancreatin
  peppermint oil
  vitamin B1
  vitamin B complex
osteopathy
qigong
reflexology
  gallbladder
  intestines
  liver
  pancreas
  stomach
traditional Chinese medicine
  (TCM)
yoga

FOOD POISONING

Ayurveda
  cumin
  coriander
  fennel tea

homeopathy
hydrotherapy
  constitutional hydrotherapy
juice therapy
  beet
  carrot
  garlic
naturopathic medicine
nutritional therapy
  acidophilus
  charcoal tablets
  citrus seed extract
  garlic capsules
  kelp
  vitamin C with
    bioflavonoids
oxygen therapy
  hydrogen peroxide IV

FRACTURE

acupuncture
biofeedback training
bodywork
cell therapy
chiropractic
fasting
guided imagery
herbal therapy
  comfrey
  horsetail
  Solomon's seal
homeopathy
  Aconite
  Arnica
  Calcarea phosphorica
  Ruta graveolens
  Symphytum
hydrotherapy
  contrast application
  ice
juice therapy
  beet

carrot
watercress
magnetic field therapy
naturopathic medicine
nutritional therapy
oxygen therapy
  hyperbaric oxygen therapy
  reconstructive therapy
reflexology
  reflex to affected area on foot
  referral area
topical treatment
  mullein
  turmeric

FROSTBITE
acupuncture
fasting
herbal therapy
  ginger tea
hydrotherapy
  immersion bath
naturopathic medicine
nutritional therapy
  vitamin B complex
oxygen therapy
  hyperbaric oxygen therapy
qigong
traditional Chinese medicine
  (TCM)
  dong quai
  peony formula

FROZEN SHOULDER
acupuncture
  Tui Na
osteopathic manipulation

FUNGAL INFECTION
aromatherapy
  geranium
  patchouli
  tea tree

detoxification therapy
diet therapy
environmental medicine
fasting
herbal therapy
  calendula oil
  garlic
  myrrh
  tea tree
homeopathy
  Belladonna
  Calendula
  Chamomilla
  Sulfur
juice therapy
  garlic
  vegetable juice
magnetic field therapy
naturopathic medicine
  tea tree
  Thuja
nutritional therapy
oxygen therapy
  hydrogen peroxide IV
  hyperbaric oxygen therapy
  ozone/oxygen mixture
topical treatment
  citrus seed extract
  crushed garlic
  honey
  pau d'arco tea
  tea tree
traditional Chinese medicine (TCM)

GALLBLADDER DISORDERS
acupuncture
cell therapy
colon therapy
detoxification therapy
environmental medicine
fasting

herbal therapy
  balmony
  chamomile
  fringetree bark
  lemon balm
  milk thistle
  wild yam
hydrotherapy
  constitutional therapy
  hot pack
juice therapy
  beet
  carrot
  cucumber
  dandelion root
  garlic
  grape
  grapefruit
  lemon
  pear
  radish
magnetic field therapy
naturopathic medicine
neural therapy
nutritional therapy
  acidophilus
  alfalfa tablets
  choline inositol
  L-taurine
  lecithin
  lipotrophic factors
  peppermint oil
  unsaturated fatty acids
  vitamin B complex
  vitamin C
  vitamin C
topical treatment
yoga

GOUT

Ayurveda
  medicated enema
bee venom therapy

HAIR LOSS

acupuncture
aromatherapy
  lavender
  rosemary
  sage
  thyme
Ayurveda
  amla
  ashwagandha
  bhringaraj oil
  brahmi oil
cell therapy
diet therapy
  whole foods diet
herbal therapy
  almond oil
  rosemary oil
homeopathy
  Arnica
  Sepia
juice therapy
  alfalfa
  beet
  carrot
  nettle
  onion
  spinach
magnetic field therapy
naturopathic medicine
nutritional therapy
  amino acid blends
  biotin
  vitamin B complex
  flaxseed oil
  iron
  protein supplements
  trace minerals
  zinc
topical treatment
  apple cider vinegar
  castor oil

olive oil
sage tea
vitamin E oil
wheat germ oil
traditional Chinese medicine (TCM)

HANGOVER
acupressure
aromatherapy
  fennel
  rose
  rosemary
bodywork
diet therapy
  lemon juice
  orange juice
  tomato juice
  whole grain breads
environmental medicine
fasting
herbal therapy
  dandelion root tincture
  digestive bitters
homeopathy
  Aconite
  Lachesis
  Nux vomica
  Sulfur
hydrotherapy
magnetic field therapy
naturopathic medicine
nutritional therapy
  glutamine
  lipotrophic formula
  vitamin B complex
  vitamin C
oxygen therapy
  liquid oxygen drops
traditional Chinese medicine (TCM)

HEADACHES
acupressure
  GB16 with B2
  GB20
  L14
acupuncture
aromatherapy
  chamomile
  eucalyptus
  lavender
  marjoram
  peppermint
  rosemary
biofeedback training
bodywork
  Alexander technique
  Feldenkrais
  polarity therapy
  Rolfing
  Trager approach
chiropractic
colon therapy
craniosacral therapy
diet therapy
  rotation diet
environmental medicine
fasting
guided imagery
herbal therapy
  bay leaves
  bromelain
  cayenne pepper
  chamomile
  coriander
  feverfew
  garlic
  ginkgo biloba
  onion
  querticin
  skullcap
  turmeric
  valerian
  willow bark
hydrotherapy
  hot bath

sauna
steam bath
hypnotherapy
juice therapy
  beet
  carrot
  celery
  cucumber
  parsley
  spinach
magnetic field therapy
nutritional therapy
  calcium
  DL-phenylalanine
  evening primrose oil
  magnesium
  MaxEPA (fish oil)
  multivitamin/mineral
  potassium
  vitamin B3
  vitamin C
  vitamin E
osteopathy
oxygen therapy
  hydrogen peroxide therapy
  hyperbaric oxygen therapy
relaxation techniques
  deep relaxation
  meditation
  progressive relaxation
  yoga
yoga

HEAVY METAL TOXICITY

Ayruveda
  aloe vera gel
  brahmi ghee nasya
  dashamoola basti
  Pancha karma
  shatavari rasayana
  tikta ghee

  yasti madhu vaman
chelation therapy
  diet therapy
  whole foods diet
fasting
homeopathy
juice therapy
  beet
  burdock
  carrot
  celery
  currant oil
  flaxseed
  garlic
naturopathic medicine
nutritional therapy
  detox program with vitamin C
  folic acid
  liver glandular
  multivitamin
  vitamin B complex
orthomolecular medicine
oxygen therapy
  IV chelation therapy
traditional Chinese medicine (TCM)

HEMORRHOIDS

acupuncture
applied kinesiology
aromatherapy
  cypress
  frankincense
  juniper
  niaouli
Ayurveda
  aloe vera
  castor oil
  ginger
  raw sugar
  sesame seeds
  shatavari

tikta ghee
triphala
Triphala guggulu
bodywork
myotherapy
cell therapy
detoxification therapy
diet therapy
 high-fiber diet
 whole foods diet
fasting
guided imagery
herbal therapy
 Aloe
 calendula
 collinsonia
 cranesbill
 ginkgo
 plantain
 St. John's wort
 witch hazel
homeopathy
 Aloe
 Berberis
 Hamamelis
 Nux vomica
 Thuja
juice therapy
 beets
 carrot
 celery
 parsley
 spinach
 watercress
light therapy
magnetic field therapy
naturopathic medicine
nutritional therapy
 aloe vera gel
 beta carotene
 essential fatty acids

folic acid
linseed oil
olive oil
rutin
vitamin A
vitamin B complex
vitamin C with bioflavonoids
vitamin E
zinc oxide
zinc
osteopathy
qigong
reconstructive therapy
reflexology
 adrenals
 diaphragm
 lower spine
 rectum
 sigmoid
topical treatment
 aloe vera
 calendula ointment
 garlic
 olive oil
 vitamin E
 witch hazel
 zinc oxide
yoga

HEPATITIS
aromatherapy
 rosemary
Ayurveda
 aloe gel
 baking soda
 brahmi ghee nasya
 Chyavan prash
 guduchi
 kutki
 shanka pushpi
 shatavari

sugarcane juice
cell therapy
colon therapy
detoxification therapy
diet therapy
  low-protein diet
  hypoglycemic regime
  whole foods diet
enemas
  chlorophyll enema
  warm enema
fasting
guided imagery
herbal therapy
  dandelion root
  fringetree bark
  licorice
  milk thistle
  Phyllanthus amarus
  wahoo
hydrotherapy
  constitutional hydrotherapy
  contrast application
juice therapy
  beet
  black currant
  burdock
  carrot
  flax
  garlic
  wheat grass
magnetic field therapy
naturopathic medicine
nutritional therapy
  adrenal glandular
  beta carotene
  betaine HCl
  evening primrose oil
  lipotropic factor
  liver glandulars
  milk thistle extract

  multienzymes
  multiminerals
  pantothenic acid
  protein (free-form amino
    acids)
  vitamin B complex
oxygen therapy
  hydrogen peroxide IV
  ozone
qigong

HERNIATED DISK
See Disk Herniation

HIATAL HERNIA
applied kinesiology
biofeedback training
breathing exercises
chiropractic
colon therapy
detoxification therapy
fasting
herbal therapy
  comfrey root
  marshmallow root
  meadowsweet
homeopathy
hydrotherapy
  contrast application
magnetic field therapy
naturopathic medicine
nutritional therapy
  aloe vera juice
  digestive enzymes
  liquid chlorophyll
  multivitamin/mineral
  pancreatin
  vitamin B complex
osteopathy
  muscle energy techniques
traditional Chinese medicine
  (TCM)

HICCUPS

acupressure
  S117
  TW17
Ayurveda
  castor oil
  honey
  mayur chandrika bhasma
biofeedback training
bodywork
  massage
  reflexology
chiropractic
environmental medicine
fasting
herbal therapy
  black cohosh
  chamomile tea
  skullcap
  vervain
homeopathy
  Acidum sulfate
  Ginseng
  Ignatia
  Lycopodium
  Magnesium phosphate
  Nux vomica
hypnotherapy
magnetic field therapy
naturopathic medicine
nutritional therapy
  charcoal tablets
  papaya enzymes
osteopathy
reflexology
  diaphragm
  stomach
traditional Chinese medicine (TCM)

HIVES

acupuncture
applied kinesiology

aromatherapy
  chamomile
  tagetes
biofeedback training
detoxification therapy
enemas
environmental medicine
guided imagery
herbal therapy
  parsley
  peppermint oil
homeopathy
  Urtica urens
hydrotherapy
  oatmeal bath
light therapy
  ultraviolet light therapy
magnetic field therapy
naturopathic medicine
neural therapy
nutritional therapy
  Alka Seltzer Gold tablets
  B complex
  beta carotene
  bioflavonoids
  bromelain
  calamine lotion
  calcium glycerophosphate
  dexpanthenol
  essential fatty acids
  hydroxocobalamin
  magnesium chloride hexahydrate
  pancreatic enzymes
  pantothenic acid
  pyridoxine hydrochloride
  unflavored yogurt
  vitamin A
  vitamin B complex
  vitamin B6
  vitamin C
  zinc oxide

orthomolecular medicine
osteopathy
oxygen therapy
  hydrogen peroxide IV
qigong
topical treatment
  coriander juice
traditional Chinese medicine
  (TCM)

HYPERTHYROIDISM

biofeedback training
diet therapy
  whole foods diet
homeopathy
  Thyroidinum
hydrotherapy
  ice packs
juice therapy
  cabbage
  carrot
  celery
  parsley
  spinach
  watercress
magnetic field therapy
naturopathic medicine
nutritional therapy
  amino acid supplements
  calcium
  choline
  iodine
  kelp
  magnesium
  multivitamin/mineral complex
  thiamine (vitamin B1)
  vitamin A
  vitamin B complex
  vitamin C
qigong
traditional Chinese medicine
  (TCM)

HYPOGLYCEMIA

applied kinesiology
biofeedback training
cell therapy
chiropractic
diet therapy
  high-fiber diet
environmental medicine
fasting
herbal therapy
  burdock
  dandelion
  licorice
hydrotherapy
  constitutional hydrotherapy
juice therapy
  beet
  burdock
  carrot
  garlic
  Jerusalem artichoke
magnetic field therapy
naturopathic medicine
nutritional therapy
  adrenal glandular
  calcium
  chromium
  magnesium
  multitrace minerals
  niacinamide
  pantothenic acid
  protein supplement
  amino acids
  vitamin B complex
  vitamin B injections
  vitamin B6
  vitamin C with
    bioflavonoids
  zinc
orthomolecular medicine
osteopathy
qigong

reflexology
   all glands
   liver
   pancreas
traditional Chinese medicine (TCM)

HYPOTHYROIDISM

acupuncture
biofeedback training
cell therapy
fasting
herbal therapy
   butternut
   cascara sagrada
   gentian
   kelp
   mugwort
   St. John's wort
   yellowdock
homeopathy
   Calcium carbonate
   Iodum
hydrotherapy
   contrast application
magnetic field therapy
naturopathic medicine
   broccoli
   brussels sprouts
   cabbage
nutritional therapy
osteopathy
qigong
traditional Chinese medicine (TCM)
yoga

INFECTION

aromatherapy
   cedarwood
   frankincense
   patchouli
   tea tree
cell therapy

craniosacral therapy
detoxification therapy
environmental medicine
fasting
guided imagery
herbal therapy
   echinacea
   garlic
   goldenseal
   myrrh
   Siberian ginseng
hydrotherapy
   constitutional hydrotherapy
juice therapy
   beet
   cantaloupe
   carrot
   celery
magnetic field therapy
naturopathic medicine
   licorice root
naturopathic medicine
nutritional therapy
oxygen therapy
   hydrogen peroxide IV
   hyperbaric oxygen therapy
   ozone
reflexology
   adrenals
   affected area
   lymph system
traditional Chinese medicine (TCM)

INFLAMMATION

acupuncture
aromatherapy
cell therapy
craniosacral therapy
detoxification therapy
diet therapy
   whole foods diet
fasting

guided imagery
herbal therapy
   calendula
   chamomile
   lemon balm
   licorice
   meadowsweet
   plantain
   St. John's wort
   wild yam
   willow bark
homeopathy
   Aconite
   belladonna
   ferrum phosphate
   sulfur
hydrotherapy
   contrast application
   ice
juice therapy
   currants
   grapes, black or red
   pineapple
   vegetable juices
light therapy
   cold (soft) laser photostimulation
   therapy
magnetic field therapy
   negative magnetic field
naturopathic medicine
nutritional therapy
   beta carotene
   bromelain
   eicosapentaenoic acid
   (EPA)
   evening primrose oil
   garlic capsules
   oily fish
   proteolytic enzymes
   vitamin C with
   bioflavonoids

vitamin A and E
   emulsion
   zinc
oxygen therapy
   hydrogen peroxide
   therapy
   hyperbaric oxygen
pancreatic enzyme therapy
reflexology

INSECT BITES

aromatherapy
   basil
   cinnamon
   garlic
   lavender
   lemon
   onion
   sage
   savory
   thyme
Ayurveda
   cilantro juice
   sandalwood
environmental medicine
flower remedies
   Rescue Remedy
herbal therapy
   aloe gel
   plantain
homeopathy
   Aconite
   Calendula
   Hypericum
   Lachesis
   Ledum
   Urtica urens
hydrotherapy
   cold compress
light therapy
naturopathic medicine

nutritional therapy
  vitamin B5
  vitamin C
  vitamin E
orthomolecular therapy
topical treatment
  charcoal
  bicarbonate of soda
  lemon juice
  vinegar
  vitamin E

INSOMNIA
aromatherapy (lavender)
herbal therapy
  alfalfa
  chamomile
  echinacea
  ginkgo biloba
  hawthorn
  kava root
  St. John's wort
  valerian
massage therapy
melatonin

JAUNDICE
aromatherapy
  hyssop
  juniper
Ayurveda
  barley soup
  coriander
  cumin
  dugdapachan bhasma
  fennel
  Gokshura guggulu
  jatamansi
  kamadudha
  mutral churna
  Punarnava guggulu

cell therapy
colon therapy
detoxification therapy
enemas
fasting
herbal therapy
  blackhaw
  cornsilk
  gravel root
  wild yam
homeopathy
  Berberis
  Sarsaparilla
hydrotherapy
  constitutional hydrotherapy
  hot pack
juice therapy
  beet
  carrot
  cranberry
  cucumber
  garlic
  horseradish
  lemon
  watermelon
light therapy
magnetic field therapy
mind/body therapy
  relaxation
naturopathic medicine
nutritional therapy
osteopathy
qigong
reflexology
  bladder
  diaphragm
  kidneys
  parathyroid
  ureter tubes
traditional Chinese medicine
  (TCM)

LARYNGITIS

acupuncture
aromatherapy
  benzoin
  frankincense
  lavender
  sandalwood
  thyme
detoxification therapy
diet therapy
  whole foods diet
environmental medicine
guided imagery
herbal therapy
  bayberry
  chamomile
  cranesbill
  echinacea tincture
  red sage
  sage
  yarrow
homeopathy
  Aconite
  Belladonna
  Causticum
  Drosera
  Spongia
hydrotherapy
  contrast application
  heating compress
juice therapy
  apple
  beet
  carrot
  celery
  cucumber
  ginger
  pineapple
light therapy
magnetic field
  therapy

naturopathic medicine
  licorice root
nutritional therapy
  acidophilus
  garlic
  vitamin A
  vitamin C
  zinc lozenges
osteopathy
oxygen therapy
  hydrogen peroxide IV
  ozonated water gargle
reflexology
  chest/lung
  diaphragm
  lymph system
  throat
  toes
topical treatment
  cold compress
traditional Chinese medicine (TCM)

LONGEVITY

acupressure
bodywork
  acupressure
  massage
  shiatsu
cell therapy
detoxification therapy
fasting
guided imagery
herbal therapy
  gingko biloba
  ginseng
  gotu kola
homeopathy
  Hydrocotyle
  Thuja
juice therapy
  apricot
  fresh fruit/vegetable juices

lemon
lime
papaya
pineapple
wheat grass
magnetic field therapy
naturopathic medicine
nutritional therapy
  coenzyme Q10
  digestive enzymes
  eicosapentaenoic acid (EPA)
  essential fatty acids
  evening primrose oil
  gamma linolenic acid (GLA)
  garlic
  green magma
  kelp
  multivitamin/mineral
    supplement
  superoxide dismutase (SOD)
  vitamin A
  vitamin B6
  vitamin C
  vitamin E
oxygen therapy
  hydrogen peroxide therapy
qigong

LUPUS

bodywork
  Rolfing
biofeedback training
cell therapy
chelation therapy
detoxification therapy
diet
  whole foods diet
environmental medicine
fasting
guided imagery
herbal therapy
  Bupleurum falcatum

echinacea
goldenseal
licorice
pau d'arco
red clover
wild yam
hydrotherapy
  constitutional hydrotherapy
juice therapy
  black currant oil
  carrot
  celery
  flaxseed oil
  garlic
light therapy
  PUVA therapy
magnetic field therapy
naturopathic medicine
nutritional therapy
  beta carotene
  calcium
  digestive enzymes
  essential fatty acids
  garlic
  L-cysteine
  L-methionine
  magnesium
  proteolytic enzymes
  selenium
  vitamin A
  vitamin B complex
  vitamin B5
  vitamin B12
  vitamin C and bioflavonoids
  vitamin E
  zinc
oxygen therapy
  hydrogen peroxide IV
  hyperbaric oxygen therapy
pancreatic enzyme therapy
qigong

reflexology
topical treatment
traditional Chinese medicine (TCM)

MENOPAUSE

diet therapy
  low-fat diet
  high-fiber diet
  vegetarian-based diet
herbal medicine
homeopathy
natural hormone therapy
nutritional therapy
  aspartate
  borage oil
  calcium
  evening primrose oil
  magnesium
  potassium
  vitamin B complex
  vitamin B6
  vitamin C and bioflavonoids
  vitamin E
traditional Chinese medicine
  (TCM)

MENORRHAGIA

herbal medicine
  lady's mantle
  partridge berry (squaw vine)
  yarrow
nutritional therapy
  iron
  vitamin A
  vitamin C with flavonoids

MONONUCLEOSIS

acupuncture
biofeedback training
cell therapy
environmental medicine
fasting
herbal therapy
  calendula
  cleavers
  echinacea
  myrrh
  wormwood
homeopathy
  Belladonna
  Phytolacca
hydrotherapy
  constitutional hydrotherapy
juice therapy
  beet
  carrot
  garlic
  green pepper
  green juices
  lemon
  onion
  orange
  pineapple
  tomato
  wheat grass
magnetic field therapy
naturopathic medicine
nutritional therapy
  acidophilus
  chlorophyll
  free-form amino acids
  glandular tissue of organs
    involved
  multivitamin-mineral
    supplement
  vitamin C
  vitamin E emulsion
  vitamin A
  vitamin B complex
osteopathy
oxygen therapy
  hydrogen peroxide therapy
qigong
traditional Chinese medicine
  (TCM)

MOTION SICKNESS

acupressure
  P6
acupuncture
aromatherapy
  peppermint oil
biofeedback training
environmental medicine
fasting
herbal therapy
  ginger
homeopathy
  Belladonna
  Cocculus
  Colchicum
  Ignatia
  Ipecac
  Nux vomica
hypnotherapy
juice therapy
  ginger
naturopathic medicine
  ginger tea
nutritional therapy
  charcoal tablets
  ginger
  magnesium
  vitamin B6
  vitamin B complex
osteopathy
reflexology
  diaphragm
  ear reflex
  neck
  spine
traditional Chinese medicine (TCM)
  ginger capsules

MUSCLE SPASM/MUSCLE CRAMP

acupressure
acupuncture

applied kinesiology
aromatherapy
  chamomile
  clary sage
  lavender
  marjoram
  rosemary
biofeedback training
bodywork
  acupressure
  Alexander technique
  Feldenkrais
  Hellerwork
  massage
  prolotherapy
  reflexology
  Rolfing
  shiatsu
  yoga
cell therapy
chiropractic
detoxification therapy
diet therapy
  whole foods diet
environmental medicine
fasting
guided imagery
herbal therapy
  cramp bark tea
  lobelia
hydrotherapy
  hot pack
  sitz bath
hypnosis
juice therapy
  beet
  carrot
  celery
  cucumber
  sweet fruit juices
light therapy
magnetic field therapy

naturopathic medicine
 Epsom salts packs
 magnesium
nutritional therapy
 aminoethanol phosphate (AEP)
 calcium
 chlorophyll
 essential oils
 evening primrose oil
 flaxseed oil
 folic acid
 magnesium
 multimineral/trace element
  formula
 niacin
 niacinamide
 potassium
 silicon
 thiamine (vitamin B1)
 vitamin B complex
 vitamin E
 vitamin A
 vitamin C
 zinc oxide
orthomolecular medicine
osteopathy
oxygen therapy
 hydrogen peroxide IV
 hyperbaric oxygen therapy
yoga

MUSCLE TENSION

herbal therapy
 echinacea
 ginkgo biloba
 hawthorn
 kava root
 St. John's wort

MYOSITIS

hydrotherapy

NAUSEA

acupressure
acupuncture
aromatherapy
 peppermint
 rosewood
biofeedback training
bodywork
 therapeutic touch
 shiatsu
colon therapy
craniosacral therapy
environmental medicine
fasting
guided imagery
herbal therapy
 ginger
 peppermint
homeopathy
 Colchicum
 Ipecac
 Nux vomica
 Pulsatilla
hydrotherapy
 constitutional
  hydrotherapy
hypnotherapy
magnetic field therapy
meditation
naturopathic medicine
 ginger tea
neural therapy
nutritional therapy
 magnesium
 vitamin B complex
 vitamin B6
osteopathy
qigong
reflexology
 diaphragm
 gallbladder

liver

stomach

NEURALGIA/ NEUROPATHY/NEURITIS

acupressure

acupuncture

aromatherapy

  Jamaican dogwood

  oat

  peppermint oil

  Siberian ginseng

  skullcap

  St. John's wort

  valerian

biofeedback training

cell therapy

chiropractic

craniosacral therapy

detoxification therapy

diet therapy

  whole foods diet

energy medicine

  Electro-Acuscope

environmental medicine

fasting

herbal therapy

homeopathy

  Aconite

  Belladonna

  Chelidonium

  Lycopodium

  Magnesium phosphate

  Phytolacca

hydrotherapy

  contrast application

juice therapy

  carrot blend

  celery

  parsley

light therapy

magnetic field therapy

naturopathic medicine

neural therapy

nutritional therapy

  brewer's yeast

  calcium

  folic acid

  lecithin

  magnesium

  niacin (vitamin B3)

  pantothenic acid

  proteolytic enzymes

  thiamine (vitamin B1)

  vitamin C and bioflavonoids

  vitamin B6

osteopathic manipulation

oxygen therapy

  hyperbaric oxygen therapy

  hydrogen peroxide therapy

relaxation

topical treatment

  Epsom salts pack

traditional Chinese medicine (TCM)

yoga

NEUROMUSCULAR DISORDERS

Feldenkrais method

  Awareness Through Movement
    (ATM)

  Functional Integration (FI)

Tragerwork

yoga

NOSEBLEEDS

acupressure

acupuncture

aromatherapy

  cypress

  frankincense

  lavender

  lemon

bodywork
  acupressure
  reflexology
  shiatsu
diet therapy
environmental medicine
fasting
herbal therapy
  oak bark
homeopathy
  Belladonna
  Chamomilla
  Hamamelis
  Hyoscyamus
  Ipecac
  Rhus tox
hydrotherapy
  ice pack
juice therapy
  beet
  carrot
  cayenne
  ginger
naturopathic medicine
nutritional therapy
osteopathy
traditional Chinese medicine (TCM)

OSTEOARTHRITIS

acupressure
acupuncture
applied kinesiology
aromatherapy
  camphor
  lemon
  marjoram
  mint
  sesame oil
bee venom therapy
bodywork
  Rolfing
  shiatsu

cell therapy
chelation therapy
chiropractic
craniosacral therapy
enzyme therapy
flower remedies
glucosamine sulfate
guided imagery
juice therapy
  beet
  cabbage
  carrot
  celery
  cucumber
light therapy
naturopathy
orthomolecular medicine
osteopathic medicine
reconstructive therapy
reflexology
yoga

OSTEOMYELITIS
hyperbaric oxygen therapy

OSTEOPOROSIS
acupuncture
Ayurveda
  amla
  ginger
  raw sugar
  sesame seeds
  shatavari
chelation therapy
chiropractic
diet therapy
  vegetarian-based diet
environmental medicine
fasting
herbal medicine
  alfalfa
  black cohosh

chasteberry
horsetail
oats
homeopathy
  Bufo
  Calcarea fluorica
  Calcarea carbonica
  Calcarea phosphorica
  Carcinosin
  Silicea
  Vermiculate
juice therapy
  beet
  carrot
  celery
  green juice
  lemon
  papaya
  pineapple
magnetic field therapy
natural hormonal
  therapy
naturopathy
nutritional therapy
  boron
  calcium
  microcrystalline hydroxyapatite
    (MCHC)
orthomolecular medicine
  copper
  dietary modification
  essential fatty acid
  zinc
osteopathic medicine
qigong
reflexology
traditional Chinese medicine
  (TCM)

PAIN

acupuncture
biofeedback

complementary alternative medicine
  (CAM)
hypnosis
osteopathic manipulation

PAIN, BACK

acupuncture
Ayurveda
  medicated enema
bodywork
  Alexander technique
  prolotherapy
  Rolfing
chiropractic
complementary alternative medicine
  (CAM)
craniosacral therapy
herbal therapy
  black cohosh
  echinacea
  ginkgo biloba
  hawthorn
  kava root
  St. John's wort
homeopathy
hydrotherapy
hypnosis
massage therapy
meditation and mindfulness
mind-body therapy
Native American
  medicine
osteopathic manipulation

PAIN, MUSCLE

massage therapy

PAIN, MYOFASCIAL

acupuncture
biofeedback
chiropractic
hypnotherapy
naturopathy

orthomolecular medicine/megavitamin
therapy
copper
dietary modification
·essential fatty acid
zinc

PAIN, NECK

acupuncture
Ayurveda
medicated enema
bodywork
Alexander technique
Rolfing
craniosacral therapy
hypnosis
mind-body therapy
osteopathic manipulation

PAIN, POSTOPERATIVE

acupuncture

PAIN, SHOULDER

acupuncture
chiropractic
osteopathic manipulation

PANCREATITIS

aromatherapy
lemon
marjoram
cell therapy
colon therapy
detoxification therapy
fasting
flower remedies
herbal therapy
homeopathy
hydrotherapy
constitutional hydrotherapy
juice therapy
beet
carrot

garlic
Jerusalem artichoke
magnetic field therapy
naturopathic medicine
nutritional therapy
acidophilus
chromium
extra niacin
L-phenylalanine
lipotrophic factors
magnesium
multiminerals
pancreas glandular
pancreatin enzymes
pantothenic acid
vitamin B complex
vitamin C
osteopathy
oxygen therapy
hydrogen peroxide IV
pancreatic enzyme
therapy
qigong
traditional Chinese medicine
(TCM)

PARALYSIS

acupuncture
Ayurveda
Kaishore guggulu
netra basti
Punarnava guggulu
triphala
Yogaraj guggulu
biofeedback training
chiropractic
craniopathy
craniosacral therapy
diet therapy
whole foods diet
environmental medicine
fasting

homeopathy
hydrotherapy
   whirlpool
magnetic field therapy
naturopathic medicine
neural therapy
nutritional therapy
   free-form amino acids
   magnesium
   niacinamide
   vitamin C
   vitamin B complex
   vitamin B6
   vitamin-mineral injections
orthomolecular medicine
osteopathy
oxygen therapy
   hyperbaric oxygen therapy
reflexology
   brain
   related reflex area
   whole spine
yoga

PARKINSON DISEASE

bodywork
cell therapy
chelation therapy
craniosacral therapy
detoxification therapy
diet therapy
   whole foods diet
fasting
flower remedies
herbal therapy
   passion flower
hydrotherapy
   constitutional hydrotherapy
juice therapy
   beet
   carrot
   cucumber

fruit juices
garlic
radish
spinach
vegetable juices
light therapy
magnetic field therapy
naturopathic medicine
nutritional therapy
   B vitamins
   calcium
   DHEA
   evening primrose oil
   free-form amino acids
   GABA (gamma aminobutyric acid)
   gerovital H-3 (GH-3)
   lecithin
   magnesium
   multivitamin/mineral complex
   neotrophin 1
   nicotinamide adenine denucleotide
      (NADH)
   vitamin E
   vitamin C
orthomolecular medicine
   niacin
   niacinamide
   vitamin B3
oxygen therapy
   hydrogen peroxide IV
reflexology
   chest/lung
   diaphragm
   all glands
   whole spine
traditional Chinese medicine
   (TCM)
yoga

PELLAGRA

magnetic field therapy
naturopathic medicine

nutritional therapy
  niacinamide
  protein supplements
  vitamin B complex
orthomolecular medicine
traditional Chinese medicine
  (TCM)

PERIODONTAL DISEASE

acupuncture
Ayurveda
  amla
  bayberry
  catechu
  coconut oil
  goldenseal
  myrrh
  neem
  sesame oil
detoxification therapy
diet therapy
  whole foods diet
  high-fiber diet
environmental medicine
fasting
herbal therapy
  chamomile
  cleavers
  echinacea
  myrrh
  prickly ash
  sage
hydrotherapy
  contrast application
juice therapy
  cantaloupe
  carrot
magnetic field therapy
naturopathic medicine
nutritional therapy
  beta carotene
  calcium

coenzyme Q10
folic acid, liquid/crystal
magnesium
vitamin A
vitamin B complex
vitamin C with bioflavonoids
vitamin E
zinc
oxygen therapy
  hyperbaric oxygen
    therapy
  ozonated water
topical treatment
  apple cider vinegar
  baking soda
  hydrogen peroxide
traditional Chinese medicine
  (TCM)

PLANTAR FASCIITIS

acupuncture

PLEURISY

acupuncture
bodywork
  Rolfing
cell therapy
detoxification therapy
environmental medicine
fasting
herbal therapy
  echinacea
  elecampane
  garlic
  mullein
  pleurisy root
homeopathy
hydrotherapy
juice therapy
  beet
  carrot
  celery

cucumber
garlic
parsley
pineapple
magnetic field therapy
naturopathic medicine
nutritional therapy
  bromelain
  essential fatty acids
  lung glandular
  proteolytic enzymes
  vitamin A
  vitamin C with bioflavonoids
qigong
reflexology
  adrenals
  chest/lung
  diaphragm
  lymph system
yoga

POISON OAK/IVY

applied kinesiology
chelation therapy
detoxification therapy
environmental medicine
herbal therapy
  mugwort
  plantain
  white oak bark
  witch hazel
hydrotherapy
  cold compress
magnetic field therapy
naturopathic medicine
nutritional therapy
  unflavored yogurt
  vitamin A
  vitamin B complex
  vitamin C
  vitamin E
  zinc/zinc oxide

oxygen therapy
  hyperbaric oxygen therapy
topical treatment
  activated charcoal powder
  aloe vera gel
  apple cider vinegar
  baking soda
  cornstarch
  goldenseal
  witch hazel
traditional Chinese medicine (TCM)

POLIO

biofeedback training
bodywork
  Feldenkrais
diet therapy
  whole foods diet
environmental medicine
fasting
hydrotherapy
  constitutional hydrotherapy
  wet sock treatment
  whirlpool bath
juice therapy
magnetic field therapy
nutritional therapy
  magnesium
  niacinamide
reconstructive therapy
traditional Chinese medicine
  (TCM)
yoga

PREMENSTRUAL SYNDROME (PMS)

acupuncture
Ayurveda
craniosacral therapy
herbal medicine
  chasteberry
  cramp bark

dandelion
skullcap
homeopathy
natural hormone therapy
nutritional therapy
  vitamin A
  vitamin B complex
  vitamin B6
  vitamin E
  zinc
traditional Chinese medicine (TCM)

PSORIASIS

acupuncture
aromatherapy
  bergamot
  lavendar
biofeedback training
bodywork
  massage
  reflexology
cell therapy
chelation
detoxification therapy
environmental medicine
fasting
guided imagery
herbal therapy
  burdock
  cleavers
  nettle
  sarsaparilla
homeopathy
  Graphites
  Psorinum
  Sulfur
hydrotherapy
  heating compress
hypnotherapy
juice therapy
  apple
  beet

burdock
carrot
cucumber
garlic
grape
yellowdock
light therapy
magnetic field therapy
mind/body therapy
naturopathic medicine
nutritional therapy
  European fumaric acid
    treatment
  evening primrose oil
  folic acid
  lecithin
  multimineral supplementation
  unsaturated fatty acids
  vitamin B6
  vitamin A
  vitamin B complex
  vitamin C with
    bioflavonoids
  vitamin B12
  zinc
orthomolecular medicine
osteopathy
oxygen therapy
  hydrogen peroxide IV
reflexology
  adrenals
  diaphragm
  all glands
  intestines
  kidneys
  thyroid
topical treatment
  avocado oil
  linseed oil
  seawater
yoga

RASH
acupuncture
Ayurveda
  black pepper
  cilantro
  coriander
  ghee
  neem oil
detoxification therapy
fasting
herbal therapy
  aloe vera
  burdock root
  coriander
  gentian root
homeopathy
  Belladonna
  Graphites
  Sulfur
hydrotherapy
  oatmeal bath
juice therapy
  beet
  carrot
  fruit
  garlic
  radish
  vegetable
  wheat grass
naturopathic medicine
nutritional therapy
  Alka Seltzer Gold tablets
  baking soda
  eicosapentaenoic acid (EPA)
  flaxseed oil
  gamma linolenic acid
    (GLA)
  vitamin A
  vitamin C
  vitamin E
osteopathy

oxygen therapy
  hydrogen peroxide
    therapy
traditional Chinese medicine
  (TCM)

RAYNAUD DISEASE
acupuncture
biofeedback training
cell therapy
chelation therapy
chiropractic
environmental medicine
fasting
guided imagery
herbal therapy
  ginger
  ginkgo
  prickly ash
homeopathy
  Secale
hydrotherapy
  constitutional hydrotherapy
juice therapy
  fruit
  vegetable
magnetic field therapy
naturopathic medicine
neural therapy
nutritional therapy
  digestive enzymes
  eicosapentaenoic acid
    (EPA)
  evening primrose oil
  folic acid
  iron
  magnesium
  niacin (vitamin B3)
  vitamin B complex
  vitamin E
orthomolecular medicine
osteopathy

oxygen therapy
  hydrogen peroxide therapy
  hyperbaric oxygen therapy
pancreatic enzyme therapy
qigong
traditional Chinese medicine (TCM)

REPETITIVE STRAIN INJURY (RSI)
acupuncture

RHEUMATOID ARTHRITIS
See Arthritis, Rheumatoid

RINGWORM
aromatherapy
  geranium
  lavender
  peppermint thyme
  rosemary
  tea tree
diet therapy
  low-sugar diet
fasting
herbal therapy
  goldenseal
  myrrh
homeopathy
  Graphites
  Sepia
juice therapy
  date
  strawberry
magnetic field therapy
naturopathic medicine
  goldenseal
  tea tree oil
  thuja oil
  thyme oil
nutritional therapy
  bee pollen
  citrus seed extract
  evening primrose oil

vitamin E
vitamin C with bioflavonoids
vitamin B complex
vitamin A
reflexology
topical treatment
traditional Chinese medicine (TCM)

SCIATICA
acupressure
  B48
applied kinesiology
aromatherapy
  birch
  chamomile
  lavender
Ayurveda
  baking soda
  Dashamoola tea basti
  ginger posder
  mahanarayan oil
  Triphala guggulu
bodywork
  acupressure
  Alexander technique
  Feldenkrais
  Hellerwork
  massage
  reflexology
  Rolfing
  shiatsu
  Trager
cell therapy
chiropractic
colon therapy
craniosacral therapy
detoxification therapy
energy medicine
  TENS unit
environmental medicine
fasting
guided imagery

herbal therapy
  black cohosh
  chamomile
  fenugreek
  juniper berries
  mugwort
  parsley
  rosemary
  skullcap
  St. John's wort
  willow bark
homeopathy
  Aconite
  Atropa belladonna
  Colocynth
  Lachesis
  Lycopodium
  Magnesium phosphate
  Rhus tox
  Ruta graveolens
  Viscum album
hydrotherapy
  contrast application
  neutral bath
magnetic field therapy
naturopathic medicine
neural therapy
nutritional therapy
  calcium
  magnesium
  manganese sulfate
  thiamine (vitamin B1)
  vitamin B complex
  vitamin E
osteopathy
pancreatic enzyme therapy
reconstructive therapy
reflexology
  hip/knee
  hip/sciatic
  lower spine
  shoulder

topical treatment
  moist/dry heat
traditional Chinese medicine (TCM)
yoga

SHINGLES

acupuncture
aromatherapy
  bergamot
  chamomile
  eucalyptus
  geranium
  lavender
  lemon
  tea tree
biofeedback training
cell therapy
detoxification therapy
diet therapy
  whole foods diet
energy medicine
  light beam generator
  TENS unit
environmental medicine
  influenza vaccine
fasting
herbal therapy
  colloidal oatmeal powder
  oat straw
  peppermint oil
  skullcap
  St. John's wort
homeopathy
  Caladium
  Rhus tox
  Sepia
hydrotherapy
  neutral bath
juice therapy
  beet
  carrot
  celery

parsley
spinach
magnetic field therapy
naturopathic medicine
  licorice root gel
neural therapy
nutritional therapy
  adenosine monophosphate (AMP)
  calcium
  L-lysine
  plain yogurt
  vitamin B complex
  vitamin B12
  vitamin C plus bioflavonoids
  zinc oxide
oxygen therapy
  hydrogen peroxide therapy
  ozone
qigong
reflexology
  diaphragm
  all glands
  whole spine
topical treatment
  apple cider vinegar
  vitamin E

SORE THROAT

acupuncture
aromatherapy
  benzoin
  clary sage
  eucalyptus
  geranium
  lavender
  sandalwood
  thyme
  turmeric
Ayurveda
  alum
  bayberry
  sage

sumac
turmeric
cell therapy
detoxification therapy
energy medicine
  light beam generator
environmental medicine
fasting
guided imagery
herbal therapy
  black pepper
  echinacea
  ginger tea
  goldenseal
  honey
  hyssop
  lavender
  licorice
  osha root
  sage
  slippery elm
homeopathy
  Aconite
  Arnica
  Gelsenium
  Hydriastis
  Ignatia
  Lachesis
  Phytolacca
hydrotherapy
  contrast application
juice therapy
  pineapple
  red potato
light therapy
  monochromatic red light
    therapy
magnetic field therapy
naturopathic medicine
neural therapy
nutritional therapy
  beta carotene

vitamin A
zinc lozenges
pancreatic enzyme therapy
reflexology
   adrenals
   cervicals
   lymph system
   toes
topical treatment
   apple cider vinegar
   honey
   lemon juice
   salt
traditional Chinese medicine
   (TCM)
yoga

SPINAL INSTABILITY

bodywork
   prolotherapy

SPINAL CORD INJURY

acupuncture

SPONDYLOLISTHESIS

chiropractic

SPRAIN/STRAIN, MUSCULOTENDINOUS

acupuncture
applied kinesiology
aromatherapy
   camphor
   chamomile
   eucalyptus
   lavender
   rosemary
biofeedback training
bodywork
cell therapy
chiropractic
craniosacral therapy
diet therapy

whole foods diet
energy medicine
fasting
guided imagery
herbal therapy
   comfrey
   horsetail
   nettle
   willow bark
homeopathy
   Ruta graveolens
hydrotherapy
   contrast application
   ice pack
juice therapy
   beet
   garlic
   radish
   vegetable juices
magnetic field therapy
Native American medicine
naturopathic medicine
neural therapy
nutritional therapy
   arginine
   bioflavonoids
   calcium
   glycine
   magnesium
   proteolytic enzymes
   valerian
   vitamin C
osteopathic manipulation
   strain-counterstrain
reconstructive therapy
reflexology
   referral area to affected
     area
   reflex area on foot
topical treatment
   dimethyl sulfoxide
     (DMSO)

STIES
applied kinesiology
detoxification
diet therapy
   whole foods diet
fasting
herbal therapy
   eyebright
   goldenseal
   red raspberry tea
homeopathy
   Graphites
   Pulsatilla
   Sulfur
hydrotherapy
light therapy
naturopathic medicine
nutritional therapy
   beta carotene
   vitamin A
   vitamin C
reflexology
   eye reflex
   neck
   toes
topical treatment
   chamomile
   hot compress
   red raspberry tea
traditional Chinese medicine (TCM)

STRAIN, BACK
chiropractic
   electrical modality
      high-volt galvanism
      interferential current
trigger point therapy

STROKE
aromatherapy
   basil
   lavender
   rosemary
biofeedback training
bodywork
   Feldenkrais
chelation therapy
diet therapy
   garlic
   onions
   whole foods diet
flower remedies
guided imagery
herbal therapy
   damiana
   elder flowers
   hyssop
   lavender
   rosemary
   Siberian ginseng
   yarrow
hydrotherapy
   constitutional hydrotherapy
hypnotherapy
light therapy
magnetic field therapy
massage
meditation
naturopathic medicine
nutritional therapy
   garlic
   ginkgo biloba
   magnesium
   omega-3 fatty acids (fish oils)
   superoxide dismutase
      (SOD)
   vitamin B complex
   vitamin B6
   vitamin C
osteopathy
qigong
reconstructive therapy
reflexology
   toes

sound therapy
traditional Chinese medicine
(TCM)
vision therapy
yoga

SUBLUXATION
chiropractic

SUNBURN
aromatherapy
  chamomile
  lavender
fasting
herbal therapy
  aloe vera gel
  calendula flowers
  St. John's wort
homeopathy
  Rhus tox
  Urtica urens
hydrotherapy
  apple cider vinegar bath
  cold compress
  colloidal oatmeal bath
juice therapy
  carrot
naturopathic medicine
  aloe vera
  vitamin E
nutritional therapy
  aloe gel
  calcium
  essential fatty acids
  magnesium
  potassium
  vitamin A
  vitamin C
  vitamin E
  zinc oxide
oxygen therapy
  hyperbaric oxygen therapy

topical treatment
  apple cider vinegar
  olive oil
  PABA cream
traditional Chinese medicine
(TCM)
  Chinese black tea

SWELLING
acupuncture
Ayurveda
  barley water
  Punarnava guggulu
  turmeric
bodywork
  lymphatic drainage massage
diet therapy
  whole foods diet
environmental medicine
fasting
herbal therapy
  ginger root
homeopathy
  Aconite
  Belladonna
  Sulfur
hydrotherapy
juice therapy
  carrot
  celery
  cucumber
  pineapple
magnetic field therapy
naturopathic medicine
nutritional therapy
  bromelain
  proteolytic enzymes
  vitamin B complex
  vitamin B6
  vitamin C and bioflavonoids
osteopathy
traditional Chinese medicine (TCM)

TENDINITIS

acupressure
acupuncture
biofeedback training
bodywork
   Feldenkrais
   Rolfing
cell therapy
chiropractic
craniosacral therapy
energy medicine
fasting
guided imagery
herbal therapy
   cramp bark
   prickly ash
   willow bark
homeopathy
   Aconite
   Belladonna
   Ruta graveolens
   Thuja
hydrotherapy
   contrast application
   Epsom salts bath
light therapy
magnetic field therapy
massage
naturopathic medicine
neural therapy
nutritional therapy
   bromelain
   calcium
   codeine liver oil
   copper
   D-phenylalanine
   essential fatty acids
   magnesium
   manganese
   selenium
   vitamin B complex
   vitamin B6
   vitamin C with bioflavonoids
   vitamin E
osteopathy
   muscle-energy techniques
oxygen therapy
   hydrogen peroxide IV
   hyperbaric oxygen therapy
reconstructive therapy
topical treatment
   apple cider vinegar
   mullein
   salt
   vinegar
yoga

TENNIS ELBOW

acupuncture

THORACIC OUTLET SYNDROME (TOS)

osteopathic manipulation

TONSILLITIS

acupuncture
aromatherapy
   benzoin
   bergamot
   geranium
   lavender
   lemon
   tea tree
   thyme
cell therapy
detoxification therapy
fasting
guided imagery
herbal therapy
   cleavers
   echinacea
   elder flower
   peppermint

yarrow
homeopathy
  Aconite
  Belladonna
  Lachesis
  Phytolacca
hydrotherapy
  contrast application
juice therapy
  apple
  beet
  carrot
  celery
  ginger
  orange
  pineapple
  tomato
magnetic field therapy
naturopathic medicine
neural therapy
nutritional therapy
  acidophilus
  bifidobacteria
  garlic
  ginger packs
  vitamin A
  vitamin C
  vitamin B complex
  zinc oxide
  zinc lozenges
osteopathy
oxygen therapy
  hyperbaric oxygen therapy
reflexology
  adrenals
  cervicals
  lymph system
  toes
relaxation
traditional Chinese medicine (TCM)
yoga

TORTICOLLIS
homeopathy

TRAUMA
craniosacral therapy
osteopathic manipulation
spiritual healing

TUBERCULOSIS
cell therapy
diet therapy
  whole foods diet
fasting
herbal therapy
  echinacea
  elecampane
  garlic
  mullein
hydrotherapy
  constitutional
    hydrotherapy
juice therapy
  almond oil
  carrot
  honey
  olive oil
  potato
light therapy
  red light
  sunlight
magnetic field therapy
nutritional therapy
  beta carotene
  citrus seed extract
  deglycyrrhized licorice
  essential fatty acids
  lipotrophic formula
  lung glandular
  multiminerals
  vitamin A
  vitamin B complex
  vitamin E

vitamin C
zinc
qigong
topical treatment
    alcohol packs (grain)
    eucalyptus oil packs
    grape packs
traditional Chinese medicine (TCM)

VARICOSE VEINS

acupuncture
aromatherapy
    cypress
    juniper
    lavender
    lemon
    rosemary
bodywork
    acupressure
    massage
    reflexology
cell therapy
chelation therapy
diet therapy
    bowel cleanse program
    whole foods diet
fasting
herbal therapy
    ginkgo
    hawthorn
    horse chestnut
    prickly ash
    witch hazel
    yarrow
homeopathy
    Hamamelis
    Pulsatilla
hydrotherapy
    cold compress
juice therapy
    beet
    carrot

celery
cucumber
parsley
spinach
turnip
watercress
magnetic field therapy
naturopathic medicine
nutritional therapy
    bioflavonoids
    calcium
    essential fatty acids
    folic acid
    lecithin
    magnesium
    proteolytic enzymes
    pyridoxine
    rutin
    vitamin B complex
    vitamin B6
    vitamin C
    vitamin D
    vitamin E
    zinc
oxygen therapy
    ozone
pancreatic enzyme therapy
reconstructive therapy
reflexology
    adrenals
    arm
    colon
    liver
traditional Chinese medicine
    (TCM)
yoga

VERTIGO

Ayurveda
    amla
    brahmi ghee nasya
    camphor

cardamom
cinnamon
ginger
grahmi
kamodudha
sesame oil
shatavari
cell therapy
chiropractic
craniosacral therapy
environmental medicine
fasting
herbal therapy
  ginger
  ginkgo
homeopathy
  Aconite
  Belladonna
  Cocculus
  Gelsemium
  Lycopodium
  Phosphorus
  Silicea
  Sulfur
hypnotherapy
magnetic field therapy
naturopathic medicine
nutritional therapy
  adrenal
  calcium
  choline
  ginger
  ginkgo biloba extract
  niacin (B3)
  rutin
  vitamin B complex
  vitamin B6
  vitamin C plus bioflavonoids
  vitamin E
osteopathy
qigong
reflexology

cervicals
ear reflex
great toes
neck
traditional Chinese medicine
(TCM)

VIRAL INFECTIONS
cell therapy
detoxification therapy
diet therapy
  whole foods diet
environmental medicine
fasting
guided imagery
herbal therapy
  echinacea
  goldenseal
  myrrh
homeopathy
  Belladonna
  Calendula
  Chamomilla
  Sulfur
hydrotherapy
  constitutional hydrotherapy
juice therapy
  beet
  carrot
  celery
  garlic
magnetic field therapy
naturopathic medicine
nutritional therapy
  acidophilus
  garlic capsules
  L-cysteine
  lysine
  pantothenic acid
  proteolytic enzymes
  raw thymus glandular
  vitamin A

vitamin B complex
vitamin C
zinc
oxygen therapy
  hydrogen peroxide IV
  hyperbaric oxygen therapy
  ozone
pancreatic enzyme therapy

VOMITING

acupuncture
  P6
aromatherapy
  black pepper
  camphor
  chamomile
  fennel
  lavender
  peppermint
  rose
colon therapy
craniosacral therapy
detoxification therapy
environmental medicine
fasting
herbal therapy
  ginger
  peppermint
homeopathy
  Ipecac
  Nux vomica
  Phosphorus
hydrotherapy
hypnotherapy
juice therapy
  ginger
  vegetable
magnetic field therapy
naturopathic medicine
nutritional therapy
  acidophilus
  deglycyrrhized licorice
  folic acid

vitamin A
vitamin B1
osteopathy
relaxation
therapeutic touch
traditional Chinese medicine (TCM)
yoga

WARTS

aromatherapy
bee venom therapy
fasting
guided imagery
herbal therapy
  dandelion
homeopathy
  Causticum
  Graphites
  Ruta graveolens
  Thuja
hypnosis
hypnotherapy
naturopathic medicine
  thuja oil
nutritional therapy
  beta carotene
  castor oil
  garlic
  L-cysteine
  vitamin A
  vitamin B complex
  vitamin C
  vitamin E
  zinc
  zinc oxide
traditional Chinese medicine (TCM)
  direct moxibustion

WHIPLASH INJURY

bodywork
  Alexander technique
  Rolfing
chiropractic

WHOOPING COUGH

aromatherapy
herbal therapy
  anise
  butterbur
  sundew
  thyme
  wild cherry bark
homeopathy
  Drosera
  Pertussinum
hydrotherapy
  constitutional hydrotherapy
  wet sock treatment
juice therapy
  carrot
  lemon
  orange
  watercress
light therapy
magnetic field therapy
naturopathic medicine
neural therapy
nutritional therapy
  acidophilus
  beta carotene
  garlic capsules
  lung glandulars
  vitamin A
  vitamin C
  zinc lozenges
osteopathy
oxygen therapy
  hydrogen peroxide IV
traditional Chinese medicine (TCM)

WORMS

acupuncture
aromatherapy
  bergamot
  camphor
  chamomile
  lavender
  melissa
  peppermint
  tea tree
  thyme
Ayurveda
  chitrak
  Indian long pepper (Piper
    longum)
  kutki
  neem
  pippali
  trikatu
  triphala
  vidanga
colon therapy
detoxification therapy
fasting
herbal therapy
  pumpkin seeds
magnetic field therapy
naturopathic medicine
nutritional therapy
  aloe vera juice/gel
  beta carotene
  deglycyrrhized licorice
  garlic capsules
  vitamin A
  vitamin C
  zinc
oxygen therapy
  hyperbaric oxygen therapy

WOUND HEALING

aromatherapy
  benzoin
  bergamot
  chamomile
  eucalyptus
  juniper
  lavender
  myrrh
  rosemary
  tea tree

Ayurveda
  ashwagandha
  coconut oil
  ghee
  licorice ghee
  tikta ghee
cell therapy
fasting
guided imagery
herbal therapy
  comfrey leaf
  echinacea
  ginkgo biloba
  goldenseal
  hawthorn
  kava root
  plantain
  St. John's wort
  witch hazel
homeopathy
  Calendula
  Hypericum
  Ledum
hydrotherapy
  ice pack
juice therapy
  beet
  celery
  garlic
light therapy
  cold (soft) laser photostimulation
    therapy
  monochromatic red light therapy
magnetic field therapy
naturopathic medicine
neural therapy
nutritional therapy
oxygen therapy
  hydrogen peroxide IV
  hyperbaric oxygen therapy
topical treatment
traditional Chinese medicine
  (TCM)
  pseudoginseng (yun nan pai yao)

Herbs (Scientific Names/Common Names; Common Names/Scientific Names)

Scientific Name	Common Name
Acacia senegal	acacia; gum arabic
Achillea millefolium	yarrow; soldier's woundwort; nosebleed; milfoil
Achillea collina	chamomile, European
Achillea millefolium	chamomile; yarrow; milfoil
Achillea lanulosa	chamomile, North American
Aconitum carmichaeli	aconite; fu tzu; monkshood; aconite fisheri
Acorus calamus	calamus; type II calamus; sweet flag; sweet sedge
Acorus americanus	North American calamus; type I calamus
Actaea arguta	baneberry
Actaea spicata	herb christopher
Adonis vernalis	adonis
Agastache rugosa	agastache; patchouli; pogostemon
Agathosma betulina	buchu
Agrimonia eupatoria	agrimony; sticklewort; cocklebur
Alchemilla xanthochlora	lady's mantle
Aletris farinosa	unicorn root
Alisma plantago-aquatica	alisma; marsh drain; water plantain
Alkanna tinctoria	alkanet
Allium cepa	onion
Allium sativa	garlic
Allium ampeloprasum	leek
Allium ascalonicum	shallot
Allium Pstulosum	scallion
Aloe barbadensis	aloe; kumari
Aloysia triphylla	lemon verbena
Amanita muscaria	fly agaric
Amanita phalloides	deadly agaric
Althaea rosea	hollyhock; althea
Amaranthus hybridus	amaranth; love lies bleeding; red cockscomb
Ammi visagna	greater ammi; toothpick ammi
Amomum villosum	amomum; grains-of-paradise; cardamom
Anemarrhena asphodeloides	anemarrhena
Anethum graveolens	dill; dillweed
Angelica polymorpha	dong quai; dang gui; tang kuei

Angelica sinensis	dong quai; tang kwei
Angelica archangelica	angelica, American
Apis mellifera	bees
Apium graveolens	celery; celeriac
Aralia racemosa	spikenard
Arctium lappa	burdock; great burdock; lappa; bardane; beggar's button
Arctostaphylos uva-ursi	uva ursi; bearberry
Arnica montana	arnica; leopard's bane
Artemisia absinthium	absinthe
Artemisia vulgaris	mugwort; moxa
Asarium heterotropoides	wild ginger; xi xin
Asclepias tuberosa	pleurisy root; butterfly weed
Aspalathus linearis	red bush tea; rooibos tea
Asparagus officinalis	asapargus; sparrowgrass
Astragalus membranaceus	astragalus; huang chi; milk vetch root; bok kay; goat thorn
Atractylodes macrocephala	pai shu; atractylodes
Atropa belladonna	belladonna; deadly nightshade
Aucklandia lappa	aucklandia; saussurea; costus root
Avena sativa	oats; oat bran; oat groats
Azadirachta indica	neem tree; azedarach; Melia; nim; margosa
Baptisia tinctoria	baptisia; wild indigo; indigoweed
Berberis vulgaris	barberry; pipperidge bush; berberry
Betonica officinalis	wood betony
Biota orientalis	biota; arborvitae
Borago officinalis	borage; burrage
Brassica alba	mustard, white
Brassica nigra	mustard, black
Bryonia alba	bryonia; wild hops
Bupleurum chinese	bupleurum; ch'ai hu
Calendula officinalis	calendula
Camellia sinensis	tea; black tea
Capparis spinosa	capers
Capsella bursa-pastoris	shepherd's purse
Capsicum frutescens	capsicum; cayenne pepper; chili pepper
Carica papaya	papaya; papain
Carthamus tinctorius	safflower; hong hua; red flower
Carum carvi	caraway
Cassia senna	senna; Tinnevelley senna
Catha edulis	khat
Caulophyllum thalictroides	blue cohosh; papoose root; squaw root

Centella asiatica	gotu kola; hydrocotyle; Indian pennywort
Centranthus ruber	red valerian
Cephaelis ipecacuanha	ipecacuanha; ipecac
Certraria islandica	Iceland moss; Iceland lichen
Cervus nippon	deer antler; lu rong; Sika red deer
Chamaelirium luteum	false unicorn; helonias
Chamaemelum nobile	chamomile; Roman chamomile; English chamomile
Chamomilla recutita	chamomile; Hungarian chamomile; single chamomile
Chelidonium majus	celandine; greater celandine
Chenopodium ambrosoides	epazote; Mexican wormseed; American wormseed
Chicorium intybus	chicory; succory
Chimaphilia umbellata	pipsissewa; prince pine; ground holly
Chionanthus virginicus	fringe tree
Chondrus crispus	Irish moss; carageenin; carageenan
Chrysanthemum morrifolium	chrysanthemum; chu hua
Cicuta maculata	water hemlock (poisonous)
Cimicifuga racemosa	black cohosh, black snake root, bugbane, rattleroot
Cinchona spp.	quinine; cinchona bark; Peruvian bark; quina, quinaquina, quinquina; Jesuits' bark
Cinnammomum camphora	camphor; gum camphor; laurel camphor
Cinnammomum cassia	chinese cinnamon bark; Chinese cinnamon twig; cassia twig
Cinnamomum zeylanicum	cinnamon
Citrus reticulata	citrus peel; chen pi; tangerine peel
Claviceps purpurea	ergot
Cnicus benedictus	blessed thistle; holy thistle; St. Benedict's thistle; Benedictine (liqueur)
Cocos nucifera	coconut; coconut palm
Codonopsis pilosula	don sen; tang shen; codonopsis root
Coffea arabica	coffee
Coix lachryma jobi	coix; Job's tears
Cola nitida	kola; cola; kola nut, kolanut; guru nut
Collinsonia canadensis	collinsonia; stoneroot
Commiphora madagascariensis	Abyssinian myrrh
Commiphora molmol	Somalian myrrh
Commiphora myrrha	myrrh; guggul
Consolida regalis	larkspur
Convallaria majalis	lily of the valley

Convolvulus spp.	bush morning glory
Convolvulus scammonia	scammany; Mexican scammany; scammony
Coptis chinensis	coptis; Chinese goldthread
Coriander sativum	coriander
Cornus officinalus	cornus; Asiatic cornelian cherry; Asiatic dogwood
Corydalis yanhusuo	corydalis
Crataegus laevigata	hawthorn
Crocus sativus	saffron
Croton tiglium	croton oil
Cryptotympana atrata	cicada (insect)
Cucurbita moschata	Canada pumpkin; crookneck squash
Cucurbita pepo	pumpkin seeds; pepo
Cucurbita maxima	autumn squash seeds
Cuminum cymium	cumin
Curcuma longa	turmeric
Cuscuta chinensis	cuscuta; Chinese dodder
Cydonia japonica	flowering quince
Cymbopogon citratus	lemongrass
Cyperus rotundus	cyperus; sedge root; nut-grass rhizome
Cypripedium calceoulus	lady slipper; nerveroot
Cytisus scoparius	broom; broom top; Scotch broom; Scotch bloom
Datura stramonium	datura; stink weed; thorn apple; jimson weed; Jamestown weed
Digitalis purpurea	foxglove
Dioscorea opposita	Chinese yam
Dioscorea paniculata	wild yam; colicroot; rheumatism root
Dioscorea villosa	colic root; American wild yam
Dioscorea floribunda	Mexican wild yam
Echinacea angustifolia	echinacea; coneflower; narrow-leaved purple cone flower; purple cone flower; prairie
Elettaria cardamomum	cardamom
Eleutherococcus senticosus	Siberian ginseng; eleutherococcus; eleuthero; ciwujia; wujiaseng
Ephedra nevadensis	Mormon tea; popotillo; Brigham tea; teamster tea; squaw tea
Ephedra sinica	ma huang; ephedra
Epimedium pimedium grandiflorum	epimedium; lusty goatherb

Equisetum arvense	horsetail
Equisetum palustre	European horsetail
Eriobotrya japonica	loquat
Eriodictyon californicum	yerba santa; holy herb; mountain balm
Erythroxylum coca	coca; cocaine
Eschscholzia californica	California poppy
Eucalyptus globulus	eucalyptus; blue gum tree
Eucommia ulmoides	eucommia bark
Eupatorium purpureum	gravel root; Joe-Pye weed; queen of the meadow
Eupatorium perfoliatum	boneset; feverwort; thoroughwort
Euphorbia spp.	eyebright; spurge
Euphorbia longana	longan berries; long yen rou; dragon's eyes
Euphrasia officinalis	eyebright; euphrasy
Evodia rutaecarpa	evodia fruit
Ferula assafoetida	asafoetida; devil's dung; gum asafetida
Foeniculum vulgare	fennel
Fucus vesiculosus	kelp; bladderwrack
Galium aparine	cleavers; clivers; goose grass; bedstraw
Ganoderma lucidum	ganoderma; ling zhi; reishi
Garcinia cambogia	garcinia; Malabar tamarind
Gastrodia elata	gastrodia; heavenly hemp
Gelsemium sempervirens	Carolina jessamine; yellow jasmine
Gentiana scabra	gentiana
Gentiana lutea	gentian; Angostura Bitters
Geranium maculatum	cranesbill root; wild geranium; storksbill; alumroot
Gillenia trifoliata	Indian physic
Ginkgo biloba	ginkgo; ginkgo nut; maidenhair tree
Glycyrrhiza glabra	licorice; gan t'sao
Gonolobus condurango	condurango
Gratiola spp.	hedge hyssop
Hamamelis virginiana	witch hazel
Harpagophytum procumbens	devil's claw; Teufelskralle; wood spider; grapple plant
Hedeoma pulegioides	pennyroyal, American
Hemidesmus indicus	false sarsaparilla; Indian sarsaparilla
Hibiscus sabdariffa	hibiscus; roselle; Sudanese tea; red tea; Jamaica sorrel

Hordeum vulgare	barley; pearl barley; prelate
Humulus lupulus	hops
Hydrangea arborescens	hydrangea; seven barks
Hydrastis canadensis	goldenseal; puccoon root; yellowroot; hydrastis
Hyoscyamus niger	henbane
Hypericum perforatum	St. John's wort
Hyssopus officinalis	hyssop
Ignatia amara	St. Ignatius bean
Ilex paraguariensis	maté
Ilex cassine	yaupon hollies
Indigofera tinctoria	indigo
Inula helenium	elecampane; scabwort; elf dock; horseheal
Ipomoea purpurea	morning glory
Iris versicolor	poison flag; wild iris; blue flag; flag lily; fleur-de-lis; liver lily
Juglans nigra	walnut, black
Juniperus communis	juniper
Lactuca virosa	lettuce opium; lactucarium; wild lettuce
Larrea tridentata	chapparal; creosote bush; greasewood
Laurelis nobilis	bay
Lavandula angustifolia	lavender; garden lavender
Ledebouriella divaricata	sileris; fang feng
Ledum palustre	marsh tea
Lentinus edodes	shiitake
Leonurus cardiaca	motherwort; lion's-tail; mother herb; IMU ch; yi mu cao
Leptandra virginica	Culver root; black root; physic root
Levisticum officinale	lovage; Maggi plant
Ligusticum chuanxiong	cnidium; chuanxiong; Chinese lovage
Ligustrum lucidum	privet fruit; ligustrum
Liquidambar spp.	sweet gum
Liriosma ovata	muira puama; potency wood
Lobelia spp.	eyebright
Lobelia inflata	lobelia; Indian tobacco; pukeweed
Lonicera japonica	Japanese honeysuckle; yin hua
Lycium chinensis	lycii; gay gee; lycium fruit
Lycopodium clavatum	club moss
Lytta (Cantharis) vesicatoria	Spanish fly; Russian fly
Magnolia lilliflora	magnolia buds
Mahonia aquifolium	barberry; Oregon grape

Malva sylvestris	malva; marshmallow; marsh mallow
Marrubium vulgare	horehound; hoarhound
Matricaria recutita	chamomile; German chamomile; Hungarian chamomile
Matteuccia struthiopteris	ostrich fern
Medicago sativa	alfalfa; lucerne
Melaleuca alternifolia	tea tree; tea tree oil
Melaleuca leucadendron	cajuput; cajeput; punk tree; white tea tree; tea tree
Melissa officinalis	lemon balm; melissa; balm
Mentha haplocalyx	field mint
Mentha piperata	peppermint
Mentha pulegium	pennyroyal, European
Mentha spicata	spearmint; garden mint
Mitchella repens	squawvine; partridgeberry
Morus alba	mulberry; white mulberry
Myrica pensylvanica	bayberry
Myrica cerifera	bayberry; candleberry; waxberry; wax myrtle
Myristica fragrans	nutmeg
Nasturtium officinale	watercress
Nepeta cataria	catnip; catmint
Ocimum basilicum	basil
Oenothera biennis	evening primrose; sundrops
Ophiopogon japonicus	Japanese turf lily; creeping lily root; dwarf lilyturf
Oplopanax horridus	devil's club
Origanum majorana	marjoram
Oryza sativa	rice; rice bran
Paeonia lactiflora	peony; shao-yao
Panax notoginseng	tienchi; notoginseng root
Panax ginseng	ginseng, Asian; jen sheng; shiu chu root; ren sheng
Panax pseudo-ginseng	san qui ginseng; tienchi ginseng; sanchi ginseng
Panax quinquefolius	ginseng, American
Papaver rhoeas	poppy, red
Papaver somniferum	poppy, opium
Parthenium integrifolium	prairie dock
Passiflora incarnata	passion flower; passionflower
Paullinia cupana	guarana
Pausinystalia yohimba	yohimbe

Periploca sepium	silk vine
Petroselinum crispum	parsley
Pfaffia paniculata	suma; para toda; Brazilian ginseng
Phoradendron leucarpum	American mistletoe
Phyllanthus emblica	myrobalan, emblic; triphala; Indian gooseberry
Physostigma venenosum	physostigma
Phytolacca americana	poke; pokeweed; pokeroot
Pimenta officinalis	pimento; pimenta; allspice
Pimpinella anisum	anise; aniseed
Pinus mugo	pine-needle oil
Pinus pinaster	Pycnogenol
Piper methysticum	kava; kava kava; kawa
Piper nigrum	black pepper
Plantago lanceolata	plantago; Englishman's foot; greater plantain; ribwort
Plantago ovata	psyllium; ispaghul
Platycodon grandiflorum	platycodon; jie geng
Podophyllum peltatum	mayapple; mandrake; vegetable calomel; devil's-apple
Polygala senega	senega snakeroot; Seneca snakeroot; senega
Polygonum multiflorum	fo-ti; he-shou-wu; ho shou wu; fleece-flower root
Polygonum bistoria	bistort; snakeweed; adderwort; dragonwort
Populus balsamifera	balm of Gilead; quaking aspen; white poplar
Poria cocos	fu ling
Prunus africana	pygeum
Prunus virginiana	chokecherry
Prunus serotina	wild cherry bark
Prunus persica	persic oil; peach kernel oil
Prunus armeniaca	apricot pit; laetrile; vitamin B17; amygdalin; ku xing ren; persica; apricot kernel oil
Ptychopetalum olacoides	muira puama; potency wood
Pueraria lobata	pueraria; ko ken; kudzu; kuzu root
Pulmonaria angustifolia	lungwort; blue cowslip
Pulsatilla nigricans	windflower
Puschkina scilloides libanotica	squill, Lebanon
Quercus spp.	acorn; oak
Quillaja saponaria	quillaja; soapbark
Ranunculus ficaria	pilewort

Ranunculus spp.	buttercup; ranunculus
Raphanus raphanistrum	wild radish
Rauwolfia serpentina	rauwolfia
Rehmannia glutinosa	rehmannia; sok day; san day; Chinese floxglove root
Rhamnus cathartica	buckthorn; common buckthorn
Rhamnus purshiana	cascara sagrada; sacred bark; chittem bark
Rheum palmatum	rhubarb; Chinese rhubarb; da huang; Turkey rhubarb; garden rhubarb
Rhus toxicodendron	poison ivy
Rhus venenata	poison sumac
Ribes nigrum	European currant
Ricinus communis	castor-oil plant; castor bean; palma Christi
Rosa canina	rose hip
Rosmarinus officinalis	rosemary
Rubus idaeus	raspberry
Rubus fruticosus	blackberry
Rumex acetosella	sheep sorrel
Rumex hymenosepalus	canaigre; wild red American ginseng; wild red desert ginseng; Indian tan plant
Rumex crispus	yellow dock; broad leaved dock; curly dock; sourdock; curled dock
Ruscus aculeatus	butcher's-broom; box holly; knee holly; Knee holy; pettier; sweet broom
Ruta graveolens	rue; garden rue
Sabbatia spp.	eyebright
Salix alba	willow; white willow
Salvia miltiorrhiza	salvia; dang shen
Salvia officinalis	sage
Sambucus niger	elder
Sambucus racemosa	red elder
Sanguinaria canadensis	bloodroot; redroot; red Indian paint; tetterwort
Sanguisorba minor	burnet; sanguisorba; salad burnet
Sanguisorba officinalis	great burnet
Santalum album	sandalwood oil; santal oil
Sargassum pallidum	sargassum seaweed
Sassafras albidum	sassafras
Satureja hortensis	summer savory; Bohnenkraut
Satureja montana	winter savory
Schisandra chinensis	schisandra

Scilla sibirica	squill, Siberian
Scutellaria lateriflora	scullcap; skullcap; blue skullcap; huang chi; scutellaria
Selenicereus grandiflorus	night-blooming cereus
Senecio cineraria	dusty miller; cineraria
Senecio aureus	life root; golden senecio; ragwort; false valerian; squaw weed
Serenoa repens	saw palmetto; sabal
Sessamum indicum	sesame oil
Silybum marianum	milk thistle; Marian thistle; St. Mary's thistle; Our Lady's thistle
Simmondsia chinensis	jojoba oil
Smilax aristolochiaefolia	sarsaparilla, Mexican
Smilax febrifuga	sarsaparilla, Ecuadorian
Smilax medica	sarsaparilla
Smilax ornata	sarsaparilla, Jamaican
Smilax regelii	sarsaparilla, Honduran
Solanum capsicastrum	false Jerusalem cherry
Spartium junceum	Spanish broom; gorse
Spiraea spp.	spirea
Spirulina maxima	spirulina; dihe; tecuitlatl; blue-green algae
Stachys officinalis	betony; wood betony
Stellaria media	chickweed; starweed
Sterculia urens	sterculia gum; karaya gum
Strophanthus gratus	ouabain
Strychnos nux-vomica	strychnine
Symphytum officinale	comfrey; knitbone
Symphytum x uplandicum	Russian comfrey
Symphytum asperum	prickly comfrey
Syzygium paniculatum	bush cherry
Syzygium aromaticum	cloves
Tabebuia heptaphylla	pau d'arco; lapacho; tabebuia; purple lapacho
Tabebuia avellanedae	pau d'arco; ipe roxo; lapacho; taheebo tea; lapacho colorado, lapacho morado
Tagetes spp.	marigold
Tamarindus indica	tamarind
Tanacetum vulgare	tansy
Tanacetum parthenium	feverfew
Taraxacum officinale	dandelion
Taraxacum mongolicum	Chinese dandelion

Terminalia bellerica	myrobalan, beleric; triphala; bhibitaki
Terminalia chebula	myrobalan, chebulic; triphala; ho-tzu ch
Teucrium canadense	common germander; pink skullcap
Theobroma cacao	coco; cocoa
Thymus vulgaris	thyme
Tilia tomentosa	silver linden
Tilia cordata	linden; linden flower; lime flowers
Toluifera balsamum	tolu; tolu balsam
Trifolium pratense	red clover
Trigonella foenum-graecum	fenugreek
Triticum aestivum	wheat; wheat bran
Tropaeolum spp.	nasturtium
Turnera diffusa	damiana
Tussilago farfara	coltsfoot; coughwort; horsehoof
Ulmus rubra	slippery elm; red elm
Uncaria tomentosa	cat's claw; una de gato
Urginea indica	Indian squill
Urginea maritima	squill; scilla, urginea; sea onion; red squill; white squill
Urtica dioica	nettle; stinging nettle
Usnea barbata	usnea; beard lichen; larch moss; old man's beard
Vaccinium oxycoccos	European cranberry
Vaccinium spp.	blueberry
Vaccinium macrocarpon	cranberry
Vaccinium myrtillus	bilberry
Valeriana officinalis	valerian
Vanilla planifolia	vanilla; Bourbon vanilla; Mexican vanilla
Vanilla tahitensis	vanilla; Tahitian vanilla
Verbascum thapsus	mullein
Verbena officinalis	vervain; blue vervain
Veronica spp.	creeping speedwell; veronica
Viburnum prunifolium	black haw, American sloe, stagbush
Viburnum opulus	cramp bark; Guelder rose; snowball tree
Vinca rosea	periwinkle
Viola odorata	violet; sweet violet
Viscum album	mistletoe, European
Vitex agnus-castus	chaste berries; vitex; monk pepper; chaste tree; hemp tree
Vitis vinifera	grape seed extract

Withania somnifera	ashwaganda
Yucca brevifolia	yucca; Joshua tree
Yucca whipplei	yucca; our-Lord's-candle
Yucca schidigera	yucca; Mohave yucca
Yucca aloifolia	yucca; Spanish bayonet; dagger plant
Yucca glauca	yucca; soapweed
Zanthoxylum americanum	prickly ash; toothache tree
Zea mays	corn silk; yumixu; stigmata maydis
Zingiber officinale	ginger; Jamaica ginger; African ginger; Cohin ginger; gan-jian
Ziziphus jujube	jujube date; da t'sao

Common Names

Scientific Names

absinthe	*Artemisia absinthium*
Abyssinian myrrh	*Commiphora madagascariensis*
acacia; gum arabic	*Acacia senegal*
aconite fisheri -*see*- aconite	
aconite; fu tzu; monkshood; aconite fisheri	*Aconitum carmichaeli*
acorn; oak	*Quercus spp.*
adderwort -*see*- bistort	
adonis	*Adonis vernalis*
African ginger -*see*- ginger	
agastache; patchouli; pogostemon	*Agastache rugosa*
agrimony; sticklewort; cocklebur	*Agrimonia eupatoria*
alfalfa; lucerne	*Medicago sativa*
alisma; marsh drain; water plantain	*Alisma plantago-aquatica*
alkanet	*Alkanna tinctoria*
allspice	*Pimenta officinalis*
aloe; kumari	*Aloe barbadensis*
althea -*see*- hollyhock	
alumroot -*see*- cranesbill	
amaranth; love lies bleeding; red cockscomb	*Amaranthus hybridus*
American sloe -*see*- black haw	
American mistletoe	*Phoradendron leucarpum*
American wormseed -*see*- epazote	
American wild yam -*see*- colic root	
amomum; grains-of-paradise; cardamom	*Amomum villosum*

amygdalin -*see*- apricot pit
anemarrhena   *Anemarrhena asphodeloides*
angelica, American   *Angelica archangelica*
Angostura Bitters -*see*- gentian
anise; aniseed   *Pimpinella anisum*
aniseed -*see*- anise
apricot pit; laetrile; vitamin B17;   *Prunus armeniaca*
    amygdalin; apricot kernel oil;
    ku xing ren; persica oil
arborvitae -*see*- biota
arnica; leopard's bane   *Arnica montana*
asafoetida; devil's dung; gum   *Ferula assafoetida*
    asafetida
asapargus; sparrowgrass   *Asparagus officinalis*
ashwaganda   *Withania somnifera*
Asiatic cornelian cherry
    -*see*- cornus
Asiatic dogwood -*see*- cornus
astragalus; huang chi; milk vetch   *Astragalus membranaceus*
    root; bok kay; goat thorn
atractylodes -*see*- pai shu
aucklandia; saussurea; costus root   *Aucklandia lappa*
autumn squash seeds   *Cucurbita maxima*
azedarach -*see*- neem tree
balm of Gilead; quaking aspen;   *Populus balsamifera*
    white poplar
balm -*see*- lemon balm
baneberry   *Actaea arguta*
baptisia; wild indigo; indigoweed   *Baptisia tinctoria*
barberry; pipperidge bush   *Berberis vulgaris*
bardane -*see*- burdock
barley; pearl barley; prelate   *Hordeum vulgare*
basil   *Ocimum basilicum*
bay   *Laurelis nobilis*
bayberry   *Myrica pensylvanica*
bayberry; candleberry; waxberry;   *Myrica cerifera*
    wax myrtle
bearberry -*see*- uva ursi
beard lichen -*see*- usnea
bedstraw -*see*- cleavers

bee	*Apis mellifera*
beggar's button -*see*- burdock	
belladonna; deadly nightshade	*Atropa belladonna*
Benedictine (liqueur)	
-*see*- blessed thistle	
berberis	*Berberis nervosa*
betony; wood betony	*Stachys officinalis*
bhibitaki -*see*- myrobalan, beleric	
bilberry	*Vaccinium myrtillus*
biota; arborvitae	*Biota orientalis*
bistort; snakeweed; adderwort;	*Polygonum bistoria*
dragonwort	
black root -*see*- Culver root	
black pepper	*Piper nigrum*
black tea -*see*- tea	
black haw; American sloe; stagbush	*Viburnum prunifolium*
black cohosh; black snake root;	*Cimicifuga racemosa*
bugbane; rattle root	
black snake root -*see*- black cohosh	
blackberry	*Rubus fruticosus*
bladderwrack -*see*- kelp	
blessed thistle; holy thistle;	*Cnicus benedictus*
St. Benedict's thistle;	
Benedictine (liqueur)	
bloodroot; redroot; red Indian	*Sanguinaria canadensis*
paint; tetterwort	
blue cowslip -*see*- lungwort	
blue gum tree -*see*- eucalyptus	
blue flag; flag lily; fleur-de-lis;	*Iris versicolor*
liver lily	
blue cohosh; papoose root;	*Caulophyllum thalictroides*
squaw root	
blue skullcap	*Scutellaria lateriflora*
blue vervain -*see*- vervain	
blue-green algae -*see*- spirulina	
blueberry	*Vaccinium spp.*
Bohnenkraut -*see*- summer savory	
bok kay -*see*- astragalus	
boneset; feverwort; thoroughwort	*Eupatorium perfoliatum*
borage; burrage	*Borago officinalis*
Bourbon vanilla -*see*- vanilla	

box holly -*see*- butcher's broom
Brazilian ginseng -*see*- suma
Brigham tea -*see*- Mormon tea
broad leaved dock -*see*- yellow dock
broom top -*see*- broom
broom; broom top; Scotch broom;   *Cytisus scoparius*
   Scotch bloom
bryonia; wild hops   *Bryonia alba*
buchu   *Agathosma betulina*
buckthorn; common buckthorn   *Rhamnus cathartica*
bugbane -*see*- black cohosh
bupleurum; ch'ai hu   *Bupleurum chinese*
burdock; great burdock; lappa;   *Arctium lappa*
   bardane; beggar button
burnet; sanguisorba; salad burnet   *Sanguisorba minor*
burrage -*see*- borage
bush cherry   *Syzygium paniculatum*
bush morning glory   *Convolvulus spp.*
butcher's-broom; box holly; knee   *Ruscus aculeatus*
   holly; Kneeholy; pettier;
   sweet broom
buttercup; ranunculus   *Ranunculus spp.*
butterfly weed -*see*- pleurisy root
coco; cocoa   *Theobroma cacao*
cajeput -*see*- cajuput
cajuput; cajeput; punk tree;   *Melaleuca leucadendron*
   white tea tree; tea tree
calamus; type II calamus;   *Acorus calamus*
   sweet flag; sweet sedge
calcium pangamate
   -*see*- pangamic acid
calendula   *Calendula officinalis*
California poppy   *Eschscholzia californica*
Camomile; Hungarian   *Chamomilla recutita*
   camommile; single camomile
camphor; gum camphor;   *Cinnammomum camphora*
   laurel camphor
Canada pumpkin; crookneck squash   *Cucurbita moschata*
canaigre; wild red American   *Rumex hymenosepalus*
   ginseng; wild red desert ginseng;
   Indian tan plant

candleberry -*see*- bayberry

capers — *Capparis spinosa*

capsicum; cayenne pepper; chili pimiento — *Capsicum frutescens*

carageenin; carageenan -*see*- Irish moss

caraway — *Carum carvi*

cardamom — *Elettaria cardamomum*

cardamom -*see*- amomum

Carolina jessamine; yellow jasmine — *Gelsemium sempervirens*

cascara sagrada; sacred bark; chittem bark — *Rhamnus purshiana*

cassia twig -*see*- Chinese cinnamon bark

castor-oil plant; castor bean; palma Christi — *Ricinus communis*

cat's claw; una de gato — *Uncaria tomentosa*

catnip, catmint — *Nepeta cataria*

cayenne pepper -*see*- capsicum

celandine; greater celandine — *Chelidonium majus*

celery; celeriac — *Apium graveolens*

ch'ai hu -*see*- bupleurum

chamomile; Roman chamomile; chamomile — *Chamaemelum nobile*

chamomile; yarrow; milfoil — *Achillea millefolium*

chamomile; German chamomile; Hungarian chamomile — *Matricaria recutita*

chamomile, North American — *Achillea lanulosa*

chamomile, European — *Achillea collina*

chapparal; creosote bush; greasewood — *Larrea tridentata*

chaste berries; vitex; monk pepper; chaste tree; hemp tree — *Vitex agnus-castus*

chen pi -*see*- citrus peel

chickweed; starweed — *Stellaria media*

chicory; succory — *Chicorium intybus*

chili pepper -*see*- capsicum

Chinese cinnamon bark; Chinese cinnamon twig; cassia twig — *Cinnammomum cassia*

Chinese floxglove root -*see*- rehmannia

Chinese goldthread -*see*- coptis

Chinese rhubarb -*see*- rhubarb
Chinese lovage -*see*- cnidium
Chinese dandelion   *Taraxacum mongolicum*
Chinese yam   *Dioscorea opposita*
Chinese cinnamon twig
   -*see*- Chinese cinnamon bark
Chinese dodder -*see*- cuscuta
chittem bark -*see*- cascara sagrada
chokecherry   *Prunus virginiana*
chrysanthemum; chu hua   *Chrysanthemum morrifolium*
chu hua -*see*- chrysanthemum
chuanxiong -*see*- cnidium
cicada (insect)   *Cryptotympana atrata*
cinchona bark -*see*- quinine
cineraria -*see*- dusty miller
cinnamon   *Cinnamomum zeylanicum*
citrus peel; chen pi; tangerine peel   *Citrus reticulata*
ciwujia -*see*- Siberian ginseng
cleavers; clivers; goose grass;   *Galium aparine*
   bedstraw
cloves   *Syzygium aromaticum*
club moss   *Lycopodium clavatum*
cnidium; chuanxiong; Chinese lovage   *Ligusticum chuanxiong*
coca; cocaine   *Erythroxylum coca*
cocaine -*see*- see coca
cocklebur -*see*- agrimony
cocoa -*see*- coco
coconut palm -*see*- coconut
coconut; coconut palm   *Cocos nucifera*
codonopsis root -*see*- don sen
coffee   *Coffea arabica*
Cohin ginger -*see*- ginger
coix; Job's tears   *Coix lachryma jobi*
cola -*see*- kola
colic root; American wild yam   *Dioscorea villosa*
colicroot -*see*- wild yam
collinsonia; stoneroot   *Collinsonia canadensis*
coltsfoot; coughwort; horsehoof   *Tussilago farfara*
comfrey; knitbone   *Symphytum officinale*
common germander; pink skullcap   *Teucrium canadense*
common buckthorn -*see*- buckthorn

condurango	*Gonolobus condurango*
coneflower -*see*- see echinacea	
coptis; Chinese goldthread	*Coptis chinensis*
coriander	*Coriander sativum*
corn silk; yumixu; stigmata maydis	*Zea mays*
cornus; Asiatic cornelian cherry;	*Cornus officinalus*
Asiatic dogwood	
corydalis	*Corydalis yanhusuo*
costus root -*see*- aucklandia	
coughwort -*see*- coltsfoot	
cramp bark; Guelder rose;	*Viburnum opulus*
snowball tree	
cranberry	*Vaccinium macrocarpon*
cranesbill root; wild geranium;	*Geranium maculatum*
storksbill; alumroot	
creeping lily root -*see*- Japanese	
turf lily	
creeping speedwell; veronica	*Veronica spp.*
creosote bush -*see*- chapparal	
crookneck squash -*see*- Canada	
pumpkin	
croton oil	*Croton tiglium*
Culver root; black root; physic root	*Leptandra virginica*
cumin	*Cuminum cymium*
curled dock -*see*- yellow dock	
curly dock -*see*- yellow dock	
cuscuta; Chinese dodder	*Cuscuta chinensis*
cyperus; sedge root	*Cyperus rotundus*
da huang -*see*- rhubarb	
da t'sao -*see*- jujube	
dagger plant -*see*- yucca	
damiana	*Turnera diffusa*
dandelion	*Taraxacum officinale*
dang gui -*see*- dong quai	
dang shen -*see*- salvia	
datura; stink weed; thorn apple;	*Datura stramonium*
jimson weed; Jamestown weed	
deadly nightshade -*see*- belladonna	
deer antler; lu rong; Sika red deer	*Cervus nippon*

devil's apple -*see*- mayapple
devil's claw; Teufelskralle; wood   *Harpagophytum procumbens*
   spider; grapple plant
devil's dung -*see*- asafoetida
devil's club   *Oplopanax horridus*
dihe -*see*- spirulina
dill; dillweed   *Anethum graveolens*
dillweed -*see*- dill
don sen; tang shen; codonopsis root   *Codonopsis pilosula*
dong quai; tang kwei   *Angelica sinensis*
dong quai; dang gui; tang kuei   *Angelica polymorpha*
dragon's eyes -*see*- longan berries
dragonwort -*see*- bistort
dusty miller; cineraria   *Senecio cineraria*
dwarf lilyturf -*see*- Japanese turf lily
echinacea; coneflower;   *Echinacea angustifolia*
   narrow-leaved purple cone
   flower; purple cone flower; prairie
Ecuadorian sarsaparilla   *Smilax febrifuga*
elder   *Sambucus niger*
elecampane; scabwort; elf dock;   *Inula helenium*
   horseheal
eleuthero   *Eleutherococcus senticosus*
eleutherococcus -*see*- Siberian ginseng
elf dock -*see*- elecampane
English chamomile
   -*see*- chamomile
Englishman's foot -*see*- plantago
epazote; Mexican wormseed;   *Chenopodium ambrosoides*
   American wormseed
ephedra; ma huang   *Ephedra sinica*
epimedium; lusty goatherb   *Epimedium pimedium grandiflorum*
ergot   *Claviceps purpurea*
eucalyptus; blue gum tree   *Eucalyptus globulus*
eucommia bark   *Eucommia ulmoides*
euphrasy -*see*- eyebright
European mistletoe   *Viscum album*
European horsetail   *Equisetum palustre*
European black currant   *Ribes nigrum*
European cranberry   *Vaccinium oxycoccos*

evening primrose; sundrops	*Oenothera biennis*
evodia fruit	*Evodia rutaecarpa*
eyebright; euphrasy	*Euphrasia officinalis*
eyebright; spurge	*Euphorbia spp.*
eyebright	*Lobelia spp.*
eyebright	*Sabbatia spp.*
false Jerusalem cherry	*Solanum capsicastrum*
false sarsaparilla; Indian sarsaparilla	*Hemidesmus indicus*
false unicorn; helonias	*Chamaelirium luteum*
false valerian -*see*- life root	
fang feng -*see*- sileris	
fennel	*Foeniculum vulgare*
fenugreek	*Trigonella foenum-graecum*
feverfew	*Tanacetum parthenium*
feverwort -*see*- boneset	
field mint	*Mentha haplocalyx*
flag lily -*see*- blue flag	
fleece-flower root -*see*- ho shou wu	
fleur-de-lis -*see*- blue flag	
flowering quince	*Cydonia japonica*
fo-ti; he-shou-wu	*Polygonum multiflorum*
foxglove	*Digitalis purpurea*
fringe tree	*Chionanthus virginicus*
fu ling	*Poria cocos*
fu tzu -*see*- aconite	
gan t-sao -*see*- licorice	
gan-jian -*see*- ginger	
ganoderma; ling zhi; reishi	*Ganoderma lucidum*
garcinia; Malabar tamarind	*Garcinia cambogia*
garden rhubarb -*see*- rhubarb	
garden rue -*see*- rue	
garden lavendar -*see*- lavendar	
garden mint -*see*- spearmint	
garlic	*Allium sativa*
gastrodia; heavenly hemp	*Gastrodia elata*
gay gee -*see*- lycii	
gentian; Angostura Bitters	*Gentiana lutea*
gentiana	*Gentiana scabra*
German chamomile -*see*- chamomile	

ginger; Jamaica ginger; African ginger; Cohin ginger; gan-jian	*Zingiber officinale*
ginkgo; ginkgo nut; maidenhair tree	*Ginkgo biloba*
ginseng, Siberian	*Eleutherococcus senticosus*
ginseng, Asian	*Panax ginseng*
ginseng, American	*Panax quinquefolius*
ginseng; jen sheng; shiu chu root; ren sheng	*Panax ginseng*
goat thorn -*see*- astragalus	
golden senecio -*see*- life root	
goldenseal; puccoon root; yellowroot; hydrastis	*Hydrastis canadensis*
goose grass -*see*- cleavers	
gorse -*see*- Spanish broom	
gotu kola; hydrocotyle; Indian pennywort	*Centella asiatica*
grains-of-paradise -*see*- amomum	
grape seed extract	*Vitis vinifera*
grapple plant -*see*- devil's claw	
gravel root; Joe-Pye weed; queen of the meadow	*Eupatorium purpureum*
greasewood -*see*- chapparal	
great burdock -*see*-burdock	
great burnet	*Sanguisorba officinalis*
greater celandine -*see*- celandine	
greater plantain -*see*- plantago	
greater ammi; toothpick ammi	*Ammi visagna*
ground holly -*see*- pipsissewa	
guarana	*Paullinia cupana*
Guelder rose -*see*- cramp bark	
guggul -*see*- myrrh	
gum camphor -*see*- camphor	
gum asafetida -*see*- asafoetida	
guru nut -*see*- kola	
hawthorn	*Crataegus laevigata*
he-shou-wu -*see*- fo-ti	
heavenly hemp -*see*- gastrodia	
hedge hyssop	*Gratiola spp.*
helonias -*see*- false unicorn	
hemp tree -*see*- chaste berries	

henbane	*Hyoscyamus niger*
herb-christopher	*Actaea spicata*
hibiscus; roselle; Sudanese tea; red tea; Jamaica sorrel	*Hibiscus sabdariffa*
ho shou wu; fo-ti; fleece-flower root	*Polygonum multiflorum*
ho-txu ch -*see*- myrobalan, chebulic	
hoarhound -*see*- horehound	
hollyhock; althea	*Althaea rosea*
holy herb -*see*- yerba santa	
holy thistle -*see*- blessed thistle	
Honduran sarsaparilla	*Smilax regelii*
hong hua -*see*- safflower	
hops	*Humulus lupulus*
horehound; hoarhound	*Marrubium vulgare*
horseheal -*see*- elecampane	
horsehoof -*see*- coltsfoot	
horsetail	*Equisetum arvense*
huang chi -*see*- scullcap	
huang chi -*see*- astragalus	
Hungarian camommile -*see*-camomile	
Hungarian chamomile - see- chamomile	
hydrangea; seven barks	*Hydrangea arborescens*
hydrastis -*see*- goldenseal	
hydrocotyle -*see*- gotu kola	
hyssop	*Hyssopus officinalis*
Iceland moss; Iceland lichen	*Certraria islandica*
IMU ch -*see*- motherwort	
Indian squill	*Urginea indica*
Indian tobacco -*see*- lobelia	
Indian gooseberry -*see*- myrobalan, emblic	
Indian tan plant - *see*- canaigre	
Indian physic	*Gillenia trifoliata*
Indian sarsaparilla -*see*- false sarsaparilla	
Indian pennywort -*see*- gotu kola	
indigo	*Indigofera tinctoria*
indigoweed -*see*- baptisia	
ipe roxo -*see*- pau d'arco	

ipecac -*see*- ipecacuanha
ipecacuanha; ipecac   *Cephaelis ipecacuanha*
Irish moss; carageenin; carageenan   *Chondrus crispus*
ispaghul -*see*- psyllium
Jamaican sorrel -*see*- hibiscus
Jamaican ginger -*see*- ginger
Jamestown weed -*see*- datura
Japanese turf lily; creeping lily root;
   dwarf lilyturf   *Ophiopogon japonicus*
Japanese honeysuckle; yin hua   *Lonicera japonica*
jen sheng -*see*- ginseng
Jesuit's bark -*see*- quinine
jie geng -*see*- platycodon
jimson weed -*see*- datura
Job's tears -*see*- coix
Joe-Pye weed -*see*- gravel root
jojoba oil   *Simmondsia chinensis*
Joshua tree -*see*- yuccca
jujube date; da t'sao   *Ziziphus jujube*
juniper   *Juniperus communis*
karaya gum -*see*- sterculia gum
kava; kava kava; kawa   *Piper methysticum*
kelp; bladderwrack   *Fucus vesiculosus*
khat   *Catha edulis*
knee holly -*see*- butcher's broom
Knee holy -*see*- butcher's broom
knitbone -*see*- see comfey
ko ken -*see*- pueraria
kola; cola; kola nut, kolanut;   *Cola nitida*
   guru nut
ku xing ren; persica; apricot kernel oil   *Prunus armeniaca*
kudzu -*see*- pueraria
kumari -*see*- aloe
kuzu root -*see*- pueraria
lactucarium -*see*- lettuce opium
lady slipper; nerveroot   *Cypripedium calceoulus*
lady's mantle   *Alchemilla xanthochlora*
laetrile -*see*- apricot pit
lapacho -*see*- pau d'arco
lapacho colorado -*see*- pau d'arco
lapacho morado -*see*- pau d'arco

lappa -see- burdock
larch moss -see- usnea
larkspur — *Consolida regalis*
laurel camphor -see- camphor
lavender; garden lavender — *Lavandula angustifolia*
leek — *Allium ampeloprasum*
lemon verbena — *Aloysia triphylla*
lemon balm; melissa; balm — *Melissa officinalis*
lemongrass — *Cymbopogon citratus*
leopard's bane -see- arrica
lettuce opium; lactucarium; wild lettuce — *Lactuca virosa*
licorice; gan t'sao — *Glycyrrhiza glabra*
life root; golden senecio; ragwort; false — *Senecio aureus*
valerian; squaw weed
ligustrum -see- privet fruit
lily of the valley — *Convallaria majalis*
lime flowers -see- linden
linden; linden flower; lime flowers — *Tilia cordata*
ling zhi -see- ganoderma
lion's-tail -see- motherwort
liver lily -see- blue flag
lobelia; Indian tobacco; pukeweed — *Lobelia inflata*
long yen rou -see- longan berries
longan berries; long yen rou; dragon's — *Euphorbia longana*
eyes
loquat — *Eriobotrya japonica*
lovage; Maggi plant — *Levisticum officinale*
love lies bleeding -see- amaranth
lu rong -see- deer antler
luceme -see- alfalfa
lungwort; blue cowslip — *Pulmonaria angustifolia*
lusty goatherb -see- epimedium
lycii; gay gee; lycium fruit — *Lycium chinensis*
lycium fruit -see- lycii
ma huang; ephedra — *Ephedra sinica*
Maggi plant -see- lovage
magnolia buds — *Magnolia lilliflora*
maidenhair tree -see- ginkgo
Malabar tamarind -see- garcinia
malva; marshmallow; marsh mallow — *Malva sylvestris*
mandrake -see- mayapple

margosa -*see*- neem tree	
Marian thistle -*see*- milk thistle	
marigold	*Tagetes spp.*
marjoram	*Origanum majorana*
marsh drain -*see*- alisma	
marsh tea	*Ledum palustre*
marshmallow, marsh mallow -*see*- malva	
maté	*Ilex paraguariensis*
mayapple; mandrake; vegetable calomel; devil's-apple	*Podophyllum peltatum*
Melia -*see*- neem tree	
melissa -*see*- lemon balm	
Mexican vanilla -*see*- vanilla	
Mexican wormseed -*see*- epazote	
Mexican sarsaparilla	*Smilax aristolochiaefolia*
Mexican wild yam	*Dioscorea floribunda*
Mexican scammany -*see*- scammany	
milfoil -*see*- yarrow	
milk vetch root -*see*- astragalus	
milk thistle; Marian thistle; St. Mary thistle; Our Lady thistle	*Silybum marianum*
mistletoe, European	*Viscum album*
Mohave yucca -*see*- yucca	
monk pepper -*see*- chaste berries	
monkshood -*see*- aconite	
Mormon tea; popotillo; Brigham tea; teamster tea; squaw tea	*Ephedra nevadensis*
morning glory	*Ipomoea purpurea*
mother herb -*see*- motherwort	
motherwort; lion's-tail; mother herb; IMU ch; yi mu cao	*Leonurus cardiaca*
mountain balm -*see*- yerba santa	
moxa -*see*- mugwort	
mugwort; moxa	*Artemisia vulgaris*
muira puama; potency wood	*Ptychopetalum olacoides*
muira puama; potency wood	*Liriosma ovata*
mulberry; white mulberry	*Morus alba*
mullein	*Verbascum thapsus*
mustard, black	*Brassica nigra*
mustard, white	*Brassica alba*
myrobalan, chebulic; triphala; ho-tzu ch	*Terminalia chebula*

myrobalan, beleric; triphala; bhibitaki	*Terminalia bellerica*
myrobalan, emblic; triphala; Indian gooseberry	*Phyllanthus emblica*
myrrh; guggul	*Commiphora myrrha*
narrow-leaved purple cone flower -*see*- see echinacea	
nasturtium	*Tropaeolum spp.*
neem tree; azedarach; Melia; nim; margosa	*Azadirachta indica*
nerveroot -*see*- lady slipper	
nettle; stinging nettle	*Urtica dioica*
night-blooming cereus	*Selenicereus grandiflorus*
nim -*see*- neem tree	
North American calamus; type I calamus	*Acorus americanus*
nosebleed -*see*- yarrow	
notoginseng root -*see*- tienchi	
nut-grass rhizome	*Cyperus rotundus*
nutmeg	*Myristica fragrans*
oak -*see*- acorn	
oats; oat bran; oat groats	*Avena sativa*
old man's beard -*see*- usnea	
onion	*Allium cepa*
Oregon grape	*Mahonia aquifolium*
ostrich fern	*Matteuccia struthiopteris*
ouabain	*Strophanthus gratus*
Our Lady's thistle -*see*- milk thistle	
our-Lord's-candle -*see*- yucca	
pai shu; atractylodes	*Atractylodes macrocephala*
palma Christi -*see*- castor-oil plant	
pangamic acid; vitamin B15; pangamate; calcium pangamate	not biological
papaya; papain	*Carica papaya*
papoose root -*see*- blue cohosh	
para toda -*see*- suma	
parsley	*Petroselinum crispum*
partridgeberry -*see*- squawvine	
passion flower; passionflower	*Passiflora incarnata*
patchouli -*see*- agastache	
pau d'arco; lapacho; tabebuia; purple lapacho	*Tabebuia heptaphylla*

pau d'arco; ipe roxo; lapacho; taheebo tea; lapacho colorado, lapacho morado — *Tabebuia avellanedae*

peach kernel oil -*see*- persic oil

pearl barley -*see*- barley

pennyroyal, European or Old World — *Mentha pulegium*

pennyroyal, American — *Hedeoma pulegioides*

peony; shao-yao — *Paeonia lactiflora*

pepo -*see*- pumpkin seeds

peppermint — *Mentha piperata*

periwinkle — *Vinca rosea*

persic oil; peach kernel oil — *Prunus persica*

persica -*see*- ku xing ren

Peruvian bark -*see*- quinine

pettier -*see*- butcher's broom

physic root -*see*- Culver root

physostigma — *Physostigma venenosum*

pilewort — *Ranunculus ficaria*

pimento; pimenta — *Pimenta officinalis*

pine-needle oil — *Pinus mugo*

pink skullcap -*see*- common germander

pipperidge bush -*see*- barberry

pipsissewa; prince pine; ground holly — *Chimaphilia umbellata*

plantago; Englishman's foot; greater plantain; ribwort — *Plantago lanceolata*

platycodon; jie geng — *Platycodon grandiflorum*

pleurisy root; butterfly weed — *Asclepias tuberosa*

pogostemon -*see*- agastache

poison sumac — *Rhus venenata*

poison flag; wild iris — *Iris versicolor*

poison ivy — *Rhus toxicodendron*

poke; pokeweed; pokeroot — *Phytolacca americana*

popotillo -*see*- Mormon tea

poppy, red — *Papaver rhoeas*

poppy, opium — *Papaver somniferum*

potency wood -*see*- muira puama

prairie -*see*- see echinacea

prairie dock — *Parthenium integrifolium*

prelate -*see*- barley

prickly comfrey — *Symphytum asperum*

prickly ash; toothache tree	*Zanthoxylum americanum*
prince pine -*see*- pipsissewa	
privet fruit; ligustrum	*Ligustrum lucidum*
psyllium; ispaghul	*Plantago ovata*
puccoon root -*see*- goldenseal	
pueraria; ko ken; kudzu; kuzu root	*Pueraria lobata*
pukeweed -*see*- lobelia	
pumpkin seeds; pepo	*Cucurbita pepo*
punk tree -*see*- cajuput	
purple lapacho -*see*- pau d'arco	
purple cone flower -*see*- see echinacea	
Pycnogenol	*Pinus pinaster*
pygeum	*Prunus africana*
quaking aspen -*see*- balm of Gilead	
queen of the meadow -*see*- gravel root	
quillaja; soapbark	*Quillaja saponaria*
quina, quinaquina, quinquina -*see*- quinine	

quinine; cinchona bark; Peruvian bark;
    quina, quinaquina, quinquina,
    Jesuits' bark
	Cinchona spp.

ragwort -*see*- life root	
ranunculus -*see*- buttercup	
raspberry	*Rubus idaeus*
rattle root -*see*- black cohosh	
rauwolfia	*Rauwolfia serpentina*
red Indian paint -*see*- bloodroot	
red squill -*see*- squill	
red tea -*see*- hibiscus	
red clover	*Trifolium pratense*
red bush tea; rooibos tea	*Aspalathus linearis*
red elm -*see*- slippery elm	
red valerian	*Centranthus ruber*
red cockscomb -*see*- amaranth	
red flower -*see*- safflower	
red elder	*Sambucus racemosa*
redroot -*see*- bloodroot	
rehmannia; sok day; san day; Chinese floxglove root	*Rehmannia glutinosa*
reishi -*see*- ganoderma	
ren sheng -*see*- ginseng	

rheumatism root	*Dioscorea paniculata*
rhubarb; Chinese rhubarb; da huang; Turkey rhubarb; garden rhubarb	*Rheum palmatum*
ribwort -*see*- plantago	
rice; rice bran	*Oryza sativa*
Roman chamomile -*see*- chamomile	
rooibos tea -*see*- red bush tea	
rose hip	*Rosa canina*
roselle -*see*- hibiscus	
rosemary	*Rosmarinus officinalis*
rue; garden rue	*Ruta graveolens*
Russian fly -*see*- Spanish fly	
Russian comfrey	*Symphytum x uplandicum*
sabal -*see*- saw palmetoo	
sacred bark -*see*- cascara sagrada	
safflower; hong hua; red flower	*Carthamus tinctorius*
saffron	*Crocus sativus*
sage	*Salvia officinalis*
salad burnet -*see*- burnet	
salvia; dang shen	*Salvia miltiorrhiza*
san day -*see*- rehmannia	
san qui ginseng; tienchi ginseng; sanchi ginseng	*Panax pseudo-ginseng*
sandalwood oil; santal oil	*Santalum album*
sanguisorba -*see*- burnet	
santal oil -*see*- sandalwood oil	
sargassum seaweed	*Sargassum pallidum*
sarsaparilla, Jamaican	*Smilax ornata*
sarsaparilla, Ecuadorian	*Smilax febrifuga*
sarsaparilla, Honduran	*Smilax regelii*
sarsaparilla	*Smilax medica*
sarsaparilla, Indian	*Hemidesmus indicus*
sassafras	*Sassafras albidum*
saussurea -*see*- aucklandia	
saw palmetto; sabal	*Serenoa repens*
scabwort -*see*- elecampane	
scallion	*Allium Pstulosum*
scammany; Mexican scammany; scammony	*Convolvulus scammonia*
schisandra	*Schisandra chinensis*
scilla, urginea -*see*- squill	

Scotch broom -*see*- broom
Scotch bloom -*see*- broom
scullcap; skullcap; blue skullcap;   *Scutellaria lateriflora*
   huang chi; scutellaria
scutellaria -*see*- scullcap
sea onion -*see*- squill
sedge root -*see*- cyperus
senega snakeroot; seneca snakeroot;   *Polygala senega*
   senega
senna; Tinnevelley senna   *Cassia senna*
sesame oil   *Sessamum indicum*
seven barks -*see*- hydrangea
shallot   *Allium ascalonicum*
shao-yao -*see*- peony
sheep sorrel   *Rumex acetosella*
shepherd's purse   *Capsella bursa-pastoris*
shiitake   *Lentinus edodes*
shiu chu root -*see*- ginseng
Siberian ginseng; eleutherococcus;   *Eleutherococcus senticosus*
   eleuthero; ciwujia; wujiaseng
Sika red deer -*see*- deer antler
sileris; fang feng   *Ledebouriella divaricata*
silk vine   *Periploca sepium*
silver linden   *Tilia tomentosa*
single camomile -*see*- camomile
skullcap -*see*- scullcap
slippery elm; red elm   *Ulmus rubra*
snakeweed -*see*- bistort
snowball tree -*see*- cramp bark
soapbark -*see*- quillaja
soapweed -*see*- yucca
sok day -*see*- rehmannia
soldier's woundwort -*see*- yarrow
Somalian myrrh   *Commiphora molmol*
sourdock -*see*- yellow dock
Spanish bayonet -*see*- yucca
Spanish fly; Russian fly   *Lytta (Cantharis) vesicatoria*
Spanish broom; gorse   *Spartium junceum*
sparrowgrass -*see*- asapargus
spearmint; garden mint   *Mentha spicata*
spikenard   *Aralia racemosa*

spirea	*Spiraea spp.*
spirulina; dihe; tecuitlatl; blue-green algae	*Spirulina maxima*
spurge -*see*- eyebright	
squaw tea -*see*- Mormon tea	
squaw root -*see*- blue cohosh	
squaw weed -*see*- life root	
squawvine; partridgeberry	*Mitchella repens*
squill, Siberian	*Scilla sibirica*
squill, Lebanon	*Puschkina scilloides libanotica*
squill; scilla, urginea; sea onion; red squill; white squill	*Urginea maritima*
St. Benedict's thistle -*see*- blessed thistle	
St. John's wort	*Hypericum perforatum*
St. Mary's thistle -*see*- milk thistle	
St. Ignatius bean	*Ignatia amara*
stagbush -*see*- black haw	
starweed -*see*- chickweed	
sterculia gum; karaya gum	*Sterculia urens*
sticklewort -*see*- agrimony	
stigmata maydis -*see*- corn silk	
stinging nettle -*see*- nettle	
stink weed -*see*- datura	
stoneroot -*see*- colinsonia	
storksbill -*see*- cranesbill	
strychnine	*Strychnos nux-vomica*
succory -*see*- chicory	
Sudanese tea -*see*- hibiscus	
suma; para toda; Brazilian ginseng	*Pfaffia paniculata*
summer savory; Bohnenkraut	*Satureja hortensis*
sweet violet -*see*- violet	
sweet broom -*see*- butcher's broom	
sweet gum	*Liquidambar spp.*
sweet sedge -*see*- calamus	
sweet flag -*see*- calamus	
tabebuia -*see*- pau d'arco	
taheebo tea -*see*- pau d'arco	
Tahitian vanilla -*see*- vanilla	
tamarind	*Tamarindus indica*
tang shen -*see*- don sen	
tang kwei -*see*- dong quai	

tang kuei -*see*- dong quai
tangerine peel -*see*- citrus peel
tansy — *Tanacetum vulgare*
tea tree; tea tree oil — *Melaleuca alternifolia*
tea tree -*see also*- cajuput
tea; black tea — *Camellia sinensis*
teamster tea -*see*- Mormon tea
tecuitlatl -*see*- spirulina
tetterwort -*see*- bloodroot
Teufelskralle -*see*- devil's claw
thorn apple -*see*- datura
thoroughwort -*see*- boneset
thyme — *Thymus vulgaris*
tienchi ginseng -*see*- san qui ginseng
tienchi; notoginseng root — *Panax notoginseng*
Tinnevelley senna -*see*- senna
tolu; tolu balsam — *Toluifera balsamum*
toothache tree -*see*- prickly ash
toothpick ammi -*see*- greater ammi
triphala -*see*- myrobalan, emblic;
    myrobalan, beleric; myrobalan,
    chebulic
Turkey rhubarb -*see*- rhubarb
turmeric — *Curcuma longa*
type II calamus -*see*- calamus
type I calamus -*see*- North American
    calamus
una de gato -*see*- cat's claw
unicorn root — *Aletris farinosa*
usnea; beard lichen; larch moss; — *Usnea barbata*
    old man's beard
uva ursi; bearberry — *Arctostaphylos uva-ursi*
valerian — *Valeriana officinalis*
vanilla; Tahitian vanilla — *Vanilla tahitensis*
vanilla; Bourbon vanilla; Mexican vanilla — *Vanilla planifolia*
vegetable calomel -*see*- mayapple
veronica -*see*- creeping speedwell
vervain; blue vervain — *Verbena officinalis*
violet; sweet violet — *Viola odorata*
vitamin B17 -*see*- apricot pit
vitamin B15 -*see*- pangamic acid

vitex -*see*- chaste berries
walnut, black   *Juglans nigra*
water hemlock (poisonous)   *Cicuta maculata*
water plantain -*see*- alisma
watercress   *Nasturtium officinale*
wax myrtle -*see*- bayberry   *Myrica cerifera*
waxberry -*see*- bayberry
wheat; wheat bran   *Triticum aestivum*
white squill-*see*- squill
white mulberry -*see*- mulberry
white poplar -*see*- balm of Gilead
white willow -*see*- willow
white tea tree -*see*- cajuput
wild red desert ginseng -*see*- canaigre
wild radish   *Raphanus raphanistrum*
wild ginger; xi xin   *Asarium heterotropoides*
wild hops -*see*- bryonia
wild red American ginseng
   -*see*- canaigre
wild cherry bark   *Prunus serotina*
wild yam; colicroot; rheumatism root   *Dioscorea paniculata*
wild iris -*see*- poison flag
wild geranium -*see*- cranesbill
wild indigo -*see*- baptisia
wild lettuce -*see*- lettuce opium
willow; white willow   *Salix alba*
windflower   *Pulsatilla nigricans*
winter savory   *Satureja montana*
witch hazel   *Hamamelis virginiana*
wood spider -*see*- devil's claw
wood betony   *Betonica officinalis*
wujiaseng -*see*- Siberian ginseng
xi xin -*see*- wild ginger
yarrow; soldier's woundwort;   *Achillea millefolium*
   nosebleed; milfoil
yaupon hollies   *Ilex cassine*
yellow jasmine -*see*- Caroline
   jessamine
yellow dock; broad leaved dock; curly   *Rumex crispus*
   dock; sourdock; curled dock
yellowroot -*see*- goldenseal

yerba santa; holy herb; mountain balm — *Eriodictyon californicum*
yi mu cao -*see*- motherwort
yin hua -*see*- Japanese honeysuckle
yohimbe — *Pausinystalia yohimba*
yucca; Spanish bayonet; dagger plant — *Yucca aloifolia*
yucca; Joshua tree — *Yucca brevifolia*
yucca; soapweed — *Yucca glauca*
yucca; our-Lord's-candle — *Yucca whipplei*
yucca; Mohave yucca — *Yucca schidigera*
yumixu -*see*- corn silk

Appendix 7
Common Phytochemicals and Common Classes of Phytochemicals

1-dehydrotrillenogenin
1-kestose
11,12-didehydrofalcarinol
11,13-dihydrohelenalin
12-hydroxystrychnine
13-hydroxylupanine
1,6-cineol
2-acetoxy-valerenic acid
2-bornanone
2-hydroxyvalerenic acid
2-kestose
2-methyl-3-butanol
2-methyl-butyric acid
2,3-dicoffeoyltartrate
27-deoxyactein
3-butylidenphthalide
3-butylphthalide
3-hydroxyglabrol
3-isobutylidendihydrophthalide
3-sn-phosphatidylcholine
3,4-dimethoxycinnamic acid
4-methoxycinnamic acid
4-terpineol
5-coffeoylchina acid
5-methoxybilobetin
7-acetoxymarrubiin
7-acetyllycopsamine
7-angeloylheliotridine
7-angeloylretronecin
7-methyl juglone
8-hydroxydroserone
A1-barrigenol
absinthin
acetyl harpagide
acetylandromedol
acetylcholine
acetylerucifoline

acetylheliosupine
achillicin
achromatin
acidis arabinogalactan
aconitine
actein
acteoside
actinidine
acutissimine A and B
adipic acid
adonitoxin
aegelinol
aesculetin
aethusanol A and B
aethusin
agasyllin
aglycone digitoxigenin
aglycone hederagenin
agnuside
agrimoniin
agrovlacine
ailanthone
ajamalicin
ajmaline
ajugalactone
ajugol
ajugoside
akuammidine
alantolactone
albumin
alginic acid
aliphatic ester
alkaloid caffeine
alkannin
alkylcyclopentenolone
allantoin
alliin

alloaromadendrene
allocryptopine
allyl mustard oil
allylalliin
allylisothiocyanate
allylpyrocatechol
aloe resin B, C and D
aloe-emodin
aloin
alpha aescin
alpha allocryptopine
alpha amyrinester
alpha bisabolol
alpha bulnesen
alpha colubrine
alpha cubeben
alpha gambogic acid
alpha guaiene
alpha guajaconic acid
alpha hederin
alpha humulene
alpha isosparteine
alpha lobeline
alpha methylpyrrylketone
alpha phellandrene
alpha santonin
alpha terpineol
alpha terpinyl acetate
alpha thujene
alpha tomatine
alpha truxillin
alstonidine
alstonine
althaein
amabiline
amarogentin
ambrette oil
ambrettolide
amentoflavone
americanine
amygdalin
anabasine

anabsin
anabsinthin
anacardic acid
anagalline
anagyrine
andromedotoxin
anemonine
anethole
angelic acid
angelicin
angustorine
anhalamine
anhalonidine
anhydrohirundigenin
anisaldehyde
anthranilate
antirrhinoside
apigenin
apigenin-7-glucoside
apiin
apiol
apoatropine
apocannoside
apovincamine
apterin
ar-curcumene
arabic acid
arbutin
arbutoside
arctigenin
arecaidine
arecoline
aristolene
arjunol acid
armepavin
arnidiol
artabsin
artemitine
artubiin
artumerone
asarone trans-isoasarone
ascaridiole

ascaridol
ascleposide
ascorbic acid
asebotoxin
asiaticoside A and B
asimilobin
asparagine
asperuloside
aspidospermine
astragaline
atlantone
atropine
aucubin
auraptene
aureusin
avenacoside A and B
avenalin
avenic acid A and B
avenin
avicularin
barbatic acid
barringtogenol
barterin
behenolic acid
belladonnine
benzaldehyde
benzoic acid
benzoylecgonin
benzyl isothiocyanate
benzyl cyanide
benzyl benzoate
benzyl cinnamoate
berbamine
berberine
bergaptene
beta aescin
beta allocryptopine
beta amyrin
beta bisobolen
beta cubeben
beta elemene
beta fagarin

beta hederin
beta-nitropropionic acid
beta oximene
beta patchoulen
beta peltatin
beta phellandrene
beta beta pinene
beta santonin
beta selinene
beta sitosterol
beta tocopherol
beta truxillin
betaine
betanin
betel phenol
bicuculline
bidemethoxycurcumin
bilobalide
bilobetin
biochanin A
biramentaceone
boldine
borneol
bornyl acetate
bornylacetate
boswellic acid
brucine
brunfelsamidine
buccocamphor
bufenolide
bulgarsenine
butyric acid
C-glycosyl-flavone
cacticine
cactine
cadenene
caffeic acid
caffeine
caffeolmalic acid
caffeoylquinic acid
calaminthadiol
californidin

caltholid
calvacin
camphene
camphor
camphor glucoronide
canadine
cantleyoside
cardol
carnosokolic acid
carnosol
carotatoxin
carpaine
carrageenine
carvacrol
carvone
caryophyllene oxide
caryophyllene
caryophyllene epoxide
cascaroside A
castalagin
castin
catapol
caulosapogenin
ceanothenic acid
ceanothusic acid
cedrol
celliamine
cellulose
cephaelin
cephalaroside
chamazulene
chavibetol
chavicol methyl ether
chavicol
chavicomethyl ether
cheiroside A
cheirotoxin
chelerythrine
chelidone
chelidonin
chelidonine
chief sapogenine

chimaphilin
chiroree acid
chlorogenic acid
chlorogenic acid sulfate
chlorogenin
cholerytrin
cholin
chondrocurarine
chondrocurine
chryoseriodictyol
chrysoeriol
chrysophanol
chymopapain A and B
cichoriic acid
cicutoxin
cineol
cinnamaldehyde
cinnamic acid
cinnamylacetate
cinnamylcinnamate
cirsilineol
cirsiliol
cirsimaritin
citral A and B
citric acid
citronellal
clavorubine
clerosterol
cnicin
colchicine
columbamine
columbin
combretin-A
condurangin
confertifoline
coniine
convallotoxin
copaene
copas
coptin
coptisine
corlumine

cornin
corynanthein
corynanthin
corytuberin
cosmosiin
costunolide
cotinine
coumaric acid
coumarin
crataegol acid
crispum apiole
crotopoxide
cryptoaescigenin
cryptochlorogenic acid
cryptofaurinol
cryptomeridiol
cryptopine
cubebol
cucurbitacin E, B, D, I and L
cucurbitacin
cucurbitin
cularine
cumarsabine
cuminaldehyde
curculone
curcumeneol
curcumin
curcumol
curlone
curzenenone
curzeren
cuskhygrine
cusparine
cycloalliin
cymarin
cynaratriol
cynarin
cynaropicrin
cynocannoside
cyperenone
cypripedi
cyrptoaescin

cytisine
D-borneol
D-camphene
D-camphor
d-carvone
d-chaulmoogric acid
D-gorli acid
D-hydnocarpic acid
D-silvestren
D-tubocurarine
daidzein
daphnetoxin
daphylloside
deglucocyclamin I and II
dehydrocostuslactone
dehydrocynaropicrin
dehydrofukinone
delphinine
alkylphthalides
demethoxycurcumin
deoxysyringoxidin
depenten
depentene
desacetylasperulosidic acid
desacetylelaterinide
desaspidin
deserpidine
desgalactotigonin
desglucohellebrin
desglucoparillin
desglucorhamnoparillin
desmethoxyyangonin
dhurrin
dicoffeoly tartaric acid
dictamdiol
dictamnine
didymin
diffractaic acid
diginin
digipurpurin
digitalonin
digitonine

digitoxin
dihydrocapsaicin
dihydrocorynanthein
dihydroguajaretic acid
dihydrosamidine
dihydroteugin
dihydroverbenalin
dihydroyohimbine
diiodothyrosine
dillapiol
dimethylaminomethylindol
dioscin
dioscorin
diosgenine diglucoside
diosmetin
diosmin
diosphenol
dioxypodophyllotoxin
dipsacan
disogenine monoglucoside
dodecanol
dracocarmin
dracoresin
dracoresinotannol
dracorhodin
dracorucin
droserone
echimidine
echinatine
eicosanoic acid
eicosanol
elaterinide
elemene
elemicin
eleutheroside I
ellagitannin
elymoclavine
emetine
emodin
emodin-physcion
ephedrine
epibaptifolin

epicatechol
epiguajpyridin
epinine
equisetumpyron
eremanthin
ergobasine
ergocornine
ergocristine
ergometrine
ergosine
ergosterol
ergotamine
ergovaline
eriodictyol
eriodictyonin
erucifoline
erysimoside
escholzine
escin
essential oil
estragole
estragon
etheric oil
euatromonoside
euatroside
eucanecine
eucovoside
eudesmol
eugenigradin
eugenol methyl ether
eugenol
eupatolid
eupatorin
eupatoriopicrin
euphroside
evernic acid
evobioside
evonine
evonoside
fagopyrin
falcarindiole
falcarinole

falcarintriol
faradiol
farnesene
farnesylacetate
fatty oil
fenchene
fenchon
fenchone
ferulic acid
feruloylsuccinic acid
fiber
ficin
fikarin
filicin
floridanine
florosenine
fluorodaturin
foenugraecin
foliamenthin
formic acid
formononetin
franganin
frangufolin
frangula amine
fraxidin
fraxin
fraxinol
friedelin
frotofagopyrin
fucane
fuchsisencionine
fucoidin
fucoidine
fuegin
fumaroprotocetraric acid
furanodienone
futranolide
gadolenic acid
galactoarabane
galacturonane
galacturonorhamane
galangin

galangol
galbaresenic acid
galegin
galiridoside
gallic acid
galloylglucose
galloylsaccharose
gamma carotene
gamma coniceine
gamma fagarine
gamma muurolen
gamma tocopherol
gardenine D
gaultherin
gedunin
gelsemicin
gelsemin
gelsevirin
gelsidin
genistein
genistin
genkwanin
genkwanin-6-methylether
gentianose
gentiobiose
gentiobiosyloleandrine
gentiopicrin
gentiopicroside
gentisic acid
geranial
geraniin
geraniol
germacrene alcohol
germacrene
gingerole
giniposidic acid
ginkgetin
ginsenoside
gitaloxin
gitoxin
glabren
glabrene

glabridin
glabrol
glechomafuran
glechomanolide
gliadin
glucobrassin
glucocaffeic acid
glucocochlearin
glucodifructose
glucoerysimoside
glucoevonogenin
glucoevonoloside
glucofrangulin A
glucofrangulin A-diacetate
glucogitaloxin
glucograngulin A
glucomannane
gluconapin
gluconasturtiin
gluconasturtin
glucoputranjivine
glucoraphanine
glucoscillarene A
glucosyloleandrin
glucotropaeolin
glucoverodoxin
glucuronide
glutaric acid
glycolic acid
glycyrrhisoflavone
glycyrrhizic acid
gnidilatidin
gossypetin
gramine
granatin
grandiflorin
grandivetin
gratiogenin
gratioside
graveobioside A and B
grayanotoxin
grindelic acid

grossheimin
guaiaverin
guaiazulene
guaiene
guajacin
guajaretic acid
guajavacine B
guvacine
guvacoline
gynocardine
gypsogen
gypsogenine
gypsoside
gyrophoric acid
hamamelitannin
harmine
haronginanthrone
harpagide
harpagoside
harunganin
hastasode
hederacoside B and C
hederagenin
hederosaponin B andC
helenalin
helianthinin
heliosupine
heliotropine
helleborin
hellebrin
hemicellulose
hemlock tannin
heptadecanoic acid
heptadecanolide
herniarin
hesperidin
hexanoic acid
hexosan
hinoki flavone
hirundigenin
histamine
homoarbutin

homoarenole
homolycorin
homoplantiginin
hordenine
hordenine
humulene
hydrangenol
hydrastine
hydrocinnamic acid
hydroxychavicol
hydroxycinnamic acid ester
hydroxycumarine
hydroxygrindelic acid
hydroxyquinone
hyoscyamine
hypaconitine
hyperforin
hypericin
hyperoside
ibotenic acid
icajine
imperatorin
integerrimine
intermedin
intybin
inulin
iodine
iovitexin
iridale
iridoide epoxy
irigenine
irigermanal
irilon
irisolone
irone
isoacteoside
isoalantolactone
isoartemisiaketon
isoavenasterol
isobergapten
isochlorogenic acid
isochondrodendrine

isocicutoxin
isocorydin
isodrimenine
isoeugenyl isovalerenate
isoeugenyl valerenate
isofucosterol
isofuranodienone
isofuranogermacren
isogentisin
isogeraniin
isoginkgetin
isoglycyrol
isohomoarbutin
isolichenan
isolicoflavonol
isoliensinine
isolindleyine
isoliquiritigenin
isolobinine
isomastic acid
isomilletone
isomorellic acid
isoorientin
isopilocarpin
isopimpinellin
isopinocamphone
isopterocarpol
isoquercetin
isoquercitrin
isoquinoline
isorhamnetin
isorhamnetin-3-glucoside
isorhoeadine
isorosmanol
isorubijervine
isosilybin
isosparteine
isosweroside
isotussaligine
isovalerenic acid
isovaleric acid
isovitexin

ixoroside
jacobine
jaconine
jateorhizine
jateorin
juglone
jujubogenine
jujuboside
kaempferide
kaempferol
kalmiatoxine
kava pyrone
kestose
khellin
knautioside
kokusaginin
kokusaginine
kryptogenin
L-hyoscyamine
L-lobeline
L-pinocarvone
L-scopolamine
lactucin
lactucopricin
lactupictin
ladroside
laminarin
laricinolic acid
lasiocarpine
laurenbiolide
lauric acid
lavandulyl acetate
ledol
ledum camphor
leicarposide
leocardin
leonuride
leucothol A
levigatin
lichenic acid
licopyranocumarin
liensinine

lignin
ligstroside
ligularenolide
ligusticumlactine
ligustilide
limnocitrin
limonene
limonin diosphenol
linalool
linalyl acetate
linamarin
linariin
lindleyine
linolenic acid
linusitamarine
linustatin
liqcoumarin
liquiritigenin
liriodenine
lithospermic acid
lobaric acid
lobelanidine
lobelanine
loganin
lotaustralin
lotusine
lucidin
lucyoside
lupanine
lupeol
luteolin
luteolin-7-glucoside
lutonarin
lycopene
lyonol A
madagascarine
madagascin
madagascinanthrone
madasiatic acid
magnoflorin
magnoflorine
magnolol

malonylginsenoside
maltol
malvin
mannitol
marindinine
marmesine
marrubiin
martynoside
masonine
mastic acid
matricarianol
matricarianolacetate
matricine
mearusitrin
mechyl alliin
mecocyanin
meconic acid
medicagen
melilotin
melilotoside
melilotosidin
menisdaurin
menispermine
menthiafolin
menthofurane
menthol
menthone
menthyl acetate
meratine
mesaconitine
methyl cardol
methyl chavicol
methyl salicylate
methyl anthranilate
methylcrotonic acid
methylcytisine
methylethylketone
methylisobutylketone
methyloctane
mezerein
milleton
monotropein

monotropitin
monotropitoside
morellic acid
mucilage
muscarine
muscimol
mussaenoside
mustard oil
myosmin
myrcene
myristicin
myristoylphoarbolacetate
myrtenol
myrtenylacetate
myrtocommulon A and B
myrtol
N-formylnornicotine
N-methyl coniine
N-methyl cytisine
N-methyltyramine
n-octylacetate
naphthadigydrodianthrones
napthoquinone
narcissin
naringin
natricin
neferine
nemorensin
neochlorogenic acid
neokestose
neolinustatin
neomenthol
neoruscogenin
nepetin
neral
neuquassin
nicotellin
nicotine
nicotinic acid amide
nicotoflorin
nicotyrin
nimbin

nologenin
nootkatone
norlobelanine
nornuciferin
norstictic
nortracheloside
notoginsenoside
novacine
nuciferin
obacunone
obacunone acid
octylbutyrate
odoroside A
oil
oleandrine
oleanolic acid
oleic acid
oleoropine
oleoroside
olivil
ononin
onopordopicrin
oreintin
orthosiphole A to E
osalic acid
oslandin
otosenin
otosenine
ouabain
oxaluric acid
oxoaconitine
oxogrindelic acid
oxypeucedanin
oxysanguinarine
oxystachydrine
p-cumaroyllupinine
p-cymene
paeonin
palmatine
palmitate
palmitin acid
palmitolactone

palustrol
palustrolid
paramenispermine
parasorbic acid
paraspidin
parillin
patchoulipyridin
patuletin
pectolinarin
pedalitin
pedunculagin
peganine
pellotin
pentadecanoic acid
pentadecanolide
pentagalloyl glucose
pentosan
pentylalliin
peperitone
persicarinpopulin
petasin
petroselic acid
phegopolin
phellandrene
phellopterin
phenol carbonic acid
phenolic acid
phenylethylamine
phenylacetaldehyde
phenylethylisothiocyanate
phloretin
phosphatidylethanolamine
phosphatidylinositol
physcion
physostigmine
phytoecdysone
phytolacanin
phytosterols
piceatannol
picrocrocin
picrosalvin
picrotin

picrotoxin
picrotoxinine
pilocarpidin
pilosin
pimpinellin
pinene
pinocamphone
pinocarvone
pipecolic acid
platyphyllin
plumbagin
podophyllotoxin
polyfructosan
polygalacturonane
polygalacturonic acid
polygalin
polygamarin
polypodosaponin I and II
pomolic acid
pontica epoxide
populin
porst camphor
potassium-strophanthoside
premarrubiin
primveroside
proazulene
procumbide
proscillaridin A
prostatin
protoanemonin
protocetraric acid
protocosin
protopin
protopine
protoverine
prunasin
pseudocarpaine
pseudoephedrine
pseudohypericin
pseudotropine
psoralen
psoromic acid

ptelein
pterocarpol
pulegone
punicalagin
purpurea glycoside A and B
purpureagitoside
pyrethrine
quassin
quebrachine
quebrachit
quercetin
quercimeritrin
quillaic acid
quinic acid
quinidine
quinine
raffinose
ramentaceone
ramentone
ranunculin
raubasine
rauhimbin
reptoside
rescinnamine
reserpine
resin
reticulin
retrorsine
rhamnazine bisulphate
rhamnazine
rhamnocitrin
rhein anthrone
rhinantin
rhodotoxin
rhoeadine
rhoeagenine
rhoifolin
ricinoleic acid
roemerin
romarinic acid
rosmadial
rosmaric acid

rosmaridiphenol
rosmariquinone
rotenone
rubijervine
ruscin
ruscocide
ruscogenin
rutin
rutoside
sabinene
sabinyl acetate
saccharose
safficinolide
safrol
salicarin
salicin
salicortin
salicylaldehyde primveroside
salicylaldehyde
salireposide
salonitenolide
samidine
sanguinarine
santalin A and B
santene
saponaretin
sarothamnoside
sarpagine
sarracenin
sarracin
sarsaparilloside
sarsapogenin
scandoside
schaftoside
sciadopytisin
scillicyanoside
scilliglaucoside
scopolamine
scopoletin
scopoletine
scopolin
scutellarein tetramethyl ether

scutellarin
secalonic acid A
secoebuloside
secoisolaricinol
sedacrin
sedamin
sedinine
sedinon
selenium
sempervirin
senecionin
senecionine
seneciphylline
senegasaponine
senegin
senkirkine
senkyunolide
sequoia flavone
serotonin
serpentinine
sesamine
silicic acid
silphinene
silphiperfolen
silybin
silybinin
silychristin
silydianin
silydianine
simarolide
simarubidin
simarubin
sinalbin
sinensetin
sinestin
skimmianin
skimmianine
skimmine
soladulcidinetetraoside
solamargine
solamarine
solasonine

sorbifolin
sparteine
spathulenone
sphondin
spinacetin
spinasterol
spinatoside
spiraeine
spiraeoside
sprintillamine
sprintillin
stachydrine
stachyose
staphisagroine
staphisine
stearic acid
stenophyllanin C
stictictic
stictinic acid
stigmasterol
strogoside
strophanthin-G
strophoside
strychnine
strychnine
styracine
styrolpyrone glucoside
succinylcyanin
supinin
supinine
sweroside
swertiamarin
swertiamarine
sylvestroside III and IV
symphytine
symphytoxide A
syringin
syringoxide
syriogenin
tadeonal
taraxacin
taraxagin

tartaric acid
taupine
taxifolin
tectoridine
terpeninol-4
terpinolene
terpinyl acetate
tetracosanoic acid
tetrahydroalstonine
tetrahydroligularenolide
tetraphylline B
tetrofuroguajacine A and B
teupolin I
teuscorodin
teuscorodonin
thamnolic acid
theaflavin acid
theaflavine
thearubigene
thebaine
thelophoric acid
theobromine
thiamin
thujone
thymol
thymonin
tinctorin
tormentolic acid
tormentoside
trachelogenin
trans-9-oxofuranoeremophilane
trans-aconitic acid
trans-isoelemicin
trans-isoeugenol methyl ether
trans-lachnophyllum ester
transcarvylacetate
tremulacin
trigloquinine
trigloylmeteloidin
trillarin
trillin
trimeric

trimethylamine
trimethylglucine
triterpenylic acid
tryptamine
tuberosum apiole
tueflin
tuescorolide
tumerone
tussilagine
tylophorin
tyramine
umbelliferone
undecane
undecanone
urezin
ursolic acid
urushiol
uzarin
uzaroside
valdiviolide
valepotriate
valeranone
valerenal
valerenaldehyde
valerenic acid
valerianine
valeric acid
vanillin
vasicin
vasicine
vasicinone
veratrin
verbanalin
verbascosaponine
verbascoside
verifuge
veronicoside
verproside
vesvalagin
vicenin-II
vicenin-1
vincadifformin

vincamine
vincetogenin
vincin
violutoside
virgaureoside A
viridifloral
visnadin
visnagin
vitamin B complex
vitamin C
vitexin rhamnose
vitexin
vomicine
warburganal
wax
weiterhin
winterin
withastramonolide
xanthoeriodictyol
xanthohumole
xanthomicrol
xanthotoxin
xanthoxyletin
xanthoxyloin
xysmarlorin
yangonine
yohimbine
zanthorrhizol
zanthotoxin
zederone
zingiberene
zingiberene
zymosterol

Common Classes of Phytochemicals

1,8-dihydroxyanthracene derivatives
acidic xylans
acylphloroglucinols
aglycones
aliphatic hydrocarbons
aliphatic alcohols

aliphatic lichen acids
alkaloids
alkanals
alkanes
alkanols
alkyl nitriles
alkyl phenoles
alkyl phthalides
allylglucosinolates
aloinosides A and B
alpha pinenes
andromeda derivatives
anthocyanins
anthocyans
anthranoids
apiogalacturonans
apocarotinoid glycosides
arabinogalactans
arabinoxylans
aristolocic acids I and II
benzophenones
benzyl isoquinoline alkaloids
benzyl esters
beta glucans
beta glycosides
beta hamamelitannins
betacyans
bicyclic sesquiterpenes
biogenic amines
bisabolol oxides
bisjatrorrhizines
C-glucosylxanthones
calcium salts
capsaicinoids
cardenolide glycosides
cardenolids
cardiac glycosides
carotenoids
carrageenans
catechin derivatives
catechin tannins
catechins

chalcones
clucosinolates
condurango glycosides
coumarin derivatives
cyanogenic glycosides
cyclamin
cyclic peptide alkaloids
cyclic peptines
cyclitols
cyclopentene fatty acids
delta cadenenes
depside ellagitannins
diarylheptanoids
dicinnamoylmethane derivatives
digalactosides
diterpenes
diterpenoid oleoresins
ellagic tannins
epicatechins
ergochromes
ester resins
esters
filicinic acids
flavano-ellagic tannins
flavanone derivatives
flavaspidic acids
flavolignans
flavone aglycones
flavones
flavonoid glycosides
flavonoids
flavonols
fructosans
furanocoumarins
furoquinolin alkaloids
galactoarabinoxylans
galactomannanes
galacturonic rhamnans
gallo tannins
gamma hamamelitannins
gamma pyrones
ginkgolic acids

ginkgolides
glucans
glucosinolates
glycoretins
glycosides
guaianolid glycosides
harpagoquinones
helenaloid sesquiterpene lactones
heteroxylans
humules
hydroquinone glycosides
hydroquinone derivatives
hydroxycoumarins
hydroxyphenylalkanones
indole alkaloids
iridoid glycosides
isoflavanone derivatives
isoflavonoids
isoquinoline alkaloids
jatrorrhizines
ketones
L-cadinenes
lactoyl flavones
lichen acids
lignane glycosides
lignans
limonoids
linolenic acid esters
liridoide monoterpenes
macrocyclic lactones
mannans
meethoxylised flavonoids
methyl xanthines
mineral salts
monogalloylhamameloses
monoterpenes
mucopolysaccharides
mustard oil glycosides
neolignans
nitrile glycosides
oligomeric procyanidins
oligomeric proanthocyanidins

oligosaccharides
p-quinones
pennogenintetra glycosides
peptides
peruresitannols
phenol glycosides
phenols
phenylethanol derivatives
phlorotannins
phosphoglycerides
phospholipids
phthalides
phytoalexins
piperidin alkaloids
polyketide alkaloids
polyketides
polysaccharides
polyynes
potassium salts
proanthocyanidins
procoumarins
proteolytic ferments
protolimonoids
purine alkaloids
pyranocoumarins
pyrrolizidine alkaloids
quassinoids
quercetin glycosides
quillaja saponins
quinolin alkaloids
quinolizidine alkaloids
rhamnoarabinogalactans
rhamnogalacturonans
rhodanides
rotenoids
saponins
sennosides
sesquiterpene lactones
sesquiterpenealdehydes
sesquiterpenes
sparteine isoflavonoids
steroid alkaloids

steroid saponins
steroids
stilbene derivatives
tannins
terpene lactones
terpene alcohols
terpineols
tetranortriterpenes
theafolia saponins
triterpene saponins

triterpene glycosides
triterpenes
triterpenoids
tuliposides
volatile oils
whitasteroids
xanthones
xyloglucans
ziyuglycosides
zyzyphus saponins

Sample Reports Featuring Acupuncture

ACUPUNCTURE TREATMENT

INFORMED CONSENT: The patient was given informed consent for this treatment. She understood the risks and benefits and elected to proceed.

PREOPERATIVE DIAGNOSIS: The patient has chronic lumbar pain because of multiple surgeries.

SUBJECTIVE: She liked the Shen Men balls. These seemed to work okay.

OBJECTIVE: What we notice on her is that her tongue has a really funny picture with a central tip that is kind of scalloped. It has also deep cracks in it. On palpation of her pulses, her kidney pulse is a little diminished primarily. Her liver pulse is maybe a little superficial, it's really hard to tell.

PROCEDURE: For her first treatment, we would like to put bilateral Shen Men balls in. We also put in an N,N+1 circuit along Shao Yin Tai Yang. We chose kidney 3 and kidney 7 and brought it down to bladder 40. We were going to do the Shu Mu system of the back, but she has a long thick scar and really all of her vertebral bodies are collapsed; I really cannot find much anatomy. I elected first to unblock that scar, so we did a scar unblocking. The needles were left in for 10 minutes with manual tonification. She tolerated this pretty well.

PLAN: We will observe her response and initiate other therapy. We might have to use Korean Hand Acupuncture to move energy along the back with her and work with the ear because of all the scarring.

ACUPUNCTURE TREATMENT

The patient is here today for her second acupuncture treatment.

INFORMED CONSENT: The patient was given informed consent for this procedure. She understood the risks and benefits and elected to proceed.

PREOPERATIVE DIAGNOSIS: The patient has fibromyalgia. She also has chronic cephalgia, neck pain, aches and pains, restless leg syndrome, and fatigue. Her biggest problem is fatigue.

SUBJECTIVE: She does not think she had any response with her last treatment. If anything, she says she is more fatigued than usual.

OBJECTIVE: Weight is 117 pounds, blood pressure 136/84, pulse 96. Her tongue is not really deviated or scalloped. Her pulses show a diminished liver and diminished kidney pulse.

We elected to put gold seeds over Shen Men, muscle relaxation, kidney, liver, and thalamus. We also decided to put in spleen 6, liver 3, gallbladder 34, kidney 3, kidney 7, and bladder 62. Really in putting the needles in, there is not much grab of these particular needles. It does not really seem to have much Qi at all going on, so for her next treatment I will probably plan to treat her on her back and do the back Shu points.

ASSESSMENT: Chronic fatigue in this authoritarian with multiple somatic complaints.

PLAN: We will observe her response to treatment and see what transpires.

ACUPUNCTURE TREATMENT

The patient is here today for her fourth electrical acupuncture treatment.

INFORMED CONSENT: The patient was given informed consent for this procedure. She understood the risks and benefits and elected to proceed.

PREOPERATIVE DIAGNOSIS: Fibromyalgia. On clinical exam, she has spleen and kidney deficiency. She has low back pain and chronic right upper quadrant pain.

SUBJECTIVE: She has been doing pretty well. Less low back pain. She has more energy than ever before.

OBJECTIVE: Blood pressure 124/82, pulse 80. Her pulses are all diminished but coming up. She has a scalloped, deviated, tremulous tongue.

We elected to do some of the back Shu points. We did the liver Shu with bladder 18, spleen Shu, bladder 20, and the kidney Shu bladder 23. We did the Mu point of the kidney and gallbladder 25 and hooked it electrically negative to positive at 5.5 Hz for 10 minutes. We also did a circuit along Shao Yin Tai Yang with kidney 3, kidney 7, and down to bladder 40. We also put in spleen 6, gallbladder 34, and gallbladder 31. We put ion gold seeds under Shen Men, kidney, liver, spleen, and thalamus. She seemed to tolerate this treatment pretty well.

ASSESSMENT: Chronic energy deficiency; chronic fibromyalgia and fatigue syndrome.

PLAN: We will observe her response to treatment.

ACUPUNCTURE TREATMENT

The patient is here today for her seventh acupuncture treatment.

INFORMED CONSENT: The patient was given informed consent for this procedure. She understood the risks and benefits and elected to proceed.

PREOPERATIVE DIAGNOSIS: She has chronic pain syndrome, right knee pain, femoral pain, low back pain, low energy, depletion of spleen, kidney, and liver.

SUBJECTIVE: She is doing about the same. Sometimes she thinks maybe the pain is a little less, but this is uncertain.

OBJECTIVE: Blood pressure 132/90, pulse 80. Her tongue shows some tense scalloping. Her pulses are relatively weak in kidney and liver.

We elected to do a circuit for liver 13 and liver 14. We put in liver 14, but it was too uncomfortable for her and we had to remove it. There was no obvious hematoma. Her symptoms kind of resolved and she really did not want me to put one back in that area. She has previously broken ribs. We did a circuit on Shao Yin and Tai Yang: kidney 3, kidney 7, down to bladder 62 prime. We put in CV 4, CV 10, CV 12, and governor vessel 24.5. On Tai Yin, we put spleen 6, spleen 9, and stomach 36. On Jue Yin Shao Yang, we did liver 3 and liver 6 to gallbladder 34. We also put in gallbladder 31. The needles were manually tonified. There were really no obvious complications.

ASSESSMENT: Chronic pain syndrome.

PLAN: Observe her response to treatment.

ACUPUNCTURE TREATMENT

The patient is here today for her 10th acupuncture treatment.

INFORMED CONSENT: The patient was given informed consent for this procedure. She understood the risks and benefits and elected to proceed.

PREOPERATIVE DIAGNOSIS: Fibromyalgia, low energy, increasing TMJ pain on the left.

SUBJECTIVE: She has learned that her father is ill, and she woke up one day and felt that she could not move and ached all over. She thought the ear seeds last time made her worse and does not want to have them today. Otherwise she is doing okay. Her energy level is alright.

OBJECTIVE: Blood pressure 122/80, pulse 80. Her pulses showed slightly weak Yin pulses in spleen, kidney, and liver, but they are almost normal. The tongue, other than being flabby, is really not deviated. It really is markedly improved. There is no more tremor or deviation.

We elected to do just a simple treatment without any auricular seeds. We did spleen 6, liver 3, gallbladder 34, kidney 3, kidney 7, and bladder 62 prime. They were manually tonified. She tolerated this procedure.

ASSESSMENT: Fibromyalgia.

PLAN: Consideration for some sort of maintenance treatment on her. We will discuss this with UR.

ACUPUNCTURE TREATMENT

The patient is here today for her eighth acupuncture treatment.

INFORMED CONSENT: The patient was given informed consent for this procedure. She understood the risks and benefits and elected to proceed.

PREOPERATIVE DIAGNOSIS: The patient has low energy, low libido, low back pain, and sometimes upper back pain.

SUBJECTIVE: She feels great. She has great energy. Her libido is great. She occasionally has upper back pain, but otherwise her low back pain is completely gone.

OBJECTIVE: Her pulses are symmetrical. Her tongue looks unremarkable. Maybe a little decreased kidney pulse.

We elected for this treatment to put in a Shu Mu system with gallbladder 25 to bladder 23, negative to positive at 5.5 Hz. We also put in kidney 3 and kidney 7 to bladder 40. We also did a lot of Ashi points on her back. Most of these were along the small intestine points. Then we took from Tl through T7 the Hua Tuo Jia Ji points. She seemed to tolerate this pretty well.

ASSESSMENT: The patient is doing quite well.

PLAN: We might just put her on a maintenance regimen since she is doing well. We will leave this up to her, but she could be done in four weeks.

ACUPUNCTURE TREATMENT

The patient is here today for her 10th electrical acupuncture treatment.

INFORMED CONSENT: The patient was given informed consent for this procedure. She understood the risks and benefits and elected to proceed.

PREOPERATIVE DIAGNOSIS: She has chronic low back pain, gastroesophageal reflux, diarrhea, and sinus problems.

SUBJECTIVE: She is doing a little better. Her back has almost improved. She is having some facial problems with sinus pain. She otherwise is doing okay. She is getting some arthritis of her hands.

OBJECTIVE: Blood pressure 120/74, pulse '72. Her tongue is not scalloped but maybe minimally. Very minimal, if any, tremor. Not much deviation. Her pulses show her kidney pulse to be pretty good. Her liver pulse is a little depleted. Spleen pulse is a little less than the kidney pulse.

Because of her facial symptoms, we elected to do spleen 6, spleen 9, large intestine 4, and stomach 36. We also put in kidney 3, liver 3, liver 6, and gallbladder 34. We put ion gold seeds in her ear over Shen Men and muscle relaxation of thalamus and kidney as well as for liver. She tolerated this treatment. We electrically tonified spleen 6 to spleen 9 at 5.5 Hz for 10 minutes.

ASSESSMENT: This is her 10th acupuncture treatment.

PLAN: We will put her on maintenance treatments.

Notes

Notes

Notes

Notes